INNOVATIONS IN HEALTH SYSTEM FINANCE IN DEVELOPING AND TRANSITIONAL ECONOMIES

ADVANCES IN HEALTH ECONOMICS AND HEALTH SERVICES RESEARCH

Series Editors: Michael Grossman & Björn Lindgren

Recent Volumes:

ADVANCES IN HEALTH ECONOMICS AND HEALTH
SERVICES RESEARCH   VOLUME 21

INNOVATIONS IN HEALTH SYSTEM FINANCE IN DEVELOPING AND TRANSITIONAL ECONOMIES

EDITED BY

DOV CHERNICHOVSKY

*Center for Health Sciences, Ben Gurion University of the Negev,
Beer Sheva, Israel*

KARA HANSON

*London School of Hygiene and Tropical Medicine,
London, UK*

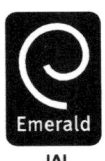

JAI

United Kingdom – North America – Japan
India – Malaysia – China

JAI Press is an imprint of Emerald Group Publishing Limited
Howard House, Wagon Lane, Bingley BD16 1WA, UK

First edition 2009

Copyright © 2009 Emerald Group Publishing Limited

Reprints and permission service
Contact: booksandseries@emeraldinsight.com

British Library Cataloguing in Publication Data
A catalogue record for this book is available from the British Library

ISBN: 978-1-84855-664-5
ISSN: 0731-2199 (Series)

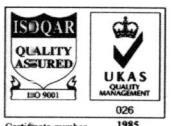

Awarded in recognition of
Emerald's production
department's adherence to
quality systems and processes
when preparing scholarly
journals for print

INVESTOR IN PEOPLE

CONTENTS

v

SECTION III: SECURING CARE

SECTION IV: MODIFYING DEMAND

SECTION V: THE UNIVERSAL INTEGRATED HEALTHCARE SYSTEM

LIST OF CONTRIBUTORS

Nelly Aguilera	Inter-American Conference on Social Security, Mexico City, Mexico
James Akazili	Navrongo Health Research Centre, Ghana Health Service, Ghana
John Ataguba	Health Economics Unit, School of Public Health and Family Medicine, University of Cape Town, Cape Town, South Africa
Peter Berman	The World Bank, Washington, DC, USA
Josephine Borghi	Health Economics and Financing Programme, Department of Public Health and Policy, London School of Hygiene and Tropical Medicine, London, UK; Ifakara Health Institute, Dar es Salaam, Tanzania
Dov Chernichovsky	Health Policy and Management Unit, Center for Health Sciences, Ben Gurion University of the Negev, Beer Sheva, Israel
Anthony Costello	Institute for Global Health and Centre for International Health and Development, University College London, London, UK
Pablo Gottret	The World Bank, Washington, DC, USA
Pieter Grobler	Medscheme Health Risk Solutions, Cape Town, South Africa

Veronica Guajardo-Barrón	Economic Analysis Unit, Ministry of Health, Mexico
Vaibhav Gupta	The World Bank, Washington, DC, USA
Cristina Gutiérrez-Delgado	Economic Analysis Unit, Ministry of Health, Mexico
Kara Hanson	Health Economics and Financing Programme, Department of Public Health and Policy, London School of Hygiene and Tropical Medicine, London, UK
Melitta Jakab	WHO Europe, Bishkek, Kyrgyzstan
Joseph Kutzin	WHO Europe, Office for Health Systems Strengthening, Barcelona, Spain
Supon Limwattananon	International Health Policy Program, Ministry of Public Health, Thailand; Faculty of Pharmaceutical Sciences, Khon Kaen University, Thailand
Dharma Manandhar	Mother and Infant Research Activities (MIRA), Kathmandu, Nepal
Gabriel Martinez	Inter-American Conference on Social Security, Mexico City, Mexico
Di McIntyre	Health Economics Unit, School of Public Health and Family Medicine, University of Cape Town, Cape Town, South Africa
Heather McLeod	Department of Public Health and Family Medicine, University of Cape Town, Cape Town, South Africa; Department of Statistics and Actuarial Science, University of Stellenbosch, Stellenbosch, South Africa

Filip Meheus

Development, Policy & Practice, Royal Tropical Institute (KIT), Amsterdam, The Netherlands

Valerie Moran

The World Bank, Washington DC, USA

Rodrigo Moreno-Serra

Department of Economics & Related Studies, University of York, Heslington, York, UK

Gemini Mtei

Ifakara Health Institute, Dar es Salaam, Tanzania

Basu Dev Neupane

Evaluation of Safe Delivery Incentive Programme, Kathmandu, Nepal

Sachiko Ozawa

Department of International Health, Johns Hopkins Bloomberg School of Public Health, Baltimore, MD, USA

Tim Powell-Jackson

Health Economics and Financing Programme, Department of Public Health and Policy, London School of Hygiene and Tropical Medicine, London, UK

Phusit Prakongsai

International Health Policy Program, Ministry of Public Health, Thailand

Clas Rehnberg

Medical Management Centre, Karolinska Institute, Stockholm, Sweden

Sergey Shishkin

State University Higher School of Economics, Moscow, Russian Federation

Susan Sparkes

The World Bank, Washington, DC, USA

Ajay Tandon

The World Bank, Washington, DC, USA

Viroj Tangcharoensathien   International Health Policy Program,
                                 Ministry of Public Health, Thailand

Suresh Tiwari   Support to Safe Motherhood
                                 Programme, Kathmandu, Nepal

Kirti Tumbahangphe   Mother and Infant Research Activities
                                 (MIRA), Kathmandu, Nepal

Adam Wagstaff   Development Research Group, The
                                 World Bank, Washington DC, USA

Damian G. Walker   Department of International Health,
                                 Johns Hopkins Bloomberg School of
                                 Public Health, Baltimore, MD, USA

Sophie Witter   Immpact, University of Aberdeen,
                                 Abeerden, UK

Winnie Yip   Health Economics Research Centre,
                                 Department of Public Health,
                                 University of Oxford, Oxford, UK

OVERVIEW

This set of chapters on health financing in developing and transitional countries is published at a critical moment. The goals of universal coverage and protection against the financial risks of ill-health, together with the recognition of the critical role of public funding in providing this protection, are shared by countries of all income levels. At the same time, there are increasing concerns about efficiency and sustainability of health systems, particularly during a period of global economic downturn, as well as about their accountability and responsiveness to clients. More than ever, pressures are mounting for health systems to use existing resources to best effect in terms of improving population health and satisfaction. For the poorest countries, there is interest in mobilizing additional funding to expand dramatically service coverage in order to meet global development targets such as the Millennium Development Goals. These new funding streams and the hope that has come with them are likely, however, to be seriously tested by the current economic crisis.

A review of recent health financing data indicates the scale and scope of the challenges. Both low- and middle-income countries appear to have increased their levels of spending on health care over the past decade, in absolute terms as well as in terms of the share of spending in gross domestic product (Table 1). While these changes appear to be reflected in their real resource availability, they are not yet captured in improvements in basic health indicators: infant mortality and life expectancy. The data are crude; yet, they give rise to questions about cost of care, efficiency of care, and health production in these two groups of countries.

Low-income countries continue to spend about a fifth of the spending level of middle-income countries. Worse, the gap between the groups appears to have increased in spite of the dramatic increase in the share of foreign aid to low-income countries. The data are consistent with the hypothesis that in both groups, but especially among the poorest countries, the increasing pressures quickly outgrow the increase in resources.

In their efforts to meet their health system goals and objectives, countries are adopting a variety of policies and approaches to their health care

Table 1. Selected Indicators, Low- and Middle-Income Countries.

Low-Income Countries			
	1995	2000	2005
Health indicators			
Life expectancy at birth (both sexes)[a]	58	59	60
Infant mortality rate (both sexes)[a]	88	82	75
Real resources			
Physicians per 10,000[b]	3.00	0.90	10.00
Hospital beds per 10,000[b]	n/a	7.50	12.29
Finance			
Total expenditure on health as a percentage of gross domestic product (GDP)[b]	4.61	4.61	5.07
Per capita total expenditure on health (Int$)[b]	49.69	56.16	74.21
Per capita governement expenditure on health (Int$)[b]	24.07	25.62	34.33
External resources for health as a percentage of total expenditure on health[b]	10.58	16.73	25.34
General government expenditure on health as a percentage of total expenditure on health[b]	43.61	40.68	45.01
Middle-Income Countries			
	1995	2000	2005
Health indicators			
Life expectancy at birth (both sexes)[a]	68	69	70
Infant mortality rate (both sexes)[a]	38	33	27
Real resources			
Physicians per 10,000[b]	5.00	11.50	15.50
Hospital beds per 10,000[b]	n/a	28.67	22.83
Finance			
Total expenditure on health as a percentage of GDP[a]	5.6	6.11	6.38
Per capita total expenditure on health (Int$)[a]	231.30	307.18	420.08
Per capita governement expenditure on health (Int$)[a]	139.27	182.31	256.56
External resources for health as a percentage of total expenditure on health[a]	5.22	6.00	7.14
General government expenditure on health as a percentage of total expenditure on health[a]	57.99	56.84	59.77

[a]Available at www.who.int/whosis. Accessed on May 11, 2009.
[b]World Bank, 2009, *World development indicators*. The World Bank, Washington, DC.

financing challenges. These efforts are increasingly accompanied by conceptual and applied research that is contributing to the development of good practice. In spite of the vast difference among countries and the various issues they face, the emerging evidence takes in all elements of health care financing: resource collection, resource pooling and allocation, provider payment, and demand-side interventions.

The aim of this volume is to assemble some of the best of this conceptual and applied research, to present it in a coherent way that reflects the structure of the system for financing health care, and to reflect on the policy implications of this research for strengthening health financing in developing and transitional countries.

Together, the 12 chapters published in this volume convey a set of core messages about the challenges of designing effective health financing systems. First, the experience across a range of countries representing differences in income level and historical legacy indicates that public sector intervention is essential to take health financing systems along the next steps to universal coverage.

The second message emerging from these chapters is the importance of seeing health financing arrangements as an integrating mechanism, bringing together multiple sources of funding with arrangements for purchasing and providing care that is effective and responsive to user needs and preferences. System design needs to consider the optimal levels of both centralization (to allow risk pooling and economies of scale in purchasing) and decentralization (to enable providers to seek innovative solutions to improving efficiency and quality and support responsiveness towards users). The incentives embodied in the design of these systems will ultimately determine whether they are able to achieve their goals.

Third, piecemeal reforms may be successful at addressing specific problems of access to care, but may introduce additional (unintended) consequences and will not bring about the fundamental changes needed to achieve both efficiency and equity goals. While the chapters in this volume present relatively positive evaluations of the experience of, for example, the use of exemptions and incentive payments to remove financial barriers to maternity care, the new problems created, such as increased exposure to the risk of catastrophic maternity expenses and the problems of fungibility and cost-shifting, serve to highlight the broader challenges of health financing. The political dynamics of such reforms are probably an important influence, with continued discussions around the optimal combination of integrated versus disease-specific programs mirrored in discussions about financing streams. But there is also a dearth of evidence about the merits of incremental versus "big bang" reforms and whether path dependence in system design implies risks for achieving long-term goals. The experiences presented in this volume support both positions: the Thai expansion of coverage took 27 years and was based on an incrementalist approach. In contrast, it could be argued that the difficulties that the United States, which has a developing health care system, has had in reforming its own system have arisen from its piecemeal approach to past reforms.

In terms of their coverage and methods, the chapters represent well the current state of knowledge and research methodology in the area of health financing. They use a variety of different research methods, ranging from contemporary program evaluation methods (Powell-Jackson et al.), state-of-the-art methods for quantitative equity analysis (Prakongsai et al.), and cross-country panel data regression methods (Wagstaff and Moreno-Serra) to mixed methods derived from case studies, household surveys, and qualitative methods (Witter, Ozawa and Walker). One chapter specifically addresses the methodological challenges of conducting health financing analysis in settings where few data are available (Borghi et al.). Collectively, they demonstrate the range of different types of evidence that can usefully contribute to better understanding of health financing arrangements.

THE CHANGING CONTEXT

The first section of this volume is concerned with the changing context for health financing in developing and transitional countries. Two chapters address contemporary issues. The first, by Cristina Gutiérrez-Delgado and Veronica Guajardo-Barrón, describes the challenges created by the "double burden" of disease in low- and middle-income countries created by the coexistence of the persistent burden of communicable disease with emerging problems of chronic and non-communicable illness. Drawing on the Mexican experience of expanding needs for anti-retroviral therapy, renal replacement therapy, and screening and prevention of cervical cancers, they present new evidence about the burden placed by these conditions on public health budgets. They also show the potential value of adopting a risk factor approach to economic evaluation of chronic disease management, presenting estimates of the financial burden imposed by four diseases strongly associated with overweight and obesity. They conclude that strengthened stewardship functions, including generating data about disease burdens and expenditure, and greater use of explicit priority setting processes, are needed to help resolve the tensions between equity and efficiency.

The second chapter, by Pablo Gottret and colleagues, analyses the challenges created by the current financial and economic crisis for health expenditure levels, service utilization, and health outcomes. In the context of the composition of health care funding today, the authors draw on evidence from earlier financial crises to provide insights into the types and magnitude of effects that might be expected, and identify from a review of World Bank lending program the forms of policy response which were particularly effective. They argue that the key objective of health policy in such circumstances must be to maintain access to essential services by the population, particularly for poor and vulnerable groups. They also identify the ways in which national policymakers have used crises as an opportunity to increase the efficiency of the health system and to improve efforts to target the poor.

NEW FINANCING SOURCES TO EXPAND COVERAGE

A set of chapters addressing alternative approaches to expanding coverage of financing arrangements makes up the second section of the volume. Three of these chapters address particular financing sources: use of general revenues to extend coverage in Thailand by Prakongsai et al, community-based health insurance in Cambodia by Ozawa and Walker, and social health insurance (SHI) in Central and Eastern Europe and Central Asia (Wagstaff and Moreno-Serra). Each of these chapters raises different questions related to the broader impact of these schemes, beyond the achievement of expanded coverage and income protection.

The Thai chapter focuses particularly on the positive impact of the universal coverage scheme on equity, demonstrating how an already pro-poor health financing system became more pro-poor after the introduction of the universal coverage scheme, which used general revenue funding to secure the access of those not covered by the two existing insurance schemes. A critical element in the Thai experience has been the accompanying changes in the arrangements for purchasing care and the importance of earlier investment in strengthening the primary health care system. Efficiency concerns have been addressed through changes to provider payment mechanisms.

Social health insurance has figured prominently in current discussions about how to achieve universal coverage, and many countries (e.g., Tanzania, Ghana, Zambia, and Kenya) are exploring options for extending their existing SHI schemes to cover informal sector workers. It also played a role in replacing budgetary allocations (e.g., countries in Eastern Europe and Central Asia). This in itself creates challenges of how to collect insurance contributions from those who are not formally employed – one reason why the Thai universal coverage scheme opted for tax funding rather than a contributory regime (see Prakongsai et al., this volume). There has, however, been concern about the potential deleterious labor market effects of SHI, with possibly immediate effects on labor costs thereby affecting the demand for labor, employment levels, and wages. Moreover, in those countries where strategies to extend coverage have resulted in parallel systems, there are concerns that SHI might also discourage formalization of the labor force. The chapter by Wagstaff and Moreno-Serra takes advantage of the variation in financing arrangements created by changes between SHI and general revenue financing in countries of Central and Eastern Europe and Central Asia. Their analysis uses panel data from 28 countries and finds that SHI increases wages, reduces employment, and increases self-employment, but no impact is found on unemployment, agricultural employment, the size of the informal economy, or foreign direct investment.

In view of fiscal space issues as well as trust in government, SHI arrangements, starting with basic voluntary schemes that imply intra-group subsidies may be indispensable. "Trust" in general is a basic requirement for health insurance, including SHI. The chapter by Ozawa and Walker focuses on the issue of trust and how trust in an insurance scheme influences the decision to enroll in community-based health insurance. While clearly a factor explaining insurance coverage levels, the authors argue that trust potentially plays a much broader role in shaping the attitudes of individuals, health care providers, and insurers and that the implications for trust of changed incentives embodied in a range of health financing arrangements should be carefully considered. Health financing arrangements can also have broader impacts on economic outcomes and performance.

The final chapter in this section has a methodological focus, setting out the challenges to studying the incidence of different health financing sources in data-limited environments. Borghi et al. draw on the experience of undertaking this analysis in three quite different contexts – Ghana, Tanzania, and South Africa. They identify the limitations of many existing household surveys for undertaking this type of equity analysis and outline how they have used supplementary surveys and data triangulation to improve the validity of their results. Their findings resonate strongly with those of Prakongsai et al. (this volume) who successfully advocated for the routine collection of household level data for undertaking equity analyses. The authors argue that a crucial link exists between ongoing monitoring and evaluation of the equity impact of health financing changes, and the political project of securing and sustaining support for such changes.

SECURING CARE

The third section of the volume addresses the critical health financing functions of resource allocation and purchasing. The chapter by McLeod and Grobler presents an analysis of the proposal to introduce a Risk Equalization Fund, a core institutional mechanism envisaged for a National Health Insurance system in South Africa. Their analysis focuses particularly on the distributional consequences of alternative reform sequencing. They present simulation evidence to show that the order in which policy measures needed to address current inequities and inefficiencies in the South African insurance system are implemented will affect different income groups differently. Their analysis echoes earlier arguments that a whole package of changes is needed to protect low-income workers in a competitive insurance environment, comprising mandatory membership, income subsidies, and risk equalization. Once more, it is clear that systemic issues must be considered for health financing reforms to have the desired impact.

A similar message is conveyed in the chapter by Yip and Hanson, which describes the range of innovative health service purchasing arrangements that have been introduced in China over recent years. Using the lens of the multiple principal–agent relationships that characterize purchasing, the authors describe the experience of purchasing health services in the context of a rural health insurance experiment and an urban employee insurance plan and purchasing of a package of preventive and promotive public health services. One component of particular interest is the experience of incorporating community representatives on the board of the health service purchaser in the rural scheme, to increase accountability in the purchaser–user relationship. While creating a structure for representation is clearly not sufficient to ensure meaningful participation and accountability, this approach has some potential to help to achieve the essential health system objectives of accountability and responsiveness. More generally, while it is too early to reach firm conclusions about the effectiveness of these schemes for increasing service quality and efficiency, it is clear that the Chinese government is seeking new ways to structure the relationships in their health system to ensure that new funds for health are well-spent.

MODIFYING DEMAND

The chapters by Witter and Powell-Jackson et al. both examine approaches to securing improved access to maternal health services in low-income settings, where problems of high maternal mortality are caused in part by low levels of professional attendance at delivery. Witter reviews the experience of applying exemptions for maternity services in Ghana and Senegal and finds evidence that exemptions are potentially a feasible and effective route for removing financial barriers to care. She concludes, however, that implementation challenges, including fungibility of resources at the facility level, and challenges of parallel funding streams mean that such a policy cannot provide a long-term solution to the problem of financing maternity care. The chapter by Powell-Jackson and colleagues evaluates the impact of the Safe Delivery Incentive Programme in Nepal, which provides cash payments both to mothers and to providers to encourage professional support at the time of delivery. Using data from one district, the authors demonstrate that the scheme has had a significant impact on uptake of delivery services, but only in communities where women's groups were active. This finding underlines the importance of effective communication to target groups in ensuring effective uptake of new financing interventions. The authors also raise concerns about the small size of the cash payment in relation to the high out-of-pocket costs of delivery and the risk that by incentivizing uptake of these services the scheme is potentially exposing households to catastrophic levels of expenditure.

FINANCING AS SYSTEMS INTEGRATION

The volume concludes with two chapters that argue that health financing reform can have an integrating effect on the health system as a whole. Kutzin and colleagues describe the reforms that have taken place in Kyrgyzstan and Moldova, showing how in both countries a centralized risk pool (called SHI) has allowed previously fragmented systems of financing and provision to be combined, with stronger risk pooling and more effective purchasing. Two key lessons emerge. First, even in a low-income setting with a large informal sector, it is possible for the creation of a new SHI fund to transform the health system, and second, that funding *sources* are not health financing *systems*: with careful attention to pooling and coverage arrangements, it is possible to introduce SHI without exacerbating fragmentation.

The chapter by Chernichovsky et al. also views the lack of sufficient coverage and income protection as a reflection of a more general problem: a lack of an integrated and coherent health system. This "developing" system, defined by the standards of the "emerging paradigm" in developed systems, cannot not live up to its potential because it cannot handle effectively policymaking and oversight, funding and allocation, organization and management of care consumption, and provision. The chapter shows that the problem can persist at any level of economic development (e.g., Tanzania, Mexico, and the United States) and can be universally rectified by adopting the standards of the "emerging paradigm." These lead to a comparatively equitable, sustainable, efficient, and responsive system.

ACKNOWLEDGMENTS

We acknowledge with thanks the contributions of colleagues who reviewed papers for the volume: Adam Wagstaff, Richard van Kleef, Owen O'Donnell, Anne Mills, William Hsiao, Eduardo Gonzales Pier, Konstantin Beck, and Oscar Picazzo. Jeremiah Groen provided excellent research assistance.

Dov Chernichovsky
Kara Hanson
Editors

SECTION I
THE CHANGING INTERNATIONAL CONTEXT

THE DOUBLE BURDEN OF DISEASE IN DEVELOPING COUNTRIES: THE MEXICAN EXPERIENCE

Cristina Gutiérrez-Delgado and
Veronica Guajardo-Barrón

ABSTRACT

Objective – *To present the challenges arising from the double burden of disease in developing countries, focusing on the case of Mexico, and to propose a strategy for addressing these challenges.*

Methodology/approach – *Mortality and morbidity data are presented for selected countries and groups of diseases. Specific examples of the pressures faced by the public health services in Mexico to provide and finance treatment for communicable and non-communicable diseases are used to illustrate the extent of the challenges in the context of a country with limited resources.*

Findings – *Public health systems in developing countries face strong pressure to provide and finance treatment for both communicable and non-communicable diseases, inevitably producing competition among diseases and conditions and requiring trade-offs between equity and efficiency goals.*

Innovations in Health System Finance in Developing and Transitional Economies
Advances in Health Economics and Health Services Research, Volume 21, 3–22
Copyright © 2009 by Emerald Group Publishing Limited
All rights of reproduction in any form reserved
ISSN: 0731-2199/doi:10.1108/S0731-2199(2009)0000021004

Implications for policy – In developing countries, addressing the challenges presented by the double burden of disease requires a multidisciplinary approach to develop and strengthen the policymaking process. This involves the use of analytical tools applied to each stage of the planning cycle, in particular the use of an explicit priority setting process together with monitoring and assessment to strengthen decision making under limited resources.

INTRODUCTION

The quest to recover and improve human health has made the field of medicine one of the most dynamic and better financed areas for research and development in human history (OMS, 2002; DeBakey, 2006). This quest has been strengthened since the mid-nineteenth century in developed countries, where the pharmaceutical and medical devices industries were created and supported as part of the long-term planning for the health sector and indeed for economic development in general (OMS, 2002).

Knowledge of human health and disease has generated two broad areas of medicine. On the one hand, there is the development of treatments for diseases once they are manifested. This area, widely taught in medical schools, is known as clinical or curative medicine. On the other hand, there is the area of prevention of diseases and promotion of healthy life styles. This area, less widespread in medical schools, is known as preventive medicine. These two areas are complementary and form the core of any integrated health system in the world (OMS, 2002; DeBakey, 2006).

During the first half of the twentieth century, rapid adoption into health systems of preventive and curative technologies to combat communicable diseases and nutritional deficiencies, as well as to improve care for maternal and prenatal conditions, led to a substantial decrease in the burden posed by these conditions in developed countries. However, adoption of these technologies in developing countries is highly dependent on three factors.

The first factor is the long-term planning that developing countries undertake for their health system. This factor is particularly relevant as many developing countries face unstable social and political conditions that make long-term planning difficult to operate and maintain. The second factor is the price of the technologies which constrains their sustainable introduction into the public health system (Jamison, Lau, & Wang, 2005). The price factor is important even if developing countries receive external funding from multilateral or philanthropic sources, given that this financial help tends to be provided for a limited period (Garrett & Schneider, 2009). The third factor is the non-financial resources required to introduce technologies into the public health sector, particularly the requirement for specialized personnel; it takes time to train such staff, and there is the further problem of retaining trained personnel in the public health system and indeed in these countries (Garrett & Schneider, 2009).

A consequence of this difference in the speed of adoption of technologies is that at the beginning of the twenty-first century, developing countries, particularly low-income countries, still face an important burden caused by communicable diseases, maternal and perinatal conditions, and nutritional deficiencies reflected in mortality and morbidity, mainly concentrated in younger age groups (Table 1).

A positive result of adopting technologies to prevent or treat communicable diseases is the increase in life expectancy at birth that has been observed worldwide, despite the slower rate of technology adoption in developing countries. This increase is particularly evident in developing countries where life expectancy has risen on average from 40 years in 1950 to 65 years in 2001 (Jamison et al., 2006). A notable exception is sub-Saharan Africa, particularly South Africa, where the human immunodeficiency virus (HIV)/acquired immune deficiency syndrome (AIDS) epidemic has caused a significant slowdown in the rate of increase for this vital index in the past 20 years (Table 2).

This increase in life expectancy has generated an increase in the number of cases of non-communicable diseases in all countries. Non-communicable diseases are mainly related to negative changes in lifestyle,[1] the effects of which are evident in the long term, affecting the quality of life of the population. As a result, the increase in life expectancy has not been translated into a direct improvement in the health and quality of life of people (Jamison et al., 2006; Lopez, Mathers, Ezzati, Jamison, & Murray, 2006).

In addition to the communicable and non-communicable disease groups, a third broad group of interest for a general analysis of the dynamics of health is formed by the injuries. However, because of their random nature, the burden placed by this group on public health systems has had only a modest growth in comparison with the growth of the non-communicable disease group (Table 1). The exceptions are countries under war conditions, which usually experience an increase in the burden of injuries for some time until gradually decreasing to near pre-war levels.

The growing burden of non-communicable diseases generates strong pressures in developing countries, which face the problem of having to provide and finance their treatment while continuing to maintain commitments to communicable diseases, nutritional deficiencies, and maternal and

GUTIÉRREZ-DELGADO AND GUAJARDO-BARRÓN

Table 1. Deaths and Disability-Adjusted Life Years (DALYs) by Level of Income and Broad Cause Group, 2004.

Development Groups	Income Groups	Concept	Age Group (years)	Broad Cause Groups					
				Communicable		Non-communicable		Injuries	
				Thousands	%	Thousands	%	Thousands	%
Developing countries	Low-income countries	Deaths	0–14	8,410	62%	580	6%	449	19%
			15–59	3,532	26%	3,106	30%	1,491	64%
			60+	1,632	12%	6,673	64%	378	16%
			Total	13,574		10,359		2,318	
		DALYs	0–14	332,459	71%	49,313	18%	28,045	33%
			15–59	125,392	27%	166,152	61%	55,318	64%
			60+	10,961	2%	57,167	21%	2,862	3%
			Total	468,812		272,632		86,225	
	Middle-income countries	Deaths	0–14	1,601	42%	347	2%	394	13%
			15–59	1,262	33%	4,023	23%	1,990	67%
			60+	985	26%	13,177	75%	571	19%
			Total	3,848		17,547		2,955	
		DALYs	0–14	71,185	56%	38,124	11%	19,088	21%
			15–59	50,202	39%	218,841	62%	66,862	74%
			60+	6,186	5%	98,230	28%	4,141	5%
			Total	127,573		355,195		90,091	
Developed countries	High-income countries	Deaths	0–14	47	9%	39	1%	17	3%
			15–59	64	12%	903	13%	277	54%
			60+	429	79%	6,153	87%	215	42%
			Total	540		7,095		509	
		DALYs	0–14	2,688	37%	6,054	6%	1,199	11%
			15–59	3,131	43%	57,349	55%	8,806	78%
			60+	1,520	21%	40,125	39%	1,217	11%
			Total	7,339		103,528		11,222	
World		Deaths	0–14	10,062	56%	966	3%	860	15%
			15–59	4,861	27%	8,035	23%	3,759	65%
			60+	3,048	17%	26,015	74%	1,164	20%
			Total	17,971		35,016		5,783	
		DALYs	0–14	406,490	67%	93,529	13%	48,348	26%
			15–59	178,826	30%	442,518	60%	131,043	70%
			60+	18,677	3%	195,604	27%	8,224	4%
			Total	603,993		731,651		187,615	

Source: Authors based on WHO (2008).
Note: The broad group "communicable" includes communicable diseases, maternal and perinatal conditions, and nutritional deficiencies.

Table 2.   Life Expectancy for Selected Countries.

Period	Sex	Country			
		South Africa	Kyrgyzstan	China	Mexico
1950–1955	Male	44.0	48.8	39.3	48.9
	Female	46.0	57.3	42.3	52.5
	Both sexes combined	45.0	52.9	40.8	50.8
1975–1980	Male	52.5	58.0	64.5	62.2
	Female	58.8	66.5	66.3	68.6
	Both sexes combined	55.5	62.3	65.3	65.0
2000–2005	Male	51.2	61.4	70.5	72.4
	Female	55.6	69.4	73.7	77.4
	Both sexes combined	53.4	65.3	72.0	74.9
2025–2030	Male	55.3	66.9	74.8	77.2
	Female	56.2	74.1	78.6	81.9
	Both sexes combined	56.0	70.5	76.6	79.6

Source: Authors based on UN (2007).

perinatal conditions. The problem of concurrent provision and financing for these two broad groups of diseases is known as the double burden of disease for developing countries.

CHALLENGES OF THE DOUBLE BURDEN OF DISEASE

The double burden of disease poses two main challenges to public health systems in developing countries. First, they must address the challenge of equity in access to treatment for communicable and non-communicable diseases as well as for injuries. Second, they must do this efficiently, understood here as maximizing health gains given limited resources (González-Pier et al., 2006a). These two objectives may conflict, creating new problems for decision makers who need to determine the best way available to reach a balance between them. The challenges are magnified in environments where health systems are fragmented, as in most middle-income countries in Latin America. The case of Mexico helps to illustrate this problem.

The Mexican population was estimated to be 105 million people in 2007 (CONAPO, 2009). Gross domestic product per capita was USD$7,972[2] that year (BANXICO, 2008). The Mexican health system is composed of three main subsystems: the social security institutions, public services, and private services.[3] Each subsystem has characteristics that create fragmentation along the lines of population covered, financing, and access to treatment (Table 3).

Mexican mortality and morbidity have been dominated by non-communicable diseases since the late 1970s (Fig. 1), soon after the introduction of community-based interventions such as the National Immunization Program (NIP)[4] in conjunction with expansion and

Table 3. The Mexican Health System in 2008.

Health Care Subsystem	Management Organization	Financing	Provider
Social security	Instituto Mexicano del Seguro Social (IMSS)	Federal government, employers, and employees	Own facilities and contracting
	Instituto de Seguridad y Servicios Sociales para los Trabajadores del Estado (ISSSTE)	Federal government and employees	Own facilities
	State social security institutions	State government and employees	Own facilities
	Petroleos Mexicanos (PEMEX), Secretaría de Defensa Nacional (SEDENA), Secretaría de Marina (SECMAR)	Employer and employees	Own facilities and contracting
Public services	IMSS-Oportunidades	Federal government	Own facilities
	System of Social Protection in Health (Popular Health Insurance)	Federal and state governments, families in income deciles III to X	State Health Services facilities
	State Health Services	State government and patient	Own facilities
Private services	Private health units	Patient	Own facilities
	Private health consortiums (networks)	Patient	Own facilities
	Insurance companies specialized in health (Health Management Organization – HMO type)	Insured population	Own facilities or contracting to private health networks

Source: Authors based on Córdova-Villalobos (2009).

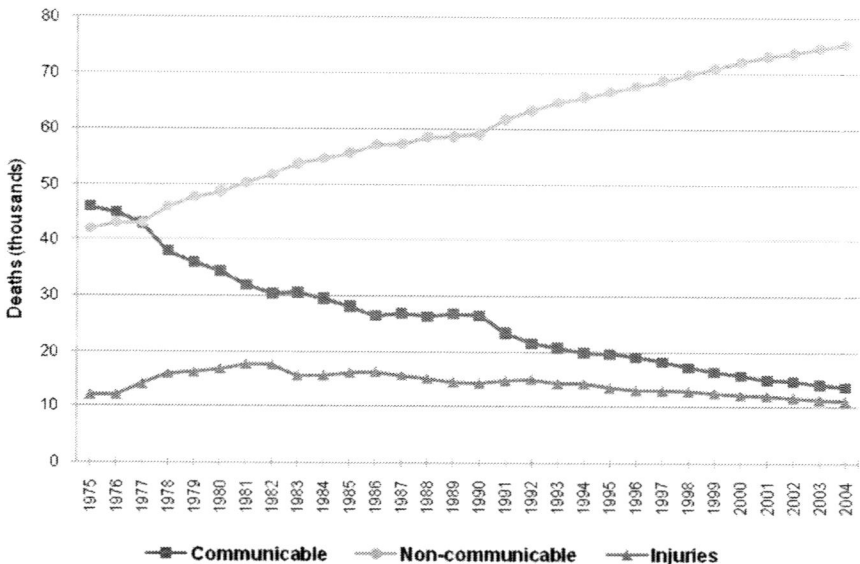

Fig. 1. Distribution of Deaths by Broad Cause Groups, Mexico, 1975–2004. *Note:* The Broad Group "Communicable" Includes Communicable Diseases, Maternal and Perinatal Conditions, and Nutritional Deficiencies. *Source:* INEGI (2009), Salud (2004).

improvement of the basic sanitary infrastructure[5] nationwide (Sepúlveda, Bustreo, & Lozano, 2006). The community-based interventions that were adopted in the early 1970s were affordable for the public health system and could be implemented using the available infrastructure and human resources (González-Pier et al., 2006a).

In the Mexican case, the burden of non-communicable disease is concentrated in a small group of chronic conditions that amount to 35% of total deaths and 17% of all lost years of healthy life.[6] In addition, road traffic accidents represent approximately 4% of deaths and lost years of healthy life, a greater share than the burden of any individual communicable disease. The concentration of the burden in a group of four chronic diseases and road traffic accidents is in line with the burden posed by their risk factors, which amount to 45% of deaths and 20.4% of all lost years of healthy life (Table 4). The specific diseases, injuries, and risk factors that are the leading causes of burden in Mexico emphasize the advanced pattern of epidemiological transition toward an aging population that is characteristic of developed countries. In the medium and long term, this transition implies

Table 4.   Leading Causes of Mortality and Disability-Adjusted Life Years (DALYs) by Disease, Injury, and Risk Factor, Mexico, 2004.

Disease	Proportion of Total for Both Sexes	Risk Factor	Proportion of Total for Both Sexes
Mortality			
Ischemic heart disease	13.3%	High blood glucose	14.40%
Diabetes mellitus	9.9%	High body mass index	12.40%
Cerebrovascular disease	6.1%	High blood pressure	10.10%
Cirrhosis of the liver	5.6%	Alcohol use	8.40%
Road traffic accidents	4.4%	Tobacco use	4.80%
DALYs			
Unipolar depressive disorders	6.4%	Alcohol use	7.50%
Road traffic accidents	4.6%	High body mass index	5.30%
Birth asphyxia and birth trauma	4.2%	High blood glucose	5.20%
Diabetes mellitus	3.6%	High blood pressure	2.40%
Ischemic heart disease	3.2%	Unsafe sex	1.90%

Source: Authors based on González-Pier et al. (2006a).

the need to create the infrastructure and train specialized personnel which at present are not available.

Despite the evidence of increasing need, treatments for non-communicable diseases have not been readily incorporated into the public health system due to the high price of technologies and the requirement for specialized facilities and personnel. In addition, new technologies in preventive medicine and in the treatment of communicable diseases place pressure on the limited resources available in the health system, generating competition for resources. Good examples of the pressure on financial resources are provided by the cases of antiretroviral (ARV) treatment for HIV/AIDS, preventive interventions against cervical cancer, and renal replacement therapies (RRP).

Antiretroviral Treatment for HIV/AIDS

HIV/AIDS is a sexually transmitted disease with no cure that affects the immune system of the person who suffers from it. Since its outbreak in the 1980s, a number of ARV drugs have been developed that aim to maintain the patient's immune system. Results show that those with good adherence to ARV treatment, combined with careful monitoring, can lead a normal life for over 15 years (King, Justice, & Roberts, 2003). The extended lifespan of

HIV/AIDS patients under ARV treatment has caused experts to contemplate whether the disease should be considered to be chronic. In 2001, following the recommendations from the World Health Organization (WHO), Mexico implemented a national program to provide ARV treatment free of charge to all people who require it, regardless of their health insurance status. In December 2007, the program covered 46,689 people, mainly men in their late 30s and early 40s. The annual average cost of providing ARV that year was USD$6,283, the highest among the countries of Latin America (Hernández-Avila, 2008). The total annual cost of the program was USD$293 million, representing 2.8% of public expenditure on health care services, making it the most expensive national program in the country[7] (Table 5). Lack of continuous monitoring[8] of patients receiving ARV is leading to the development of earlier resistance to conventional ARV, forcing a change to more expensive second-line ARV treatment and generating an unsustainable increase in the total cost of the program. In 2008, the Ministry of Health negotiated with pharmaceutical suppliers to reduce the price of patented ARVs to address the disparity in the average cost of ARV among comparable economies of Latin America.

Table 5. Financial Burden of Treatment for Three Diseases, Mexico, 2007.

Disease	Intervention	Target Population	Annual Unit Cost (USD)	Annual Total Cost (Million USD)	Percentage of Public Expenses for Health Care Services
HIV/AIDS	Antiretroviral treatment	46,689	6,283	293.4	2.8%
Cervix uteri cancer	HPV vaccine	863,582	237	205.0	1.9%
	Hybrid capture screening	5,607,471	12	66.4	0.6%
	Papanicolaou screening	7,337,520	8	56.5	0.5%
End-stage renal disease	Peritoneal dialysis	80,231	9,439	757.3	7.1%
	Hemodialysis	20,058	16,423	329.4	3.1%
	Renal transplant	5,050	37,479	189.3	1.8%

Note: HPV, human papilloma virus.
Source: Authors calculations based on Guajardo-Barrón, Gutiérrez-Delgado, and Rivera-Peña (2009), Gutiérrez-Delgado, Baéz-Mendoza, González-Pier, Prieto de la Rosa, & Witlen (2008), Gutiérrez-Delgado (2006), and SHCP (2009).

The results were mixed as some firms did not offer any reduction in their prices, while others offered reductions of up to 30%. That same year the Ministry of Health decided to include the cost of the tests required for continuous monitoring in the total cost of the program. In parallel, the Ministry decided not to purchase the newest and most expensive patented ARVs until a cost-effectiveness analysis for the Mexican situation could be performed. Results of these measures to try to control the total cost of the program are likely to be seen in the medium term, although the Ministry of Health is aware that there will be pressure from patients to include the newest ARVs.

Screening and Prevention of Cervical Cancer

In Mexico, cervical cancer is the most frequent cancer in women over 25 years; it represents the 11th highest cause of death among women with 4,270 deaths in 2005 and a mortality rate of 8 cases per 100,000 women. Cervical cancer is partially preventable and treatment can produce complete recovery if the disease is detected in its early stages. Its prevalence is higher among marginalized women who never have access to screening.[9] New preventive technologies against cervical cancer have been developed since the 1980s, among them the hybrid capture (HC) test for screening for human papilloma virus (HPV) and a vaccine against the four most frequent types of HPV.[10] As both technologies are substantially more expensive than the preventive screening by Papanicolaou (Pap) smear provided through the National Cervical Cancer Screening Program (NCCSP), the Ministry of Health undertook a health technology assessment to assess the combination of interventions that maximizes health outcomes given limited resources (UAE & CENETEC, 2008). The strongest financial restriction is imposed by the price per dose of the HPV vaccine, which was originally offered to the Ministry at USD$80, making it the most expensive vaccine in history and impossible to integrate into the NIP.[11] The financial burden of purchasing the vaccine to cover around 863,000 women of 12 years of age represents 1.9% of public health service expenditure for 2007 (Table 5). The results of the health technology assessment recommended strengthening the NCCSP through a gradual introduction of the HC test that would represent a financial impact of 0.6% of public health service expenditure for 2007, potentially covering 5.6 million women aged 30–64. Results also show that the vaccine is not offering enough evidence of long-term efficacy: the protection provided by immunization should last for at least 20 years without waning, but evidence from clinical trials suggested protection of only six years. In addition, the average cost-effectiveness ratio of the vaccine is eight times higher than the Pap or HC tests, making it not cost-effective in the Mexican case unless the price per dose drops to USD$16.40 (Gutiérrez-Delgado, Báez-Mendoza, González-Pier, Prieto de la Rosa, & Witlen, 2008). However, lobbying by the two manufacturers to introduce the vaccine into the NIP led to the inclusion of the vaccine in the Mexican Norm for Diagnostics, Prevention, and Treatment of Cervical Cancer in 2007, as well as in the Positive List of Medicines and other Medical Materials.[12] This was followed in 2008 by successful lobbying of the Chamber of Deputies, in charge of assigning the annual budget for health care, to allocate funds to develop a HPV vaccine pilot program to be applied in the 125 poorer municipalities in the country[13] (CNEGSR & INSP, 2008). Results from the pilot program show that if introduced to the NIP, the vaccine can be implemented with a smaller number of doses than recommended by the producers (CONAVA, 2009). The long-term results of eventually introducing this vaccine to the NIP remain to be seen. The main concern of the Ministry of Health is the impact that it would have on coverage of Pap or HC tests in the NCCSP, as the vaccination does not remove the need for screening, and if immunized women are not properly informed, they can develop false expectations about their probability of developing cervical cancer[14] (Prieto de la Rosa, Gutiérrez-Delgado, Feinholz-Klip, Morales-González, & Witlen, 2008).

Provision of Renal Replacement Therapy for Chronic Renal Disease

Chronic renal disease (CRD) is a condition developed as a complication of other, primarily chronic diseases such as diabetes mellitus, hypertension, or glomerulonephritis and less frequently derived from genetic conditions as polycystic kidney disease.[15] CRD is partially preventable if the diseases that cause it are well controlled, implying lifestyle changes among the population over 50 years of age. Once a person develops CRD, the only way to be kept alive is through any of the three RRT available: peritoneal dialysis (PD), hemodialysis (HD), or kidney transplant (KT). Of the three therapies, KT is the only one that offers almost total recovery, the best quality of life, and the longest survival time.[16] The number of people who suffer from CRD is estimated to be approximately 100,000 nationally.[17] Among those suffering from the disease, only the ones covered by social security institutions (Table 3) have access to any of the therapies without paying out-of-pocket.

The costs of RRT impose a major financial burden on the social security institutions that offer them.[18] In contrast with other countries, institutions in Mexico offer PD as the most frequent RRT. The annual cost of PD is about 40% less than the corresponding cost of HD while survival results are similar for both types of therapies (González-Pier et al., 2006b). The infrastructure for KT in Mexico is incipient and the culture of organ donation weak, making this therapy an option for only a small number of patients. Overall, the cost of providing RRT to all of those estimated to be in need would represent 12% of public health service expenditure for 2007, a level of spending which could not be sustained in the long term without causing major funding problems for the rest of the health system (Table 5). As a response to pressure from producers and patients, the System of Social Protection in Health (Table 3) is discussing whether it would be possible to finance RRT for patients under 18 years of age, as financing these therapies for the entire covered population is unaffordable. However, the decision about whether to restrict the eligible population poses ethical and social dilemmas, as setting limits to RRT based on age is controversial among both clinicians and patients. In addition, it is evident that the public services do not have the infrastructure and human resources to provide the services even among this restricted population (Table 3). These constraints, which require both financing and time to overcome, are two strong limitations that the System of Social Protection in Health should bear in mind before reaching a decision.

The Costs of Obesity and Overweight

The increasing financial burden of treatment of non-communicable diseases such as CRD is raising awareness in Mexico, and worldwide, of the need to strengthen the delivery and uptake of preventive measures that in the long term can reduce the non-communicable disease burden. One strategy that is widely discussed is to address their risk factors (OECD, 2008). In 2008, the Mexican Ministry of Health developed an analysis of the financial burden posed by selected non-communicable diseases. The study included diseases for which obesity and overweight are the most important risk factors.

Obesity and overweight are considered the most important risk factors for developing chronic diseases including diabetes mellitus type 2, hypertension, cardiovascular diseases, some types of cancer, and osteoarthritis. The treatment required for these diseases places a major burden on the finances, human resources, and infrastructure available in any health care system.

In Mexico, the prevalence of obesity and overweight is increasing rapidly (Olaiz et al., 2003; Olaiz-Fernández et al., 2006). In 2006, the prevalence of obesity among adult women was 34.5%, and among men was 24.2%. The prevalence of overweight was higher among men (42.5%) compared with 37.4% for women (Olaiz-Fernández et al., 2006). These results indicate that obesity and overweight are a major public health problem in Mexico.

Estimates of the financial impact of this risk factor in the Mexican population were calculated by Guajardo-Barrón, Gutiérrez-Delgado, & Arzoz-Padrés (2009a). These estimates concentrated on the financial implications of providing treatment for selected diseases that have obesity as their main risk factor.

Fig. 2 shows the lost income for premature death due to diabetes mellitus type 2, cardiovascular diseases, breast cancer, and colon-rectal cancer attributable to obesity and overweight for the period 2000–2017. The estimated lost income under the base scenario for 2008 was USD$1,931 million, affecting 45,504 families that probably face a situation of catastrophic and impoverishing health expenditures. A wide range of scenarios were estimated for 2017, which vary between USD$2,338 million and USD$7,776 million per year, affecting 68,471 families.

Fig. 3 shows the estimated annual total cost of treatment for diabetes mellitus type 2, hypertension, breast cancer, and osteoarthritis attributable to obesity and overweight. Estimates show that in 2008 the total cost was USD$3,250 million under the base scenario. This amount represents 33.2% of the Mexican public health services budget in that year. The present value of cost estimates for 2017 fluctuates between USD$5,993 million and USD$7,791 million, which would represent between 61.2% and 79.5% of the public health services budget in 2008.

These results demonstrate the urgent need to implement preventive measures to reduce the rate of growth of this risk factor in Mexico. International experience shows that a combination of preventive measures should be implemented to address obesity and overweight (OECD, 2008). However, the results of any strategy to modify this risk factor will only be observed in the long term.

ADDRESSING THE DOUBLE BURDEN OF DISEASE

To address the double burden of disease in developing countries, it is essential to create and strengthen the multidimensional cycle of rational policymaking in health. This cycle, composed of planning, formulation,

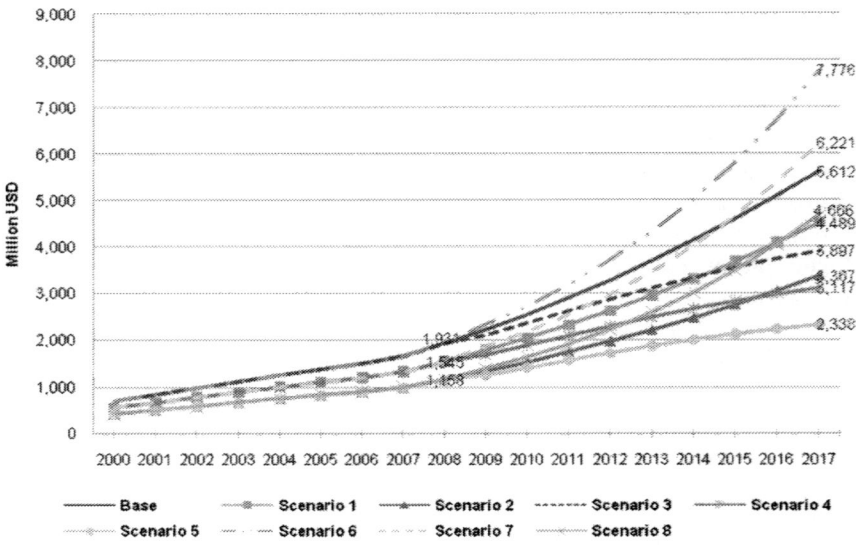

	Assumptions	
Scenario	Income	Projected income
base	no change	no change
1	- 20%	no change
2	- 40%	no change
3	no change	- 5%
4	- 20%	- 5%
5	- 40%	- 5%
6	no change	+ 5%
7	- 20%	+ 5%
8	- 40%	+ 5%

Fig. 2. Lost Income from Premature Death due to Four Non-Communicable Diseases Strongly Related to Obesity and Overweight, Mexico, 2000–2017. *Note:* The Non-Communicable Diseases Considered in the Analysis are Diabetes Mellitus Type 2, Cardiovascular Diseases, Breast Cancer, and Colon-Rectal Cancer. *Source:* Guajardo-Barrón, Gutiérrez-Delgado, & Arzoz-Padrés (2009a).

implementation, monitoring, and assessment, requires a series of processes and analytical tools that complement and reinforce each other to achieve a balance between the two main challenges of health systems under limited resources: equity and efficiency.

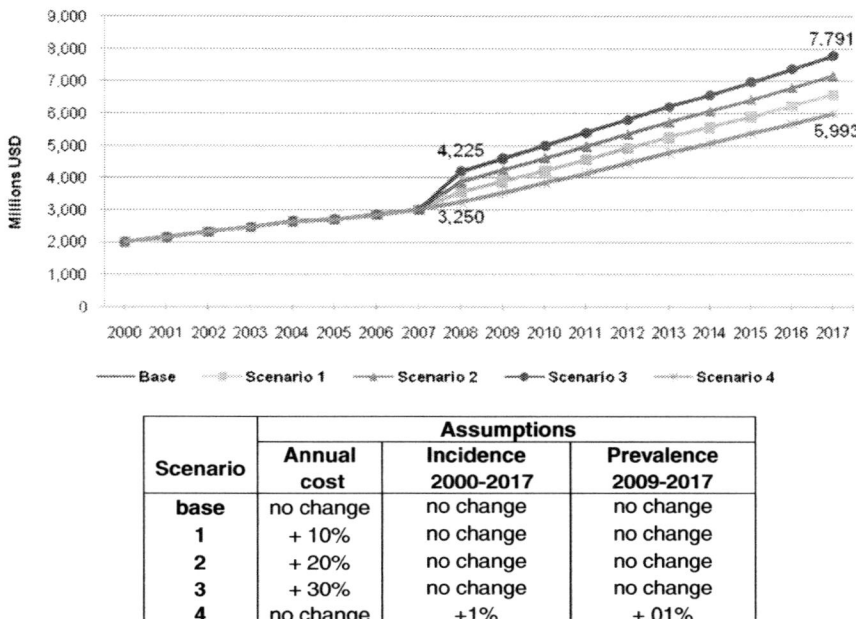

Scenario	Assumptions		
	Annual cost	**Incidence 2000-2017**	**Prevalence 2009-2017**
base	no change	no change	no change
1	+ 10%	no change	no change
2	+ 20%	no change	no change
3	+ 30%	no change	no change
4	no change	+1%	+.01%

Fig. 3. Estimated Annual Total Cost of Treatment for Four Non-Communicable Diseases Strongly Related to Obesity and Overweight, Mexico, 2000–2017. *Note:* The Non-Communicable Diseases Considered in the Analysis are Diabetes Mellitus Type 2, Hypertension, Breast Cancer, and Osteoarthritis. *Source:* Guajardo-Barrón, Gutiérrez-Delgado, & Arzoz-Padrés (2009a).

Under this wider context, developing countries should be aiming to develop and strengthen the public systems that capture data. The relevant systems will include vital statistics, administrative processes (preventive and health care services registered in electronic clinical records, purchasing and inventories, infrastructure, and human resources), monitoring and assessment processes, and periodic surveys (national health surveys, income surveys, and specific panel surveys). Data provided by these systems will provide the basis for other more complex processes of priority setting, which, in turn, provide information through the different stages of the policymaking cycle.

In Mexico, several public institutions are charged with systematically capturing these basic data. Among these institutions are the National Institute of Geographical and Statistical Information (INEGI), the National

Population Council (CONAPO), the Treasury (SHCP), and the Ministry of Health through the National System of Health Information (SINAIS). From 2003, the Law of Access to Public Information makes it possible for anyone to access public data, allowing the cycle of rational policymaking to be developed at the macro, meso, and micro levels.

At the start of the rational policymaking cycle, the use of a priority setting process aims to provide an equitable, transparent, and contestable way to manage pressures from interest groups while defining the needs that will receive the limited resources available. As the priority setting process implies a trade-off between different health system goals, which in turn reflect general values of society, it is always best to develop and use it in an explicit way (Daniels & Sabin, 2002; Baltussen & Niessen, 2006; Baltussen, 2006).

In Mexico, the most recent effort to institutionalize an explicit priority-setting process is found in the context of deciding the order in which a group of more than 60 complex diseases classified as catastrophic expenses by the General Health Council would be financed by the System of Social Protection in Health (González-Pier, Barraza-Lloréns, Gutiérrez-Delgado, & Vargas-Palacios, 2006c). This priority setting process incorporates two groups of general considerations. One group is composed by analytical criteria amenable to quantification through the use of tools such as clinical and epidemiological modeling, cost-effectiveness analysis, budget availability, and implementation analysis. Another group is composed of qualitative concerns that must be addressed through a deliberative process to reach consensus, when possible by different stakeholders (CSG, 2009). Results of this joint process are to be produced in the coming years.

The monitoring and assessment process complements the priority setting process by closing the policymaking cycle. This process provides valuable information on whether priority interventions are available to their target populations and allows re-assessment and refinement of priorities in health as evidence become available (González-Pier et al., 2006a).

In the Mexican context, public institutions providing health care services are subject to an annual performance assessment that involves the measuring of different indicators to assess whether the institutions are reaching their targets for that year. In the case of the Ministry of Health, the results of the performance assessment are published in an annual report available online through the website of the Ministry (Salud, 2008). The publication of results from the assessment is aimed to improve accountability, which is key in the institutionalization of a fair process in the health sector (Daniels & Sabin, 2002).

IMPLICATIONS FOR POLICY

Most developing countries are already advanced along the epidemiological transition toward non-communicable diseases, which generates increasing pressure on the limited resources available for their health care systems. The most relevant policy implications derived from the Mexican case highlight the importance of creating and strengthening a rational policy-making cycle. The cycle requires the development and use of proven analytical tools to understand the challenges posed by the double burden of disease in a country with limited health system resources. These tools include the establishment of public data systems as well as processes for priority setting and assessment that together will allow the re-assessment of health priorities as new evidence become available.

NOTES

1. The negative changes in life style include incorrect nutrition patterns, physical inactivity, addictions, and stress, among other risk factors.

2. Exchange rate 11 Mexican pesos per U.S. dollar.

3. The public health sector is composed of social security institutions and public services as both subsystems receive public funds from the federal and state governments.

4. The Mexican immunization program is one of the most comprehensive worldwide. It includes the basic immunization scheme for children under 5 years of age (with coverage rates consistently above 95%), vaccines for young adults (rubeola, sarampion), and for the elderly (pneumoccocus, influenza). Mexico is the fourth biggest purchaser of vaccines worldwide.

5. The basic sanitary infrastructure comprises electricity, potable water and dwelling networks, paved roads, and the construction of primary care units.

6. Lost years of healthy life are measured through disability-adjusted life years (DALYs). This measure is recommended by the WHO and widely used in the WHO-CHOICE project.

7. In 2007, the total cost of the biggest and most important national program in the health sector, the National Immunization Program, which covers almost 9 million children less than 5 years of age, was USD$273 million.

8. The monitoring consists of periodic tests for CD4 counts and viral load that together cost USD$197 (exchange rate 11 Mexican pesos per U.S. dollar at December 2007). The Mexican norm mandates that the test must be performed at least twice per year meaning an annual cost of USD$395 per patient.

9. Although 80% of women will develop natural immunization against the HPV, the remaining 20%, particularly those with deficiencies in their immune system would be prone to pre-cancer injuries provoked by a persistent HPV infection. If the injury is not detected by screening and treated, it will evolve to cervical cancer in a period of 20 years.

10. Eighteen types of HVP (the oncogenic subgroup out of 100 types of HPV) are related to 99% of cases of cervical cancer. The vaccines developed so far address four of the oncogenic subgroup.

11. If included at the original price offered the annual budget for the National Immunization Program would need to double.

12. Public health care providers are legally bound to purchase only products on the Positive List and to provide the services included in the Mexican Norms.

13. The operation of pilot programs is the traditional way pharmaceutical have found to force the introduction of their products into the public health care system. The pilot program for the HPV vaccine is not exceptional, as its operation is already forcing the Ministry of Health and the social security institutions such as IMSS to introduce gradually the HPV vaccine to a restricted group of beneficiaries.

14. In this respect, producers have developed a publicity campaign that is generating misinformation among the female population, as they are emphasizing benefits that the vaccine does not produce.

15. In Mexico, CRD mortality statistics for the period 2004–2007 show that about 50% of the cases were related to diabetes mellitus, almost 30% of the cases were derived from hypertension, and less than 3% were generated by genetic conditions.

16. Even after transplant, patients should be under lifetime immune-suppression therapy to minimize the probability of rejection of the transplanted kidney. On average, survival time after transplant is 15 years.

17. In Mexico, there is no renal data registry; thus, estimates of Mexicans with CRD are based on information from the U.S. Renal Data System. The estimates fluctuate between 75,000 and 108,000, depending on the prevalence rate used.

18. The financial burden of RRT is so great that IMSS, the biggest social security institution, includes it into its Programa de Administración de Riesgos Institucionales (PARI – Management of Institutional Risk Program).

ACKNOWLEDGMENTS

We acknowledge helpful comments from Kara Hanson. Cristina Gutiérrez-Delgado receives financial support from the Consejo Nacional de Ciencia y Tecnología (CONACyT).

REFERENCES

Battussen, R. (2006). Priority setting of public spending in developing countries: Do not try to do everything for everybody. *Health Policy, 78*, 149–156.

Battussen, R., & Niessen, L. (2006). Priority setting of health interventions: The need for multi-criteria decision analysis. *Cost Effectiveness Resources Allocation, 2006*(4), 14.

Banco de México – BANXICO. (2008). Política monetaria e inflación. Available at www.banxico.gob.mx. Accessed March 2009.

Centro Nacional de Equidad de Género y Salud Reproductiva – CNEGSR e Instituto Nacional de Salud Pública – INSP. (2008). *Programa Madre-Hija*. México: Secretaría de Salud.

Consejo de Salubridad General – CSG. (2009). *Manual para la definición y priorización de intervenciones que ocasionan gastos catastróficos*. México: Secretaría de Salud.

Consejo Nacional de Población – CONAPO. (2009). Proyecciones de la población en México 2005–2050. Available at www.conapo.gob.mx. Accessed March 2009.

Consejo Nacional de Vacunación – CONAVA. (2009). Primera Sesión Ordinaria, Resultados de la primera fase del programa piloto Madre-hija, México.

Córdova-Villalobos, J. (2009). *La salud de los mexicanos 2007–2012, Colección Memoria – Platino, Academia Mexicana de Cirugía*. México: Editorial Alfil.

Daniels, N., & Sabin, J. (2002). *Setting limits fairly*. New York: Oxford University Press.

DeBakey, M. (2006). The role of government in health care: A societal issue. *The American Journal of Surgery, 191,* 145–157.

Garrett, L., & Schneider, K. (2009). Global health: Getting it right. In: A. Gatti & A. Boggio (Eds), *Health and development: Toward a matrix approach*. New York: Plagrave MacMillan.

González-Pier, E., Barraza-Lloréns, M., Gutiérrez-Delgado, C., & Vargas-Palacios, A. (2006c). *Sistema de Protección Social en Salud. Elementos conceptuales, financieros y operativos. Colección Biblioteca de la Salud*. México: Fondo de Cultura Económica – FCE; Secretaría de Salud; Fundación Mexicana para la Salud – FUNSALUD; e Instituto Nacional de Salud Pública – INSP.

González-Pier, E., Gutiérrez-Delgado, C., Stevens, G., Barraza-Lloréns, M., Porras-Condey, R., Carvalho, N., Loncich, K., Dias, R., Kulkarni, S., Casey, A., Murakamu, Y., Ezzati, M., & Salomon, J. (2006a). Priority setting for health interventions in Mexico's system of social protection in health. Health system reform in Mexico 2. *The Lancet Series, 368*(November 4), 1608–1618.

González-Pier, E., Gutiérrez-Delgado, C., Barraza-Lloréns, M., Porras-Condey, R., Salomon, J., Carvalho, N., Casey, A., Dias, R., Ezzati, M., Feehan, M., Hogan, D., Kulkarni, S., Lee, D., Loncich, K., Murakami, Y., Sridharan, L., & Stevens, G. (2006b). *Priority-setting for health interventions in Mexico: 2006 final report*. Mexico: Mexican Ministry of Health and Harvard University.

Guajardo-Barrón, V., Gutiérrez-Delgado, C., & Arzoz-Padrés, J. (2009a). *Documento técnico para la estimación del impacto financiero en la salud de la población Mexicana derivado de la obesidad y el sobrepeso*, Documento de Trabajo 2/2008, Unidad de Análisis Económico, Secretaría de Salud, México.

Guajardo-Barrón, V., Gutiérrez-Delgado, C., & Rivera-Peña, G. (2009b). Mecanismos de integración del sector salud mexicano: Análisis de flujos de efectivo del fondo para el financiamiento público de los servicios de alta especialidad, Documento de Trabajo 1/2008, Unidad de Análisis Económico, Secretaría de Salud, México.

Gutiérrez-Delgado, C. (2006). Impacto financiero de las terapias renales sustitutivas en México, Documento de Trabajo 1/2006, Unidad de Análisis Económico, Secretaría de Salud, México.

Gutiérrez-Delgado, C., Báez-Mendoza, C., González-Pier, E., Prieto de la Rosa, A., & Witlen, R. (2008). Relación costo-beneficio de las intervenciones preventivas contra el cáncer cervical en mujeres mexicanas. *Salud Pública de México, 50*(2), 107–118.

Hernández-Avila, M. (2008). *Financial sustainability of universal access to antirretrovirals in Mexico*. Mexico: HIV/AIDS Conference.

Instituto Nacional de Información Estadística y Geográfica – INEGI. (2009). Indicadores sociodemográficos de México 1930–2000. Available at http://www.inegi.org.mx. Accessed March 2009.

Jamison, D., Breman, J., Measham, R., Alleyne, G., Claeson, M., Evans, D., Jha, P., Mills, A., & Musgrove, P. (2006). *Disease control priorities in developing countries, second edition, disease control priorities project.* New York: The World Bank and Oxford University Press.

Jamison, D., Lau, L., & Wang (2005). Health's contribution to economic growth in an environment of partially endogenous technical progress. In: G. Lopez-Casanova, B. Rivera & L. Currais (Eds), *Health and economic growth: Findings and policy implications.* Cambridge: MIT Press.

King, C., Justice, A., & Roberts, M. (2003). Long-term HIV/AIDS survival estimation in the highly active antiretroviral therapy era. *Medical Decision Making, 23*(1), 9–20.

Lopez, A., Mathers, C., Ezzati, M., Jamison, D., & Murray, C. (2006). *Global burden of disease and risk factors, disease control priorities project.* New York: Oxford University Press.

Olaiz, G., Rojas, R., Barquera, S., Shamah, T., Aguilar, C., Cravito, P., López, P., Hernández, M., Tapia, R., & Sepúlveda, J. (2003). *Encuesta Nacional de Salud 2000. Tomo 2. La salud de los adultos.* Cuernavaca, Morelos, México: Instituto Nacional de Salud Pública.

Olaiz-Fernández, G., Rivera-Dommarco, J., Shamah-Levy, T., Rojas, R., Villalpando-Hernández, S., Hernández-Avila, M., & Sepúlveda-Amor, J. (2006). *Encuesta Nacional de Salud y Nutrición 2006. Cuernavaca.* México: Instituto Nacional de Salud Pública.

Organización Mundial de la Salud – OMS. (2002). Macroeconomía y Salud: Invertir en salud en pro del desarrollo económico, Informe de la Comisión de Macroeconomía y Salud. Ginebra, Suiza.

Organization for Economic Co-operation and Development – OECD. (2008). The economics of prevention, directorate for employment, labour and social affairs, health committee, DELSA/HEA (2008) 13.

Prieto de la Rosa, A., Gutiérrez-Delgado, C., Feinholz-Klip, D., Morales-González, G., & Witlen, R. (2008). Implicaciones éticas y sociales de la introducción de la vacuna contra el virus del papiloma humano en México: Reflexiones sobre una Propuesta de Intervención, Acta Bioethica, year XIV, No, 2.

Secretaría de Hacienda y Crédito Público (SHCP). (2009). Cuenta de la Hacienda Pública Federal 2007, Ejercicio Funcional Programático Económico del Gasto Programable Devengado para los Ramos incluidos en el análisis. Available at http://www.hacienda.gob.mx. Accessed March 9, 2009.

Secretaría de Salud – Salud. (2004). Boletín de información estadística 2004, Mexico.

Secretaría de Salud – Salud. (2008). Rendición de Cuentas en Salud 2007. Secretaría de Salud: Mexico. Available at www.salud.gob.mx. Accessed March 2009.

Sepúlveda, J., Bustreo, F., & Lozano, R. (2006). Improvement of child survival in Mexico: The diagonal approach. *The Lancet,* October 25, DOI: 10.1016/S0140-6736(06)69569-X.

Unidad de Análisis Económico – UAE & Centro Nacional de Excelencia Técnica en Salud – CENETEC. (2008). Evaluación de tres intervenciones preventivas contra el cáncer cervico-uterino, reporte final, Secretaría de Salud, México.

United Nations Secretariat – UN. (2007). World population prospects: The 2006 revision and world urbanization prospects: The 2005 revision, population division of the department of economic and social affairs. Available at http://esa.un.org/unpp. Accessed March 6, 2009.

World Health Organization – WHO. (2008). *The global burden of disease 2004 update.* Available at http://www.who.int/healthinfo/statistics. Accessed March 9, 2009.

PROTECTING PRO-POOR HEALTH SERVICES DURING FINANCIAL CRISES: LESSONS FROM EXPERIENCE ☆

Pablo Gottret, Vaibhav Gupta, Susan Sparkes, Ajay Tandon, Valerie Moran and Peter Berman

ABSTRACT

Objective – This chapter assesses the extent to which previous economic and financial crises had a negative impact on health outcomes and health financing. In addition, we review evidence related to the effectiveness of different policy measures undertaken in past crises to protect access to health services, especially for the poor and vulnerable. The current global crisis is unique both in terms of its scale and origins. Unlike most previous instances, the current crisis has its origins in developed countries, initially the United States, before it spread to middle- and lower-income countries. The current crisis is now affecting almost all countries at all levels of income. This chapter addresses several key questions aimed at helping

☆The findings, interpretations, and conclusions expressed in this chapter are those of the authors and do not necessarily reflect the views of the Board of Executive Directors of the World Bank or the governments they represent.

Innovations in Health System Finance in Developing and Transitional Economies
Advances in Health Economics and Health Services Research, Volume 21, 23–53
© **Published by Emerald Group Publishing Limited**
ISSN: 0731-2199/doi:10.1108/S0731-2199(2009)0000021005

inform possible policy responses to the current crisis from the perspective of the health sector: What is the nature of the current crisis and in what ways does it differ from previous experiences? What are some of the key lessons from previous crises? How have governments responded previously to protect health from such macroeconomic shocks? How can we improve the likelihood of positive action today?

Methodology/approach – *The chapter reviews the literature on the impact of financial crises on health outcomes and health expenditures and on the effectiveness of past policy efforts to protect human development during periods of economic downturn. It also presents analysis of household surveys and health expenditure data to track health seeking behavior and out-of-pocket expenditures by households during times of financial crisis.*

Findings – *Evidence from previous crises indicates that health-related impacts during economic downturns can occur through various channels. The impact in households experiencing reductions in employment and income could be manifest in terms of poorer nutritional outcomes and lower levels of utilization of health care when needed. Households may become impoverished, reduce needed health services, and experience reductions in consumption as a result of health shocks occurring during a time when their economic vulnerability has increased. Women, children, the poor, and informal sector workers are likely to be most at risk of experiencing negative health-related consequences in a crisis. Real government spending per capita on health care could decline due to reduced revenues, currency devaluations, and potential reductions in external aid flows. Low-income countries with weak fiscal positions are likely to be the most vulnerable.*

Implications for policy – *Past crises can inform policy-making aimed at protecting health outcomes and reducing financial risk from health shocks. Evidence from previous crises indicates that broad-brush strategies that maintained overall levels of government health spending tended not to be successful, failing to protect access to quality health services especially for the poor. It is particularly vital to ensure access to essential health commodities, which in many low-income countries are imported, in the face of weakening exchange rates. Focused efforts to sustain the supply of lower-level basic services, combined with targeted demand-side approaches like conditional cash transfers may be more effective than broader sectoral approaches. Low-income countries may need specific short-term measures to ensure that health outcomes do not suffer.*

BACKGROUND

From a macroeconomic perspective, it is an understatement to say that 2008–2009 has been extremely challenging for almost all countries across the world. For some of the poorer countries, the worst global economic contraction since the Great Depression comes on top of the earlier difficulties posed by higher food, fuel, and commodity prices. The initial impacts were felt in the financial, credit, housing, and export markets and are now reaching other economic sectors. Ministers of Finance and Central Bankers around the world, especially from developed countries, have reacted to the crisis with unprecedented rescue packages. The fiscal stimulus in G-20 countries in 2009 is projected to amount to 1.5% of GDP (IMF, 2009). Additional measures have been taken by developing countries. For example, China has announced a 4 trillion Yuan (585 billion US dollars) two-year economic stimulus package to boost growth and domestic demand (Hanson, 2009).

These support and stimulus packages are likely to have important fiscal implications which could have unintended adverse impacts on government sector priorities, including for the health sector. One key imperative is that the rescue and stimulus spending plans not come at the expense of resources for human development, especially programs targeted for the poor. It is equally important that the developed countries maintain the commitments that have made over the past few years to support efforts to reach the millennium development goals (MDGs). These issues are especially critical, given that the evidence from prior crises suggests that government expenditures on health in developing countries are vulnerable during periods of fiscal stress and that donor funding can be very volatile, even in robust economic times. At the same time, economic downturns are often periods when household out-of-pocket health expenditures, especially on medicines, tend to decline. Potential reductions in health expenditures could therefore negatively impact progress toward meeting both the overall as well as the health-specific MDGs.

This chapter reviews the impact of previous financial crises and the impact of the policy measures undertaken in response to these crises on health outcomes and health financing. Learning from past experience should help us to make improved decisions during the present crisis. The chapter draws on existing literature on the impact of financial crises on health as well as more generally on the economy. This review notes the impact of previous financial crises in Latin America and Asia over the 1980s and late 1990s on the real incomes of workers and households and their distribution, and school enrolment. On the policy response side, the chapter warns that social expenditures are procyclical, and that during adjustments, the less pro-poor social expenditures are more likely to be protected. The chapter also emphasizes that crises can have serious consequences for human development, including short-term nutritional deprivations that may increase child mortality, as well as long-lasting negative effects on cognitive ability and physical growth.

The chapter also attempts to assess past experiences of the World Bank with regard to protecting human development in light of economic downturns. The World Bank has supported countries undergoing financial crises, especially in Latin America, Asia, Eastern Europe, and the former Soviet Union through different types of financial and other assistance programs. An important component of this support included adjustment loans that had provisions to protect pro-poor expenditures, including expenditures on health, from declining. The question we seek to answer is whether such provisions were successful in protecting these expenditures and more importantly, whether the expenditures that were protected were actually pro-poor to begin with. If not, it would be important to know what actions on behalf of national governments and donors during this financial crisis could be taken to improve protection for the poor. It is not the purpose of this chapter to make an exhaustive review of World Bank operations in the sphere of health during financial crises. Rather, the aim is to draw some practical lessons from previous operations to gain some understanding about what to replicate and what to avoid in dealing with the current financial crisis.

The chapter draws on a review of existing research and on the analysis of household surveys and other data to track health outcomes and expenditure behavior during times of financial crisis. Most of the analyses of past contractions have focused on middle-income countries. But today, much of our attention on health outcomes is on the low-income countries, especially those of Sub-Saharan Africa whose progress is critical for global achievement of the MDGs. There is little evidence on how previous crises affected these countries, which raises the question of the relevance of past experience to the current threats faced by the low-income countries. Despite this caveat, we believe the lessons learned on protecting pro-poor expenditures are probably highly relevant across a range of poor and middle-income countries.

ECONOMIC CRISES AND HEALTH

Economic crises can have significant negative consequences for health, especially for the poor. Large economic contractions could squeeze public and private resources thereby impacting the availability of health funding and eventually health outcomes. In particular, the poor are especially susceptible to irreversible damages to their health status as a result of economic contractions. Fig. 1 sets out some of the most important pathways linking economic crisis to health outcomes.

Increases in unemployment, declining foreign aid/foreign direct investment (FDI), declining tax revenues, and a lower demand for exports can be expected to result from the current economic crisis. Economic downturns usually result in a significant rise in unemployment, and the current crisis is already witnessing layoffs across the developing and developed world. The current crisis, which originated in the developed countries, has already resulted in a slowdown of growth in most developing countries. Governments in developing and developed countries alike are also likely to witness a fall in government revenues as tax collections dip. Economic uncertainty and domestic problems could force donors to scale back their aid commitments and developing countries to reduce social spending.

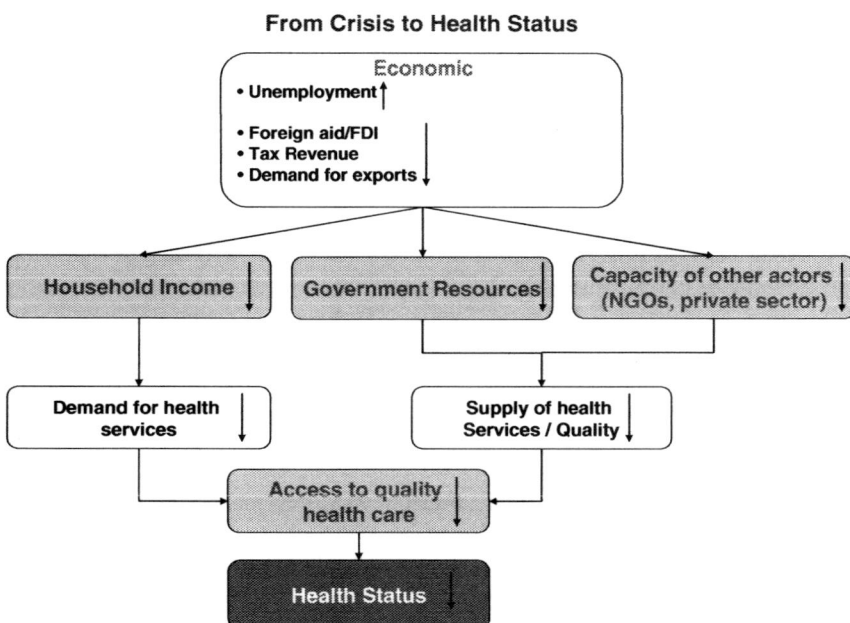

Fig. 1. From Crisis to Health Status.

Household incomes, government resources, and the economic resource capacity of other actors also tend to decline during any crisis. As economic activity slows down and unemployment rises, both labor and non-labor incomes tend to decline. Poorer households are likely to suffer the most as they have less room to readjust and cushion their expenditures, often forcing a decline in demand for health services. Crises can also significantly weaken the public sector, and its ability to supply quality health services; often, delivery of certain services also may be stopped – budget cuts could force public hospitals to freeze hiring of nurses and doctors, for instance. Other actors including NGOs, who typically attract fewer donors during a financial crisis, are also likely to face significant financial constraints during economic crises.

These factors limit individuals' and households' access to quality health care, and consequently, could have an impact on population health outcomes. The poor, and other marginalized groups such as girls and the elderly, are especially likely to suffer during crises as they typically have less control over resources. The non-poor and other groups have in the past captured the public sector to the detriment of the poor. Even if outcomes do not change much in the aggregate, it is likely that the health status of the poor and other marginalized groups will regress if preemptive measures are not taken.

HOW DOES THE CURRENT CRISIS COMPARE WITH PREVIOUS CRISES?

We begin with a brief overview of how the current crisis differs from previous prominent examples. It is important to highlight some of the key differences to understand the implications for the current financial crisis. We focus here on the crisis in Argentina (2001), East Asia (1997–1998), Russia (1997–1998), Peru (1988–92), and Mexico (1980s and 1990s).

One key difference is that previous crises primarily originated in developing countries. The East Asian financial crisis started in April 1997 with the depreciation of the Thai baht, which then triggered a domino effect on the currencies of Indonesia, Korea, Malaysia, and the Philippines. Additionally many countries at the time were plagued by large fiscal and external deficits that inhibited their ability to enact countercyclical government expenditure. The Government of Argentina's foreign debt alone totaled approximately 50% of GDP in late 2001, with $30 billion due in 2002 (Feldstein, 2002).

Fig. 2 shows the contractions in GDP from previous crises for Indonesia, Thailand, Argentina, and Mexico. In all four countries, economic growth not only decreased dramatically, but became negative. The Argentinean economy, for instance, lost 20% of its GDP between 1999 and 2002 (World Bank, 2003b). As a result of the 1997–1998 financial crisis, GDP in Indonesia contracted by 13.1% and by 10% in Thailand in 1998 (Macfarlane Burnet Centre for Medical Research, 2000).

In contrast with the situation during previous crises, the current financial crisis has originated in developed economies. The United States and Europe have been the first hit, with US GDP falling by 6.2% (annualized) in the fourth quarter of 2008 (http://www.bea.gov/newsreleases/national/gdp/gdpnewsrelease.htm) and GDP expected to decline by 4–6% in the Euro area in 2009 (World Bank, 2009b). The IMF estimates as of January 2009 that growth in emerging and developing countries will fall from 6.25% in 2008 to 3.25% in 2009. As shown in Fig. 3, the fall in GDP growth is expected to be less severe in emerging and developing economies than in advanced economies, where growth is expected to become negative.

Some countries are in better fiscal positions now than during the early stages of previous crisis, but more countries are affected. As of 2008, emerging and developing countries on average had positive general government fiscal balances and were in a better fiscal position than advanced economies (Fig. 4). In reaction to the crisis, some governments have announced expansionary fiscal packages to boost their economies (IMF, 2009). These policy levers were not necessarily available during previous crises. But as the crisis expands, it affects more countries that are less able to mobilize significant domestic or international financing to produce much stimulus.

Trade is slowing down and reduced demand for exports from developed country markets is hurting developing countries. World trade volumes are projected to contract 2.1% in 2009 and there are fears that a prolonged crisis in developed countries may give way to increasing calls for protectionism (World Bank, 2009a). In November and October 2008, exports from low-income countries to the United States were down approximately 6% relative to the same time period in 2007, and approximately 3% from middle-income countries (World Bank, 2009a). Although some of these declines reflect a fall in commodity prices, low-income countries are likely to continue to face adverse market conditions for exports to high-income countries.

The importance of FDI has increased in most developing countries in recent years. As shown in Fig. 5, FDI is playing an increasingly important role in the economies of both low- and middle-income countries. Between 2005 and 2007, FDI totaled approximately 2.8% of GDP in low- and

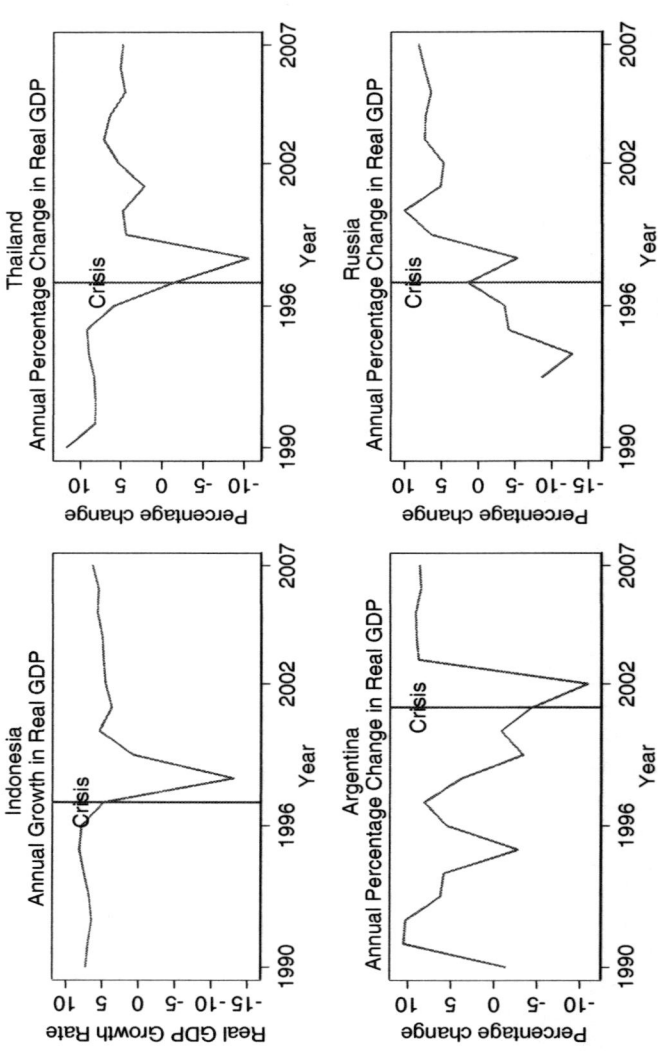

Fig. 2. GDP Growth in Indonesia, Thailand, Argentina, and Russia, 1990–2007. *Source:* IMF, World Economic Outlook, October 2008.

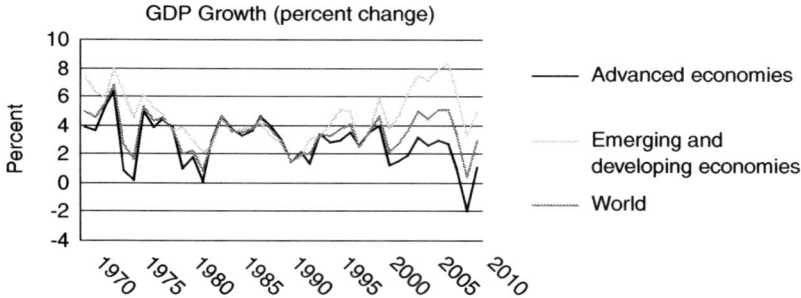

Fig. 3. Trends and Projections of GDP Growth, 1970–2010. *Note:* Projections are for 2009 and 2010. *Source:* IMF (2009).

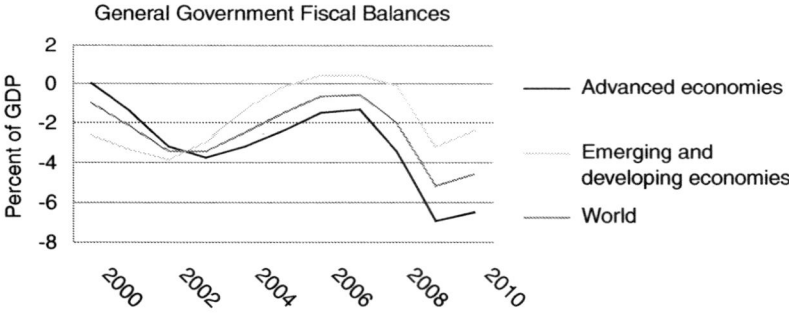

Fig. 4. General Government Fiscal Balances, 2000–2010. *Note:* Projections are for 2009 and 2010. *Source:* IMF (2009).

middle-income countries (World Bank, 2009a). Declines in FDI and private international capital flows triggered by the financial crisis are already having a strong impact in developing countries. FDI flows in 2008 saw a 10% decline from 2007. This was highlighted by the UN Conference on Trade and Development (UNCTAD) in its World Investment Report 2008 (UN Conference on Trade and Development, 2008).

Remittances constitute an increasingly important source of foreign exchange and direct support to households in many developing countries. In 2008 alone, remittances totaled $283 billion (World Bank, 2009a). Between 2005 and 2007, the median value of remittances to low-income countries was 3.2% of GDP. In some countries, this number was above 20%.[1] Recession in developed countries and resulting rises in unemployment and decreased demand may decrease these remittances substantially.

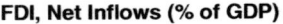

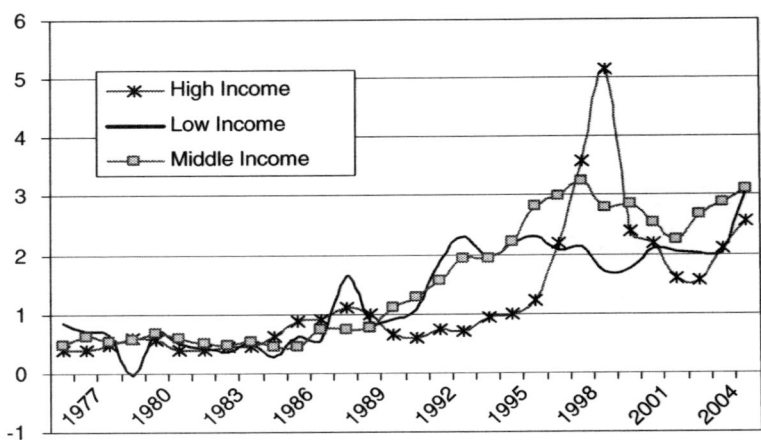

Fig. 5. Foreign Direct Investment (1977–2007).

World Bank projections in November 2008 suggested that remittances to developing countries could decrease by between 1% and 6% in 2009.

Increased reliance on development assistance for health (DAH) in recent years puts poor countries at greater risk of being affected by what happens in developed countries. In 1996, only seven countries received DAH, which comprised 30% or more of total health expenditure. By 2006, this number had grown to 23 (WHO, 2008). Currently, in Rwanda and Ethiopia, over 50% of total government budgeted health expenditure is financed by donors, and off-budget donor funding for health accounts for more than 100% of government health expenditures. Although these large increases in external assistance for health have allowed governments to expand service provision, this has also made many countries dependent on these flows to sustain expenditure levels and service delivery to their populations, especially the poor and most vulnerable. It is yet to be seen how the financial crisis will affect aid flows. Research has shown that there is an ambiguous relationship between economic growth in donor countries and subsequent aid flows to developing countries (Mold, Olcer, & Prizzon, 2008), and this is clearly an area of concern.

In addition to key differences from previous crises, there remain elements that tend to be common across all financial crises. Unemployment, for instance, is projected to increase dramatically in both the developed and developing world. The International Labor Organization projects that global unemployment could increase by 18–30 million in 2009 (International Labor Organization, 2009). Additionally, in the worst case scenario approximately 200 million workers, particularly in developing countries, could be pushed into extreme poverty.

Slower growth and shrinking trade will likely halt progress made by developing countries in reducing poverty. Estimates suggest that slower growth in Indonesia will force some 1.6 million Indonesians, who otherwise would have escaped poverty, to remain below the national poverty line in 2009. In 2010, 2.7 million Indonesians will remain in poverty who would otherwise have escaped (Lin, 2008). This slowdown in poverty reduction is expected to be compounded by the already severe impacts of the food and fuel crisis. Current estimates suggest that between 130 and 155 million people were pushed into poverty in 2008 as a result of increased food and fuel prices (World Bank, 2009a). Coupled with these numbers are estimates that as a result of lower economic growth, 46 million people who would have otherwise exceeded this limit will remain below the $1.25 per day poverty line (World Bank, 2009b).

As noted above, reduced trade flows and remittances along with downward pressures on FDI and donor assistance are channels through which the severe economic and financial difficulties in Europe, the United States, and Japan are being transmitted to less developed countries in ways that were not so significant in past crises. Nevertheless, although previous financial crises may have been different in nature, lessons can be derived with specific reference to health expenditures, utilization, and outcomes. These are discussed subsequently.

IMPACT OF THE PREVIOUS CRISES ON HEALTH EXPENDITURES

The previous section looked at the general economic impact of financial crisis. In this section, we focus more specifically on the impact on government health expenditures. Evidence from Latin America shows that public expenditure, particularly in the social sectors, tends to be procyclical in countries with large fiscal deficits (Ravallion, 2008; Braun & Di Gresia, 2003). Governments tend to expand social expenditures during times of economic expansion and decrease them during recession (Braun & Di Gresia, 2003). For instance, in Mexico the 4.9% fall in GDP per capita between 1994 and 1996 was mirrored by a 23.7% fall in targeted spending per poor person (Hicks & Wodon, 2000).[2] During times when the population is suffering due to stagnant or decreasing economic growth, social spending on health and education, including certain safety net programs, is at risk of being cut.

The experience of Argentina during the 1980s and 1990s highlights this point. Data shows that the elasticity of social spending with respect to total government spending from 1980 to 1997 is 2.14 and statistically significant (Ravallion, 2002b).[3] Therefore, a 1% decrease in total government spending is – on average – mirrored by a 2.14% decline in social spending. Conversely, Ravallion (2002b) finds that the elasticity of social spending to total spending during times of fiscal expansion was 0.14 and was not statistically significant. Thus, it is critical to look separately at the elasticity of social spending during recessions and expansions. During times of macroeconomic shocks and negative GDP growth, expansionary fiscal policy can help to compensate for declines in income through public spending, especially for vulnerable portions of the population (Braun & Di Gresia, 2003). However, between 1994 and 1996, targeted social spending in Mexico and Argentina actually contracted, concurrently with declines in GDP.

There is evidence that Argentina was able to reverse some of its procyclical social spending trends during the 2001 financial crisis. Although total government health spending per capita contracted in real terms and the total government budget contracted by 25% (Figs. 6 and 7), national spending on public health programs actually expanded by 70% in real terms – from $90 million pesos in 2001 to $150 million pesos in 2002 (Braun & Di Gresia, 2003; World Bank, 2003a). These increases were particularly focused on strengthening maternal and child health programs and programs targeted at specific diseases, including vaccinations. The Government of Argentina effectively prioritized this targeted health spending, despite overall fiscal and economic contractions.

Evidence from previous crises in Thailand, Indonesia, Argentina, and Russia highlights the procyclical declines in health spending in both real local currency units (LCUs) and at the average US dollar exchange rate (the latter highlights the impact of the sharp devaluations that take place during a crisis) (Figs. 6 and 7). Total, out-of-pocket, and public health spending per capita fell in real LCUs, and fell at a much sharper rate in US dollar terms than in LCUs. In the case of Indonesia, Thailand, and Russia, it took many years for health spending to reach pre-crisis levels again. In the case of Argentina, total and public health spending per capita have yet to reach pre-crisis levels in US dollar terms. Devaluations result in a rise in prices in local currencies of imported commodities, including drugs. Declines in government and out-of-pocket expenditure levels, combined with the increased utilization and demand for government services discussed later in this

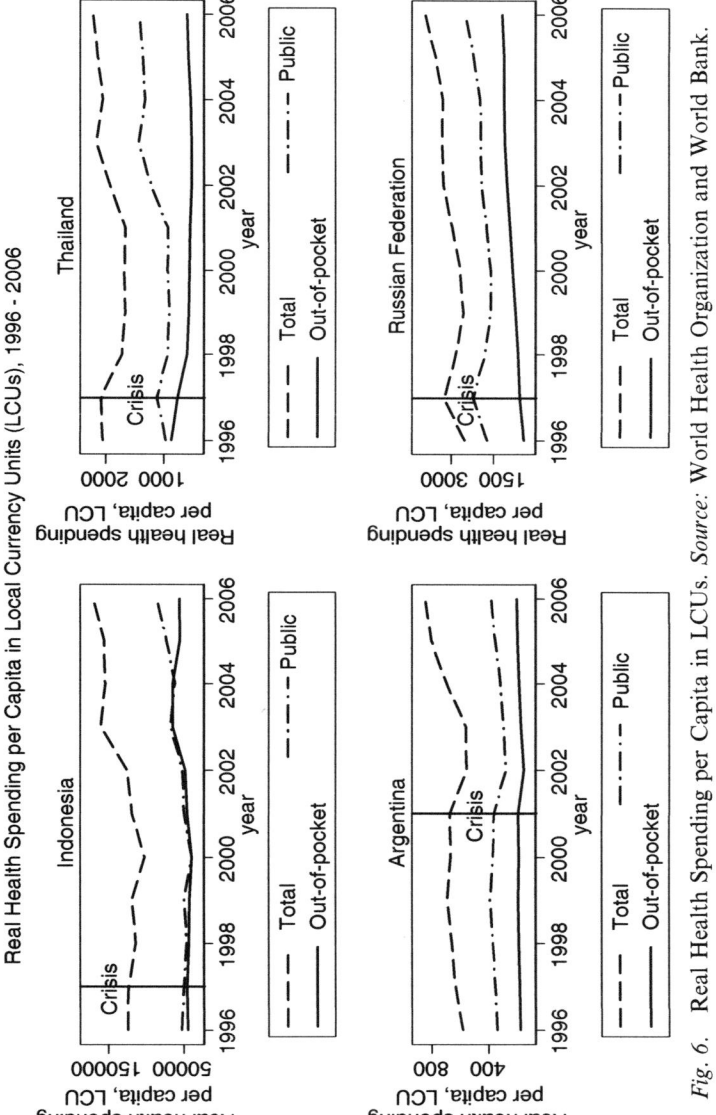

Fig. 6. Real Health Spending per Capita in LCUs. *Source:* World Health Organization and World Bank.

PABLO GOTTRET ET AL.

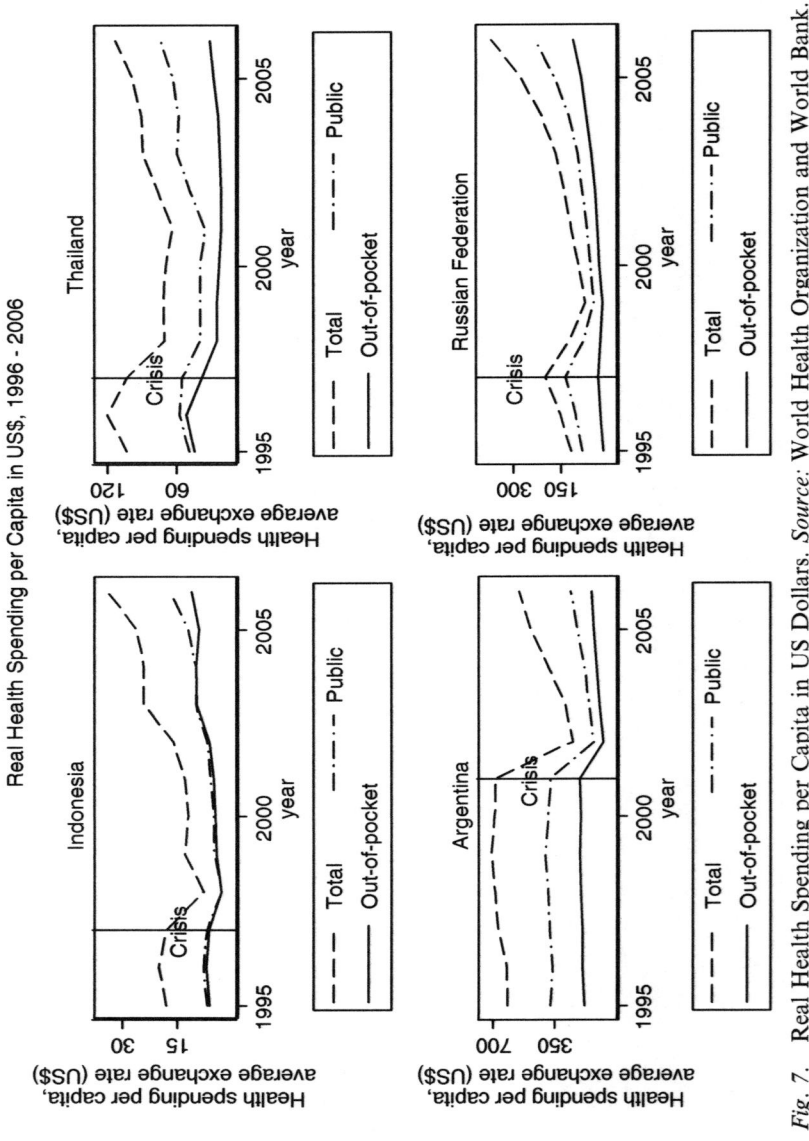

Fig. 7. Real Health Spending per Capita in US Dollars. *Source:* World Health Organization and World Bank.

chapter, emphasize the squeezing effect these crises can have on the financing of health service delivery. As a result, households may spend less of their income on health and other social services and look to publicly funded and provided sources. However, in the case of Argentina, Indonesia, Thailand, and Russia, the decreases in real public health spending per capita also inhibited the ability of governments to provide services.

One often-considered policy response is to protect health spending as a share of GDP, or as a share of the budget. For instance, in response to the economic crisis in 1999, the Government of Georgia tried to maintain spending on health at 7.3% of the total government budget, as part of its lending agreement with the World Bank. Not only did government health spending decline in real terms that same year, it also did not meet the 7.3% target, according to WHO data. Evidence suggests that efforts to protect government health expenditure as a proportion of GDP, or as a proportion of total government expenditure, may not be sufficient, as government expenditures per capita in real terms may still decline substantially. In Argentina and Indonesia, despite increases in the share of health in government expenditure (Fig. 8), government health spending per capita declined due to a fall in both GDP and overall government expenditure as a percentage of GDP. The decline in government health spending per capita in Thailand was driven by the decrease in health's share of government expenditure and an overall GDP decline. The situation in Russia was particularly severe, with government expenditure as a percent of GDP and government health expenditure as a percent of overall government expenditure both declining.

Non-salary expenditures may see the sharpest declines. In many countries, a large proportion of government health expenditure goes to pay salaries. Given the difficulty in downsizing the civil service, non-salary expenditures, used to pay for drugs and other variable inputs, as well as investments, may decline substantially and impact the quality of care. During the 1997 East Asian financial crisis, the percentage of the Thailand Ministry of Public Health budget going to salaries increased from approximately 39% in 1995 to 47% in 1999 (Wibulpolprasert, 1999). In the Thailand case, the investment portion of the health budget fell from approximately 39% of total health expenditure in 1995 to 11.5% in 1999. Even if health workers are protected, the quality of health care will decline in the absence of critical inputs such as equipment and medicines, due to reductions in variable budgets. Such a situation may be further exacerbated if the price of imported drugs and other supplies increases due to currency devaluation. Subsequent to the 1997/1998 financial crisis in Indonesia, the decrease in utilization of health services was

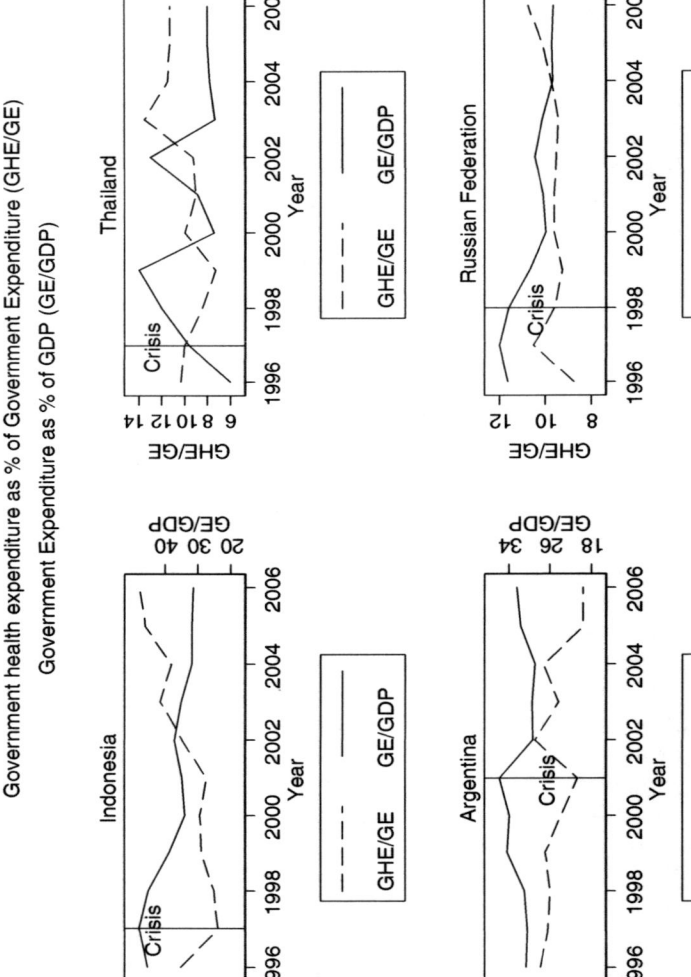

Fig. 8. Government Health Expenditure as Percent of Government Expenditure. *Source:* World Health Organization.

more pronounced for public facilities than for their private counterparts, primarily as a result of the severe shortage of drugs and other medical supplies in public facilities and the detrimental impact on quality of care (Frankenberg, Beegle, & Sikoki, 1998; Knowles, Pernia, & Racelis, 1999).

Governments need to put into place safeguards to protect health expenditures in real terms, particularly for those services and programs utilized by the poor and most vulnerable. Time-series data for Argentina shows that "social spending in general, and targeted social spending in particular, took a heavy hit at times of fiscal austerity" (Ravallion, 2002b). Trabajar, an externally financed workfare scheme introduced in response to a macro crisis, was far better targeted than other social spending. However, even here, a small but relatively well-protected share of its benefits went to the non-poor (Ravallion, 2002b). In reviewing social programs from Argentina, Bangladesh, and India, Ravallion (2002a) also found that targeting tends to improve as the program expands. This is certainly true of Argentina, where targeting improved significantly in later workfare programs. The workfare component of the Jefes de Hogar (Heads of Household) Program[4] addressed some of the weaknesses of earlier programs by expanding coverage and increasing spending on the social safety net (SSN)[5] (World Bank, 2002).

Argentina's response during the 2001–2002 is also illustrative of how government protection of priority health programs can protect essential services used by the poor and the most vulnerable. Although total health spending during the period was reduced, the national government protected spending on priority health programs. National spending on public health programs (including transfers to provinces) increased by 70 percent in real terms – from 90 million pesos in 2001 to 150 million pesos in 2002. This increase is largely attributable to the strengthening of the maternal and child health program and the program for preventing and controlling specific diseases and risk factors (which include the purchase of vaccines). The health allocation in 2003 reflected a continued priority accorded to these programs (World Bank, 2003a).

Additional evidence from India and Bangladesh confirms that aggregate cuts in social programs tend to be associated with worse targeting and the deterioration of benefit incidence (Ravallion, 2002a). In India, based on the difference between the average and marginal odds of participation in three key poverty reduction programs – public works schemes, the Integrated Rural Development Program, and a food rationing scheme[6] – higher aggregate outlays of various social programs are associated with more pro-poor benefit incidence and conversely, as budgets are cut, the targeting of the programs also deteriorates. The marginal odds of participation tended to fall more steeply than average odds of participation for richer income quintiles, pointing to a capture by the rich of the benefits and a greater vulnerability of the poor to lose out to budget cuts. Bangladesh's Food-for-Education Program, whose goal is to keep children of rural poor families in school through the distribution of food, provides a similar result. Ravallion (2002a) found that, as allocations were raised, the participation rate for the poor in the program increased faster than for the non-poor. This finding again suggests that targeting weakens with a contraction in the program. Other authors find similar results in Indonesia. These results suggest that during a financial crisis, policy makers need to be particularly cognizant that the non-poor are likely to capture the benefits of social programs as budgets contract.

In many countries, social spending is not specifically targeted and not inherently pro-poor (Tandon & Zhuang, 2006). For instance, services such as pensions, unemployment compensation, and higher education cannot necessarily be categorized as pro-poor and therefore the protection they offer during a financial crisis may not be effective at reaching those most vulnerable to fall below the poverty line or worse (Ravallion, 2002b).

The next section summarizes evidence on the impact of financial crisis on health service utilization rates as well as on population health outcomes.

IMPACT OF PREVIOUS CRISES ON HEALTH UTILIZATION AND OUTCOMES

Financial crises often disproportionately impact the ability of the poor to afford health services. This can occur due to a variety of reasons. During financial crises, real wages tend to fall and unemployment tends to rise, driving down labor earnings. Non-labor incomes also fall because of declines in economic activity and changes in the relative prices of the goods and services produced by the poor. Thus, demand for, and utilization of, health services may experience a decline during periods of economic distress. Apart from being unable to afford treatment at health facilities and hospitals, the poor may be forced to forego consumption of essential drugs as local currency devaluation results in an unaffordable increase in the local currency price of drugs. During the East Asia crisis, prices of drugs rose significantly in Indonesia, and prices of some generic drugs, which were generally affordable to the poor, rose sharply during 1997–1998; some antibiotics doubled in price (Kashiwagi & Sjaf, 1999).

As mentioned earlier, the public sector also scales down its activities, including social programs, during crises. When government health expenditures decline, the quality of services in public facilities declines. Available services may be captured by the non-poor. Thus, without specific interventions, the poor are disproportionately affected in terms of utilization of health services. For example, in Argentina, from the end of 2001 to the middle of 2002, preventive health care for children dropped 38% in the general population, but 57% in the poorest households (World Bank, 2003a).

Financial crises have a significant adverse impact on nutrition. Poor households are often forced to switch from more expensive to cheaper and often less nutritional foods, resulting in weight loss and severe malnutrition[7] (World Bank, 2008b). Even though the crisis itself may last for a few years, the impact on maternal and child health may be permanent. Children who experience short-term nutritional deprivations can suffer long-lasting effects including retarded growth, lower cognitive and learning abilities, lower educational attainment, and lower earnings in adulthood (Ravallion, 2008). These problems may be more acute for developing countries, particularly Africa and low-income Asia, where health outcomes such as infant mortality and malnutrition rise as GDP growth declines during recessions (Ferreira & Schady, 2008).

Worsening nutritional outcomes were observed during the East Asia crisis. A survey of public health facilities in Thailand reported a 22% increase in anemia among pregnant women during the East Asia crisis, which is suggestive of a switch to less nutritious foods (Knowles et al., 1999). In Indonesia, prevalence of micronutrient deficiencies (especially vitamin A) in children and women (of reproductive age) increased during the crisis period (Macfarlane Burnet Centre for Medical Research, 2000). Also, the share of women whose body mass index is below the level at which risks of illness and death increase rose by a quarter, and the average weight of children under age three declined in Indonesia in 1998 (World Bank, 2001).

Women and children often bear the brunt of the impact on health. Most crises tend to affect these groups disproportionately because of their lack of control over resources and gender-based discrimination.[8] As mentioned earlier, there is some evidence that households have been forced to cut back on both food quantity (caloric intake) and quality (dietary diversity) during a crisis, and girls and women usually suffer more as they are unable to protect the nutrient intake that they particularly need (IFPRI, 2008). Mortality of girls may be much more sensitive to changes in economic circumstances than that of boys: one multicountry study reported that infant girls may experience almost three times higher increased mortality than boys for a given change in per capita GDP, des- cribed by the authors as "a remarkable difference by any standard"

(Baird, Schady, & Friedman, 2007). This highlights the vulnerability of marginalized groups during crises.

Over 1 million excess infant deaths may have occurred in the developing world during 1980–2004 in countries experiencing economic contractions of 10% or higher (Baird et al., 2007). Although the impact may vary across countries, it appears that crises either result in a worsening of health outcomes for infants and children, or a slowing down of health improvements.

In Latin America, the pace of decline in the infant mortality rates (IMR) decreased in some countries because of the financial crisis during the 1980s (Lustig, 1995). During these crisis years, child mortality increased by an average of 7–10% in Mexico[9] (Ferreira & Schady, 2008). However, children and women are not the only groups at risk; the young and elderly are also susceptible. For example, mortality rates for the very young and the elderly increased or declined less rapidly in Mexico during the crisis years as compared with non-crisis years (Cutler, Knaul, Lozano, Méndez, & Zurita, 2002). Peru provides further evidence of the impact that crises can have on children. The economic crisis during 1998–2002 resulted in a 2.5% point increase in infant mortality, with 18,000 more children dying than in the absence of the crisis (Ferreira & Schady, 2008). Though causality cannot be proved, the contraction of public health spending may have contributed to the increase in infant mortality.[10]

There is limited evidence that child health outcomes suffer less in countries where expenditure on health is protected. Past crises have resulted in cuts in expenditures on health, lower utilization of health services, and deterioration of child and maternal nutrition and health outcomes. However, it is difficult to establish whether these nutrition and health outcomes deteriorated less in countries that protected health expenditures from cuts, since the counterfactual is largely absent and establishing causality is difficult. Government health expenditures were cut in Indonesia following the 1998 crisis, but the effect of this was somewhat mitigated by increased donor assistance to the health sector. This may have contributed to Indonesia's somewhat better performance in health outcomes, compared to other countries during crisis time. The contrast between Argentina's policy actions after the 1993 crisis, which largely led to protecting non pro-poor expenditures, and the 2001 crisis, with strong protection of expenditures on nutrition, maternal and child services, and essential drugs, may help explain some of the improved child and maternal outcomes seen in Argentina after 2002.

The next section discusses the response to previous crises by governments and policymakers to protect vulnerable populations from worsening health outcomes.

RESPONSE TO PREVIOUS CRISES BY GOVERNMENTS AND POLICYMAKERS

Social health insurance programs and SSNs can serve as effective instruments in protecting health service utilization during crises. In Indonesia, the Health Care Subsidies (Health Card) program was an important component of the SSN, introduced by the government as a response to the economic crisis in 1997.[11] Under this program, a number of services were offered free to card holders, including (1) outpatient and inpatient care, (2) contraception for women of child bearing age, (3) prenatal care, and (4) birth assistance. Although similar schemes already existed at the time, the coverage and scope of the program were changed and expanded as part of the SSN program. The program was part of an overall effort to address the impact of the crisis, which included a rise in the price of items such as food and medicine. It was somewhat effective in increasing the utilization of health services, where direct subsidies were provided for basic health services for the poor (World Bank, 2008a). Evidence suggests that though targeting was pro-poor in the distribution of the health card, there was considerable leakage to the non-poor. Utilization of the health card for outpatient care was also pro-poor (Sparrow, 2008).

The Thailand government also expanded existing social insurance programs as a response to the financial crisis. As part of this expansion, increased support was provided to the Public Assistance Scheme for low-income families. Government subsidy to the Voluntary Health Card (VHC) was also doubled from 500 baht to 1,000 baht per card.[12] Health centers and district hospitals reported a large increase in distribution of free health care cards between 1997 and 1998, and this may have contributed significantly to the increased use of public facilities,[13] thus mitigating the impact of the crisis on demand for health services by the poor (Pongsapich & Brimble, 1999).

Other examples of effective policy interventions include conditional cash transfer (CCT) programs. Expanding the coverage and increasing the benefit levels on CCTs has been one of the many responses to economic crises, particularly in Latin America. Mexico was able to redress the adverse welfare impacts of the recent rise in food prices by implementing a one-time top up payment to Oportunidades[14] participants (Ravallion, 2008). Payment to the poorest families increased by 24.3% in 2008. Although this additional payment did not fully compensate the poor for the increase in food prices, it did help avoid a detrimental effect on the poor[15] (Food and Agricultural Organization, 2008).

CCTs have been an extremely cost effective mechanism for financially constrained governments. On average, safety net expenditures in developing countries fall in the range of 1–2% of GDP, although there is significant variation across countries. Some of the more successful programs such as Mexico's Oportunidades or Brazil's Bolsa Familia, cost approximately 0.4% of GDP (World Bank, 2008b). However, CCTs are not always responsive to changes in the need for assistance, and can be prone to capture. Thus, it is critical that governments reassess eligibility when a crisis occurs. Finally, CCTs do not, in themselves, improve the supply or quality of services. If vaccines are not available at the health center, the baby will not be vaccinated, even if the CCT encourages the mother to bring the child to the clinic. Thus, demand-side incentives such as CCTs must be accompanied by adequate access to and supply of services to be effective. This is even truer in times of crisis, when budget support for service delivery may be under stress.

Financial crises have been used as an opportunity to improve the efficiency of public health systems. In Thailand, for instance, the Ministry of Public Health (MoPH) launched the "Good Health at Low Cost" strategy in the post-crisis period. This involved drug management reform (procuring a higher proportion of essential drugs, and support for greater use of generic drugs as currency devaluation increased the relative price of the more expensive patented formulations), and savings from a reduction of operating/capital costs and material costs[16] (Macfarlane Burnet Centre for Medical Research, 1999). As part of the reformulation of the MoPH budget, capital costs were reduced from 38.7% of the total budget in 1997 down to 11.5% in 2000 (Wibulpolprasert, 1999).[17] At the same time, budgets were protected for essential services and programs such as HIV/AIDS.

In addition, public works programs have often been used by governments as a safety net. Public spending on labor-intensive public works projects, such as building rural roads, can combine the benefits of an aggregate fiscal stimulus with those of income support for poor groups. Indonesia and Korea introduced such programs during the East Asian financial crisis; as did Mexico in the 1995 peso crisis; Peru during its recession of 1998–2001; and Argentina in the 2002 financial crisis. India has used public works programs to provide safety nets for many years. Research suggests that such programs do provide income gains for participants. Programs like Argentina's Trabajar provide effective household income support and also show that if correct incentives are in place for targeting work to poor areas, such programs may serve to compensate somewhat for what made those areas poor in the first place. This further demonstrates that protecting government spending in sectors other than health can complement essential health expenditures. Preventing people from slipping into poverty could be critical in protecting health outcomes, as the ability of the poor to afford health services is the most at risk during crises.

RESPONSE TO PREVIOUS CRISES BY HOUSEHOLDS

This section discusses how households are forced to change health utilization behavior in response to financial crisis, and how they might respond to such periods of economic distress. During a crisis, households may no longer be able to afford health insurance or might become ineligible for it. In most developing countries, pension, health, and unemployment insurance systems generally cover only formal sector workers. Thus, only a small proportion of the poor are insured. If unemployment increases, covered households may lose insurance as it is often tied to formal employment and layoffs during a crisis may result in a large pool of unemployed and uninsured individuals. The absence of health insurance, combined with the inability to finance health services through out-of-pocket payments, may result in reduced utilization of health services. For example, a 2002 World Bank survey revealed that one negative consequence of the 2001–2002 Argentinean crisis was that by mid-2002, 13% of households reported that they had canceled their health insurance (World Bank, 2003a). The reduction in insurance coverage was three times greater among poor households relative to non-poor households. As a result, 57% of poor households reported a reduction in the utilization of preventative health services by their children (World Bank, 2003a).

Users may switch from the private health sector to the public health sector as their ability to pay for health services is impacted. For example, in Thailand, the private sector faced significant demand reductions, and doctors from the private sector turned to the public sector for employment (WHO, 2009). Increased government support to the public assistance and VHC schemes, and measures such as a reduction in private hospital entitlements in the Civil Service Medical Benefit Scheme, facilitated a transition to the public health sector. In Argentina, household incomes shrank during the 2001–2002 crisis and households modified their demand for health services. The 2002 World Bank survey also revealed that, in comparison to end of 2001, by mid-2002, 38% of households reported greater use of public health centers instead of private services (World Bank, 2003a).

Households may have to bear additional costs and be forced to reduce their utilization of health services if public health systems are unable to respond because of reduced budgets and increased demand. In Argentina, public hospitals in Buenos Aires Province were unable to cope with a surge in demand as a result of the 2001–2002 crisis (World Bank, 2003a).

WHAT SHOULD DONORS DO? EVIDENCE FROM PAST RESPONSES TO CRISES

The evidence on the effectiveness of support to countries to protect pro-poor health expenditures and health service delivery for poor and vulnerable populations during financial crises is mixed. World Bank programmatic lending operations in countries affected by financial crises in the 1990s and 2000s were reviewed to assess past experience and derive good practices for all donors to consider to support quality health services for the poor during the current financial crisis. We reviewed these loans to see whether loan agreements included support for health expenditures, with an additional focus on whether pro-poor expenditures and services were identified as priorities.

Our findings suggest that successful projects financed the initiation or expansion of sustainable safety nets that tied essential health services to identified funding on a per capita basis, along with an appropriate system of monitoring and evaluation. For instance, the primary objective of a loan to Brazil by the World Bank in 1999 was to maintain expenditures on basic education, medical care, and nutritional services.[18] Specifically, budget protection in health was included, based on floors set on per capita spending at the state and municipal level for a defined benefit package. Successful projects also avoided placing conditions on short-term financial assistance that involved long-term institutional reforms (which require an investment or capacity building instrument). Additionally, projects worked better when government efforts to expand the breadth and depth of coverage of an existing safety net, or to introduce a new, more sustainable safety net, were supported. This includes the Bolsa de Familia in Brazil referenced earlier.

Despite some strong evidence of good practice, many of the projects reviewed suffer from insufficient evidence relating to baseline data and measurable indicators. The project data tended to concentrate on the source of financing, rather than analyzing the potential effect of such financing on service delivery, or health outcomes. Likewise, the evaluations focused on indicators such as percentage of government expenditure allocated to health or other social programs which, as we have seen earlier, may not provide sufficient evidence about the beneficiaries. Few evaluations investigated whether the programs that were supported were pro-poor to begin with. As the World Bank and other donors respond to the current crisis, the focus should be to help finance a specific set of services for the poor/vulnerable, protect expenditures on a per capita basis and in real terms, and where possible, the focus should be on expanding existing, well-targeted, and sustainable safety nets. Baseline indicators are needed as the foundation for rigorous post-crisis evaluation.

CONCLUSIONS AND RECOMMENDATIONS

The global financial crisis is impacting almost all developed and developing countries. Slower growth is forecasted for most emerging and developing economies. Developed country economies are contracting and this may impact foreign aid contributions, FDI, remittances, and global trade. Highly donor-dependent countries are especially vulnerable to aid cuts. Currency devaluations in developing countries will result in higher domestic prices of imported goods, including drugs. These price increases in LCUs may decrease access to essential medicines, as well as increase the pressure on potentially shrinking government health budgets. The timing of the current crisis, on the heels of the food crisis, puts the poor at even greater risk.

This chapter uses country examples from previous crises to highlight the potential negative impacts on health expenditures, health utilization rates, and health outcomes. It highlights mechanisms by which financial crises might impact the health sector, provides examples where impacts have been fairly severe, and identifies some effective policy responses. Because this crisis is different from previous crises and because much of the evidence available from earlier events relates more to middle income countries than to the poorest countries, there is a need for more and better evidence and sensitive prospective monitoring going forward.[19]

The chapter argues that a fundamental objective of public health policy during a crisis is to maintain/improve access to essential services by the population, and especially the poor and vulnerable. This is not at odds with the potential reduction in health expenditures during a financial crisis as governments struggle with tightening budgets. Past experience shows that some countries took advantage of the crisis to improve the efficiency of their public health systems and were able to protect those services that are essential to the welfare of the poor. Thus, a combination of efficiency improvements, being selective in cutting of certain types of expenditures, and income-support mechanisms can allow governments to maintain services that are critical to the most poor and vulnerable.

Previous crises in Asia and Latin America show the negative impact that crises can have on access to health and nutrition services and health outcomes. Women and children are especially vulnerable. During crises, households may demand fewer health services and opt for lower quality and quantity of nutrition. Government capacity is also affected. This may result in deteriorating health outcomes, especially marked in the poorest quintiles of the population.

Measures to protect public "pro-poor" expenditures have worked better when they: (i) were aimed at financing a specific set of services that are used by the poor/vulnerable; (ii) protected expenditures on a per capita basis and in real terms rather than only ratios such as percent of GDP, or government expenditure; (iii) financed expansion of existing safety nets, or facilitated introduction of a sustainable and well targeted safety net with clearly defined beneficiary populations; and (iv) supported appropriate monitoring and evaluation mechanisms. Experience suggests that certain policies should not be supported: (i) general input or commodity subsidies; (ii) general conditions that earmark expenditures for the whole sector; (iii) conditions that only protect expenditures without identifying the services, or the target population to be protected; and (iv) conditions that protect financing or services that are not pro-poor in the first place.

Although maintaining government health expenditures as a proportion of total government expenditure may be a worthwhile objective, it does not guarantee that pro-poor services will be protected. Real government health expenditures per capita declined in all the reviewed countries immediately after the crisis. This decline occurred even as many countries tried to protect government health expenditures as a proportion of total government expenditures. Development partners need therefore to focus on protecting pro-poor health expenditures, rather than overall expenditures. Interventions that boost household income so as to enable the poor to maintain access to essential health services may also be an option if mechanisms are in place to manage such expenditures. Evidence suggests that if well designed, low cost social insurance programs and CCTs can be successful in reaching the poor with minimum leakage, and can also be extremely cost effective.

Finally, given that the fall in the quantity and quality of nutrition is one of the most serious human development consequences of an economic/ financial crisis, pro-poor expenditures must focus specifically on ensuring adequate nutrition. Pro-poor public spending on health, education, and social protection will need to be protected to ensure that nutrition-related outcomes, and others, do not deteriorate.

NOTES

1. Kyrgyzstan, Moldova, Tajikistan, Haiti, Honduras, and a number of small island economies.
2. Targeted social spending includes government spending aimed at establishing or strengthening systems of social protection that mitigate the potential impact of crises before they occur and assist the poor to cope with the shocks after that have happened (Hicks & Wodon, 2000).
3. Social spending includes education, health, water and sewage, housing and urban development, social assistance, and labor programs.
4. A SSN launched by the Government of Argentina in April 2002 to alleviate the impact of rising unemployment due to the sharp worsening of the economic crisis. The Jefes de Hogar Program provides a stipend of 150 Argentine pesos/month to an unemployed head of a household in exchange for participation in 4 h of work in community services, small construction or maintenance activities, or training, including finishing basic education, or as a temporary employee of a private company.
5. For a more detailed discussion on the targeting component of the Jefes de Hogar (Heads of Household) Program, see World Bank (2002).
6. Ravallion (2002a, 2002b) and Lanjouw, Pradhan, Saadah, Sayed, and Sparrow (2001) used the marginal odds ratio of participation (MOP) to infer the incidence by quintile of an increase or decrease in public spending on a given program. The MOP is defined as the increment to the program participation of a given expenditure quintile associated with a change in the aggregate participation in the program. The average odds participation ratio is the quintile-specific participation rate relative to the participation rate of the entire population and can vary from MOP in its results (Lanjouw et al., 2001).
7. It is estimated that higher food prices in 2008 may have already increased the number of children suffering permanent cognitive and physical injury due to malnutrition by 44 million (World Bank, 2008b).
8. Including extensive time burdens; threats or acts of violence; and limited legal benefits and protections, decision-making authority, and control of financial resources (IFPRI, 2008).
9. Cutler et al. (2002) concluded that the three crisis periods resulted in increases in child mortality of 9.2% (1982–1984 crisis), 10.3% (1985–1989), and 6.9% (1994–1996).
10. Paxson and Schady showed that public health expenditure fell from approximately 80 Peruvian soles per capita in 1988 to 30 soles in 1990 (Ferreira & Schady, 2008).

11. A nationwide health program was introduced by the Indonesian government in August 1998, as part of the larger Indonesian SSN – Jaring Pengaman Sosial (JPS) (Sparrow, 2008).

12. Under this scheme, free health cards were distributed to the unemployed and low-income families.

13. VHCs accounted for two-thirds of the outpatients visiting public health facilities.

14. During the Tequila financial crisis of 1994, the Government of Mexico realized that it lacked an effective safety net for the country's poor. In 1997, it responded with a program called "PROGRESA" (later called Oportunidades), which was oriented toward the poor and replaced simple cash transfers with subsidies to household investments in human capacity development. It worked more effectively because it relied on the active participation of women to improve their own and their families' education, health, and nutrition status (Coady, Filmer, & Gwatkin, 2005).

15. The number of beneficiaries increased by 1 million and the total number of Mexicans assisted by the program reached 5 million households (one out of four Mexican families) in 2008. Payment to the poorest families also increased to an average of 665 pesos per month (from an average of 535 pesos per month).

16. This included measures such as reducing expenses on electricity, water, and telephone in public hospitals and minimizing capital costs. No new capital investment projects were undertaken in 1998 and 1999 except to complete existing obligations (Macfarlane Burnet Centre for Medical Research, 1999).

17. Capital costs were reduced from 38.7% of the total budget in 1997 down to 27.3% in 1998, 15.5% in 1999, and 11.5% in 2000 (Wibulpolprasert, 1999).

18. Brazil Social Protection Special Sector Adjustment Loan (BSPSSAL).

19. Some new work to develop such monitoring and more in-depth country analysis is now in the planning phase in partnership with other development agencies.

ACKNOWLEDGMENT

We are thankful to colleagues across the World Bank for comments on early drafts of this chapter.

REFERENCES

Baird, S., Schady, N., & Friedman, J. (2007). *Infant mortality over the business cycle in the developing world*. World Bank Policy Research Working Paper no. 4346. World Bank, Washington, DC.

Braun, M., & Di Gresia, L. (2003). *Towards effective social insurance in Latin America: The importance of countercyclical fiscal policy*. Annual Meetings of the IADB and Inter-American Investment Corporation, Milan, Italy.

Coady, D., Filmer, D., & Gwatkin, D. (2005). *PROGRESA for progress: Mexico's health, nutrition, and education program.* Development Outreach, May 2005. Washington, DC: World Bank.

Cutler, D. M., Knaul, F., Lozano, R., Méndez, O., & Zurita, B. (2002). Financial crisis health outcomes, and ageing: Mexico in the 1980s and 1990s. *Journal of Public Economics, 84*(1), 279–303.

Feldstein, M. (2002). Argentina's fall: Lessons from the latest financial crisis. *Foreign Affairs, 82*(2), 8–14.

Ferreira, F., & Schady, N. (2008). *Aggregate economic shocks, child schooling and child health.* Development Research Group. Poverty and Human Development and Public Services Teams. Washington, DC: World Bank.

Food and Agricultural Organization. (2008). *Country responses to the food security crisis: Nature and preliminary implications of the policies pursued* (December 2008). Rome, Italy: Agricultural Policy Support Service, Food and Agricultural Organization.

Frankenberg, E., Beegle, K., & Sikoki, B. (1998). Health, family planning and well-being in Indonesia during an economic crisis: Early results from the Indonesian family life survey. *Rand Labor and Population Program Working Paper Series 99-06.* The Rand Corporation, CA, USA.

Hanson, T. (2009). *Why China's stimulus plan will change the world.* MSNBC. Available at http://www.msnbc.msn.com/id/29692478/. Accessed on March 16, 2009.

Hicks, N., & Wodon, Q. (2000). Economic shocks, safety nets, and fiscal constraints: Social protection for the poor in Latin America. Paper presented at the XII Seminario Regional de Política Fiscal, Santiago, Chile.

IFPRI. (2008). *Helping women respond to the global food price crisis.* Policy Brief no. 007. October 2008, Washington, DC.

IMF. (2009). Global economic slump challenges policies. *World Economic Outlook Update,* January 28, 2009, Washington, DC.

International Labor Organization. (2009). *Global employment trends.* January 2009, Geneva, Switzerland.

Kashiwagi, E., & Sjaf, A. (1999). The impact of economic crisis on hospital and health center management in Indonesia especially on drug supply and use. Presented at Bappenas-JICA Interim Discussion on the Survey Finding on the Impact of the Economic Crisis, March 3, 1999, Health Research Center, University of Indonesia, Jakarta.

Knowles, J., Pernia, E., & Racelis, M. (1999). *Social consequences of the financial crisis in East Asia.* Manila, Philippines: Asian Development Bank.

Lanjouw, P., Pradhan, M., Saadah, F., Sayed, H., & Sparrow, R. (2001). *Poverty, education and health in Indonesia: Who benefits from public spending?* Policy Research Working Paper no. 2739. World Bank, Washington, DC.

Lin, J. (2008). *Extraordinary times: The effect on poverty.* Note prepared for induction program for World Bank Executive Directors. Washington, DC: World Bank.

Lustig, N. (1995). *Coping with austerity: Poverty and inequality in Latin America* (March). Washington, DC: Brookings Institution Press.

Macfarlane Burnet Centre for Medical Research. (1999). *The impact of the Asian financial crisis on the health sector in Thailand.* Commissioned by the Australian Agency for International Development, Melbourne, Australia.

Macfarlane Burnet Centre for Medical Research. (2000). *Impact of the Asian financial crisis on health*. Commissioned by the Australian Agency for International Development, Melbourne, Australia.

Mold, A., Olcer, D., & Prizzon, A. (2008). *The fallout from the financial crisis (3): Will aid budgets fall victim to the credit crisis?* (Policy Insights no. 85, December 2008). Paris: OECD Development Center.

Pongsapich, A., & Brimble, P. (1999). Assessing the social impacts of the financial crisis in Thailand. Presented at the Finalization Conference, Assessing the Social Impact of the Financial Crisis in Selected Asian Developing Countries, June 17–18, 1999, Asian Development Bank, Manila.

Ravallion, M. (2002a). Who is protected? On the incidence of fiscal adjustment. Paper presented at the Conference on Macroeconomic Policy and Poverty at the IMF on March 14, 2002, World Bank, Washington, DC.

Ravallion, M. (2002b). Are the poor protected from budget cuts? Evidence for Argentina. *Journal of Applied Economics, 5*(1), 95–121.

Ravallion, M. (2008). *Bailing out the worlds poorest*. Policy Research Working Paper no. 4763. October, 2008. Development Research Group, Director's Office, The World Bank, Washington, DC.

Sparrow, R. (2008). Targeting the poor in times of crisis: The Indonesian health card. *Health Policy and Planning, 23*(3), 188–190Oxford University Press, Oxford.

Tandon, A., & Zhuang, J. (2006). Inclusiveness of economic growth in the people's republic of China: What do population health outcomes tell us?. *Asian Development Review, 23*(2), 53–69.

UN Conference on Trade and Development. (2008). *World Investment Report 2008*. Geneva, Switzerland.

WHO. (2008). WHO Statistical Information System, Geneva.

WHO. (2009). Health amid a financial crisis: A complex diagnosis. *Bulletin of the World Health Organization, 87*(1), 4–5.

Wibulpolprasert, S. (1999). Globalization and access to essential drugs: Case study from Thailand. Paper Presented at the Meeting on Globalization and Access to Essential Drugs, November 25–26, 1999, Amsterdam, The Netherlands.

World Bank. (2001). *"Managing economic crises and natural disasters" in World Development Report 2000/01*. Washington, DC: The World Bank.

World Bank. (2002). Project appraisal document for Jefes De Hogar (Heads of Household) Program in Argentina. Sector Management Unit for Human Development, Country Management Unit for Argentina, Chile, Uruguay and Paraguay, Latin America and Caribbean Region. The World Bank, Washington, DC.

World Bank. (2003a). The health sector in Argentina: Current situation and options for improvement. Human Development Department, Argentina, Chile, Paraguay, and Uruguay Country Management Unit, Latin America and the Caribbean Region. The World Bank, Washington, DC.

World Bank. (2003b). *Argentina – crisis and poverty 2003: A poverty assessment. Poverty reduction and economic management, Latin America and the Caribbean region*. Washington, DC: World Bank.

World Bank. (2008a). *Introducing health cards to cushion the impact of financial crisis on the poor.* Reaching the Poor Policy Brief Series. Washington, DC: World Bank.

World Bank. (2008b). Global financial crisis and implications for developing countries. November 8, 2008. World Bank background paper prepared for G-20 Finance Ministers Meeting São Paulo, Brazil.

World Bank. (2009a). *Global economic prospects: Commodities at the crossroads.* Washington, DC: World Bank. December 2008. ISBN: 0-8213-7799-X.

World Bank. (2009b). *Low-income countries and the financial crisis: Vulnerabilities and policy options.* Policy Note. Washington, DC: The World Bank.

SECTION II
EXPANDING COVERAGE AND
ITS FUNDING

THE EQUITY IMPACT OF THE UNIVERSAL COVERAGE POLICY: LESSONS FROM THAILAND

Phusit Prakongsai, Supon Limwattananon and Viroj Tangcharoensathien

ABSTRACT

Objective – *This chapter assesses health equity achievements of the Thai health system before and after the introduction of the universal coverage (UC) policy. It examines five dimensions of equity: equity in financial contributions, the incidence of catastrophic health expenditure, the degree of impoverishment as a result of household out-of-pocket payments for health, equity in health service use and the incidence of public subsidies for health.*

Methodology – *The standard methods proposed by O'Donnell, van Doorslaer, and Wagstaff (2008b) were used to measure equity in financial contribution, healthcare utilization and public subsidies, and in assessing the incidence of catastrophic health expenditure and impoverishment. Two major national representative household survey datasets were used: Socio-Economic Surveys and Health and Welfare Surveys.*

Findings – *General tax was the most progressive source of finance in Thailand. Because this source dominates total financing, the overall outcome was progressive, with the rich contributing a greater share of*

Innovations in Health System Finance in Developing and Transitional Economies
Advances in Health Economics and Health Services Research, Volume 21, 57–81
Copyright © 2009 by Emerald Group Publishing Limited
All rights of reproduction in any form reserved
ISSN: 0731-2199/doi:10.1108/S0731-2199(2009)0000021006

their income than the poor. The low incidence of catastrophic health expenditure and impoverishment before UC was further reduced after UC. Use of healthcare and the distribution of government subsidies were both pro-poor: in particular, the functioning of primary healthcare (PHC) at the district level serves as a "pro-poor hub" in translating policy into practice and equity outcomes.

Policy implications – *The Thai health financing reforms have been accompanied by nationwide extension of PHC coverage, mandatory rural health service by new graduates and systems redesign, especially the introduction of a contracting model and closed-ended provider payment methods. Together, these changes have led to a more equitable and more efficient health system. Institutional capacity to generate evidence and to translate it into policy decisions, effective implementation and comprehensive monitoring and evaluation are essential to successful system-level reforms.*

BACKGROUND

Equity in health has been recognized by policy makers as an important objective of health systems, and has recently received greater attention from international organizations. Slow progress in achieving health equity has been observed in a range of developing countries. Various developing countries in Asia and Latin America have employed universal coverage (UC) in access to healthcare as both a means and an end (Tangcharoensathien, Wibulpolprasert, & Nitayarampong, 2004; Frenk, 2006). Development partners have also been supportive of the concept of UC and World Health Assembly Resolution 58.33 encouraged member states to work towards UC.

Objectives of the UC policy are to ensure universal access to effective health services regardless of a person's income or social status, and to protect household income and assets from medical care costs (Kutzin, 2000; Mills, 2007). In low- and middle-income countries, key constraints in achieving UC include limited government health resources, inadequate health service infrastructure, lack of political will and poor administrative and technical capacity of governments (Nitayarumphong, 1998; Mills, 2007).

To achieve UC in developing countries, there is a need for a substantial increase in the public share of financing for health, through either general revenue or social health insurance contributions, replacing the current dominant role of household direct payments. Concerns have been raised over the small tax base and limited government capacity to collect taxes in low- and middle-income countries. However, raising additional general tax revenue has been shown to be feasible and successful in a number of developing countries such as Bolivia, Armenia, Bulgaria, Estonia and Slovakia (Wagstaff, 2007).

Description of the UC Scheme

By early 2002, Thailand achieved UC of healthcare for the whole population by introducing a tax-funded health insurance scheme, the so-called "UC scheme", to cover the approximately 47 million people who were not beneficiaries of the Civil Servant Medical Benefit Scheme (CSMBS) or the Social Security Scheme (SSS). It took almost three decades for Thailand to achieve UC, beginning in 1975 with the creation of a social welfare scheme for the poor (the Low Income Scheme). In addition to the Low Income Scheme, successive governments applied a piecemeal approach to extending health insurance to the non-poor (Tangcharoensathien, Teokul, & Chanwongpaisarn, 2005b) by creating a public-subsidized voluntary insurance scheme (the Voluntary Health Card Project) in 1983[1] (Tangcharoensathien, Supachutikul, & Lertiendumrong, 1999; Srithamrongsawat, 2002). In addition, the coverage of formal sector private employees under the mandatory tripartite payroll tax arrangements of Social Health Insurance (SHI) was gradually extended from larger firms with more than 20 employees in 1990 to the smallest firms with more than one employee in 2002. Despite government attempts to expand health insurance coverage through several targeted approaches, evidence indicates that approximately 30% of Thais were uninsured before implementation of the UC policy (Wibulpolprasert, 2005). Therefore, the Thai government decided to start implementing the UC policy in 2001 and achieved UC in 2002. Table 1 describes the current scheme. Note that SHI does not cover dependants of the contributory members. When UC was launched, the SHI dependants were covered by the UC scheme.

The Thai UC scheme comprises a comprehensive benefit package that includes ambulatory care, hospitalization, disease prevention, health promotion and many expensive medical services such as radiotherapy and chemotherapy for cancer treatments, surgical operations and healthcare for accidents and emergency illnesses. Prescription drugs are also free of charge. UC beneficiaries are guaranteed universal access to health services by registering with a primary care network, from which they can obtain health

Table 1. Characteristics of Three Public Insurance Schemes (2002).

Insurance Scheme	Population Coverage		Financing Source	Mode of Provider Payment	Access to Service
Social Health Insurance	Private sector employees, excluding dependants	16%	Tri-partite contribution, shared by employer, employee and the government	Inclusive capitation for outpatient and inpatient services	Registered public and private competing contractors
Civil Servant Medical Benefit Scheme	Government employees plus dependants (parents, spouse and up to two children age <20)	9%	General tax, non-contributory scheme	Fee for service, direct disbursement to mostly public providers	Free choice of providers, no registration required
Universal coverage	The rest of the population not covered by SHI and CSMBS	75%	General tax	Capitation for out-patients and global budget plus DRG for inpatients	Registered contractor providers, notably district health system

Source: Authors' synthesis.

services when needed. If the registered hospital cannot provide appropriate treatment, patients are transferred to a higher-level health facility such as a provincial or regional hospital, and sometimes a university hospital. Although the UC benefit package is quite comprehensive, some expensive medical care, for example, renal replacement therapy for end-stage renal disease has been excluded due to the high costs of certain procedures and the limited government health resources[2] (Jongudoumsuk, 2002; Tangcharoensathien et al., 2005a).

The UC scheme promotes use of primary care at the district level by shifting health service delivery from tertiary care hospitals to primary care provider networks through the contracting method for which registration of beneficiaries with a provider network is required. A contractual agreement is made between the government and a Contractor Unit for Primary care or "CUP" as the main provider for its registered population. The CUP comprises all health centres in a district along with a primary care unit located in the district hospital. Patients can access either health centres or district hospitals in this network, and referral to provincial or regional hospitals is covered if care beyond the clinical capacity of the CUP is needed. The CUP receives a capitation budget for ambulatory care according to the number of people registered and reimburses the expenses for inpatient care based on diagnostic-related group (DRG) weights from a pooled inpatient budget. As a result, evidence suggests that government health resources have tended to shift from urban hospitals to primary care facilities, and more public healthcare subsidies have been allocated to rural areas (Jongudoumsuk, 2002). In addition, the promotion of primary care is likely to increase access to healthcare services of the poor in the countryside (Vasavid, Tisayatikom, Patcharanarumol, & Tangcharoensathien, 2004).

Evidence on Health Inequity

Over decades, Thailand has experienced an improvement in population health. A recent study reported a substantial drop in the under-five mortality rate, from 58 in 1980 to 30 in 1990 and 23 in 2000 (Hill et al., 2007). Thailand's success in reducing childhood deaths was accompanied by a narrowing rich–poor mortality gap over the past decade (Vapattanawong et al., 2007). Even though the poor suffer from higher child mortality than the rich, the concentration index for child mortality reduced from -0.20 in 1990 to -0.12 in 2000 reflecting a reduction in the difference between rich and poor. The relative risk of mortality for a child under five between the

20% poorest and the 20% richest reduced from 2.8 in 1990 to 1.8 in 2000, a 55% reduction. Universal access to primary healthcare (PHC) services, even before the UC era, has been one of the key determinants of Thailand's success in improving population health over the past 30 years (Rohde et al., 2008).

This chapter assesses the health equity achievement of the UC scheme in Thailand. Equity is measured in five dimensions: (1) equity in financing contribution, (2) incidence of catastrophic health expenditure, (3) impoverishment as a result of out-of-pocket (OOP) payment for health by households, (4) equity in utilization of services and finally (5) incidence of public expenditure on health. Where applicable, before and after UC comparisons provide the additional assessment of the impact of the UC scheme on equity in the Thai healthcare system.

METHODS

We applied standard techniques for equity analysis in health that are appropriate for data obtained from household surveys (O'Donnell, van Doorslaer, & Wagstaff, 2008b). These methods have been used to measure health equity through empirical studies using large-scale survey datasets available in certain countries in Asia-Pacific (O'Donnell et al., 2007; O'Donnell et al., 2008a; Van Doorslaer et al., 2006; Van Doorslaer et al., 2007) and other regions. Disparities across socioeconomic groups in three sets of healthcare-related variables, including payments and utilization, and government subsidies received by household members, are the main focus of this analysis.

Equity in financial contribution to healthcare was measured by determining the level of payments from various sources (indirectly through direct and indirect taxes, social insurance contributions, private insurance premiums; and directly through OOP payments) that are incurred by the poor as compared with the better-off. For determining equity in healthcare utilization, the frequency of ambulatory visits and hospital admissions was compared across socioeconomic groups. The total healthcare cost incurred in government facilities (as a product of visit or admission frequencies and corresponding unit costs by level of care) net of household's OOP payments gives a measure of health subsidy paid by the government and is used for benefit incidence analysis.

Depending on data availability, ranking of the households by living standards in the measurement of equity in health financing was based on monthly consumption expenditure per adult-equivalent, using Deaton's formula (Deaton, 1997), where the Socio-Economic Survey (SES) was used for this assessment. The ranking by living standards for healthcare utilization and incidence of government subsidy was derived from estimated household income, in cash and in kind, reported in the Health and Welfare Survey (HWS) as there is no consumption expenditure in this instrument and only a short income question was available.

This chapter analyzed equity in health financing, healthcare utilization and government subsidy using the concentration index (CI). This index, ranging from -1 to 1 captures the extent to which the amount of health payment and utilization are concentrated among the poor as compared with the better-off. A CI of 0 means a perfectly equitable distribution of the health variables across households or population ranking. A negative CI indicates a pro-poor distribution of the health variables, whereas the positive CI reflects a pro-rich distribution or concentration among the better-off. For example, where the CI for under-five mortality is typically negative, it means that the poor shoulder a higher mortality burden than the rich; the positive CI for financial contribution reflects progressivity whereby the rich pay more than the poor, which is the societal goal.

In this chapter, health catastrophe is defined as OOP payment for self-medication, ambulatory visit and hospitalization that exceeds 10% of total household expenditure (Russell, 1996; Wagstaff & van Doorslaer, 2003). Healthcare-induced impoverishment is defined as the additional poverty arising from household payments for health, calculated using the national poverty lines in each year specific to geographic regions and rural–urban areas.

Data Sources

Data were obtained primarily from two nationally representative household surveys, the SES and HWS. The National Statistical Office (NSO) conducts these two national surveys on a regular basis, SES every two years over a 12-month (January–December) period and HWS every one or two years in April, using face-to-face, structured interviews with household members, where proxy respondents are not allowed for health modules. Both surveys have sample sizes of approximately 30,000 households, and use a multi-stage, random sampling technique to represent approximately 15–16 million households in Thailand across five geographic regions including Greater Bangkok.

For the determination of equity in financial contribution to health and identification of catastrophic expenditure and impoverishment from health spending, the 2000, 2002, 2004, and 2006 rounds of SES provided information on the monthly average household payment by each particular expenditure item, including healthcare and other consumption expenses. Fractional composition of health financing sources at the country level over the same periods was derived from the National Health Account (NHA) developed by the International Health Policy Program (IHPP) of the Ministry of Public Health (MOPH).

An estimation of CI for healthcare utilization and government spending relied on quantification of visits and admissions and amount of payment to health facilities available in HWS 2001 and 2003. The reference period for utilization and healthcare payments made by household members was the last two weeks (in 2001) or last month (in 2003) for ambulatory visits and the last 12 months for hospitalization. Unit costs by level of health facility were estimated from routine reports on inputs and activities of the MOPH-affiliated health centres and hospitals, with the application of cost weights to allocate total costs between inpatient and outpatient services.

RESULTS

Equity in Financial Contribution

Compared to other lower-middle income countries, Thailand spends a relatively low share of its gross domestic product (GDP) on health. In 2002, health spending amounted to 3.5% of GDP, or Int$266 per capita, lower than the average among the lower-middle income country group of Int$304 or 5.6% of GDP (Gottret & Schieber, 2006). Given the level of health achievement (Rohde et al., 2008) and health spending, the health system in Thailand is relatively efficient and able to achieve good health at low cost.

The design of UC embraces several objectives: equitable and better access to functioning PHC, notably access to an effective district health system by rural people who are mostly poor; efficiency gains through the use of PHC with proper referral care to support it; and gains in responsiveness through the application of a purchaser–provider split, whereby the MOPH and private health facilities are service providers, and the National Health Security Office (NHSO) and Social Security Office (SSO) are purchasers on

Table 2. Financing Sources for Healthcare and their Progressivity.

Financing Sources	2002		2004		2006	
	CI[a]	Fraction[b]	CI[a]	Fraction[b]	CI[a]	Fraction[b]
Direct tax	0.8221	0.20	0.8162	0.21	0.7687	0.23
Indirect tax	0.5594	0.38	0.5958	0.37	0.5512	0.33
Social insurance contribution	0.4975	0.06	0.4561	0.07	0.4492	0.08
Private insurance	0.3785	0.09	0.4221	0.09	0.4188	0.08
Direct payment	0.4883	0.27	0.4626	0.26	0.4705	0.28
Total	0.5719	1.00	0.5822	1.00	0.5593	1.00

[a]Concentration Index (CI) based on Socioeconomic Survey (SES: 2002, 2004 and 2006). CI ranges from −1 to +1, the closer to 1 the more progressive the financial contribution.
[b]Fraction of health expenditures by source was derived from Thailand National Health Account (figures in 2006 were estimated from 2005 data).

behalf of their members (Tangcharoensathien, Prakongsai, Limwattananon, Patcharanarumol, & Jongudomsuk, 2007c). A monopsonistic purchaser can encourage the market towards efficient use of resources while ensuring quality of care.

In 2005, three years after UC was introduced, household OOP payment for health fell to 27.6% of total health expenditure, down from 34% in 2000; public sources were 64% (general government revenue 55.7%, SHI 8%). Donors play no role in financing healthcare in Thailand.

The results of our analysis of equity in financial contribution are shown in Table 2. Between 2002 and 2006, the proportion of total expenditure made up from direct tax payments increased from 20% to 23%, whereas the share from indirect tax payments fell from 38% to 33%. The proportion from household direct payments remained unchanged, at 27–28%. Direct tax was the most progressive funding source, where the rich paid proportionally more than the poor, followed by indirect tax and SHI contribution. Private insurance premiums and household OOP payment were both more regressive. General tax finance (direct, indirect tax and other government revenues) was therefore progressive. As indicated in Table 2, the dominant share of general tax as a source of total health expenditure in Thailand resulted in an overall progressive system. The overall CI remained virtually unchanged over the three observations: 0.5719 in 2002, 0.5822 in 2004 and 0.5593 in 2006.

The main reason why the SHI contribution was less progressive was the ceiling placed on the assessment of contribution, which is 15,000 baht (approximately US$428) per month. This ceiling is not indexed and has not been revised since the inception of SHI in 1990, resulting in consistent movements towards less progressivity as workers' wages have increased.

With the whole population covered by three separate public insurance schemes, the design of the reforms had to address the harmonization of the benefit package and the level of government subsidies. When SHI members retire at the age of 60 or lose their job, they are automatically enrolled by the UC scheme. Similarly, when UC members are employed in private sector firms, they are enrolled in the contributory SHI scheme and leave the UC scheme.

As a result of the pro-poor policy interventions and the piecemeal extension of financial protection to new groups, particularly the Low Income Scheme and the Voluntary Health Card Scheme, Fig. 1 shows a consistent closing of the equity gap in terms of OOP payment by households expressed as a percentage of household income between the pre-UC period (1992–2000) and the post-UC period (2002–2006). The ratio of OOP shares (the "equity gap") between deciles one and ten decreased from 6.4 times in

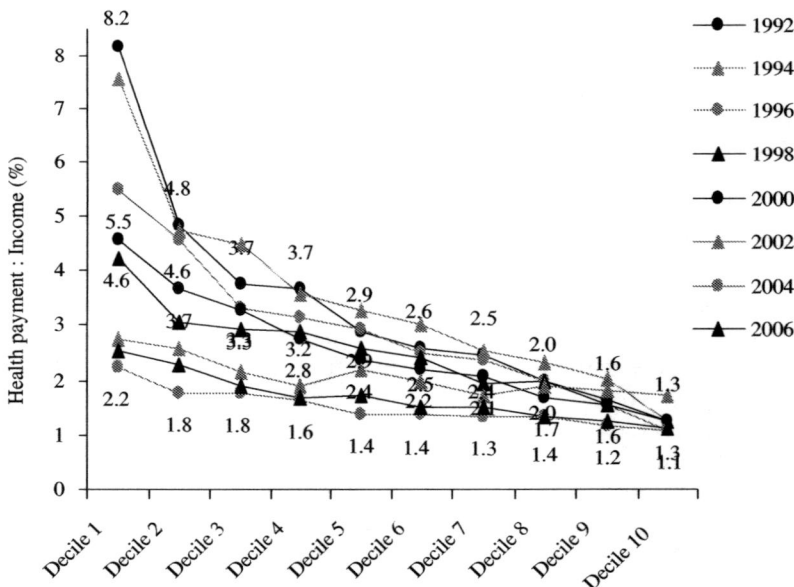

Fig. 1. Household Health Expenditure as % of Household Income by Income Deciles Before UC (1992–2000) and After UC (2002–2006). *Source:* Socioeconomic Survey 1992–2006 (National Statistical Office, 2007).

1992 to 2.3 times in 2006. The largest decreases in OOP share were observed among lower income deciles, notably deciles 1–4.

Incidence of Catastrophic Health Expenditure

The UC scheme provides both breadth and depth of coverage: breadth in terms of whole population coverage, and depth in terms of the benefit package that provides comprehensive financial protection. It includes outpatient services, inpatient services, high cost care, disease prevention and health promotion. The initial co-payment of 30 baht (US$0.86) per ambulatory visit or per admission, from which the poor were exempted, was terminated in 2006. There is neither deductible nor ceiling on financial coverage, though a limited number of services are not covered such as aesthetic surgery.

However, the UC beneficiaries are required to register with a CUP to be entitled to use free health services. A typical provider is the district health system, including the MOPH district hospital and its affiliated health centres. Referral to provincial hospitals for special investigations and treatment ensures access to quality of care beyond the services provided through the district health system. Beneficiaries bypassing the primary care or district hospital level, or using services outside the registered providers without referral, are liable for full payment.

As a result of these system design features, the evidence indicates a minimal incidence of catastrophic health expenditure.

Catastrophic health expenditure is defined as a level of OOP payment for health which exceeds 10% of total consumption expenditures of the household (Russell, 1996; Wagstaff & van Doorslaer, 2003). Table 3 indicates that before UC in 2000, the incidence of catastrophic health spending among households covered by the Low Income Scheme and the Voluntary Health Card was 4.7%, ranging from 7.1% in the richest quintile to 2.7% in the poorest quintile. Households using inpatient care, especially in private hospitals, experienced catastrophic expenditures most often (Limwattananon, Tangcharoensathien, & Prakongsai, 2007). The incidence of catastrophic health spending at district hospitals was lower.

In the UC era, the incidence of catastrophic health expenditure among UC beneficiaries fell to 3.2% in 2002, 2.6% in 2004 and finally to 1.9% in 2006. This is a remarkable achievement despite the low level of total health expenditure in Thailand. As a result of breath and depth of coverage, the poorest quintile benefited most from the UC scheme in preventing health catastrophe: the incidence among this group was 1.7% in 2002, and 1.6%

Table 3. Pre-post UC Incidence of Catastrophic Expenditure
Households.

	All Households (%)	LIC/VHC (%)	UC Scheme (%)
Before UC (2000)			
Quintile 1	4.0	2.7[a]	
Quintile 5	5.6	7.1[a]	
All quintiles	5.4	4.7[a]	
Post UC (2002)			
Quintile 1	1.7		1.7
Quintile 5	5.0		6.1
All quintiles	3.3		3.2
Post UC (2004)			
Quintile 1	1.6		1.6
Quintile 5	4.3		5.2
All quintiles	2.8		2.6
Post UC (2006)			
Quintile 1	0.9		0.9
Quintile 5	3.3		3.0
All quintiles	2.0		1.9

Source: NSO SES (various years).
[a]Members of Low Income Scheme and Voluntary Health Card in 2000 who were transferred to
be covered by UC scheme in 2002; they are the same population.

and 0.9% in 2004 and 2006, respectively. The richest quintiles still faced a
higher risk of catastrophic health expenditure, with incidence decreasing
from 6.1% in 2002 to 3% in 2006, as they bypassed the registered providers
and used private hospitals instead.

Impoverishment Arising from Health Expenditure

Healthcare-induced impoverishment is defined as the additional poverty
arising from household payment for health, calculated using national
poverty lines. Fig. 2 indicates that inpatient service use was the major cause
of impoverishment due to OOP payment, but this has reduced significantly
from 11.9% in 2000 to 4.3% in 2002 and 2.6% in 2004. Use of outpatient
services had little effect on impoverishment.

Equity in Healthcare Utilization

The use of registered providers, notably services provided by the district
health system is the main determinant of equitable use of health services.

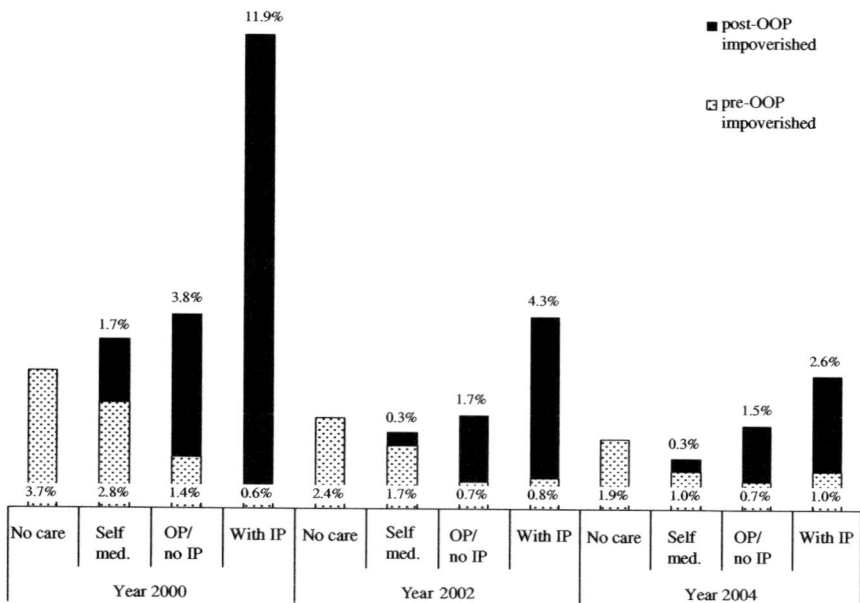

Fig. 2. Poverty Incidence by Type of Healthcare – All Households Before (2000) and After UC (2002 and 2004). *Source:* Limwattananon et al. (2007).

Owing to its geographical proximity, the district health system is a "close-to-client service" where the majority of the poor who reside in rural areas can use these services at lower travel cost. In addition, the district health system is well equipped and staffed by qualified physicians and a team of professional nurses, pharmacists, dentists and other allied public health workers.

Fig. 3 demonstrates that even before the introduction of UC, utilization of ambulatory services was pro-poor. However, in 2003 when UC was fully operating, there was a significant increase in outpatient service use by the poorest quintile, and this increase was much larger than in the richest quintile.

The CI in Table 4 also indicates a pro-poor distribution of outpatient utilization before UC, which became more pronounced after UC, particularly at health centres and district hospitals. Utilization in provincial and regional hospitals was also pro-poor, though to a lesser extent. In 2001 the CI for outpatient use was −0.0898, and after UC in 2003 this became more pro-poor, with a CI of −0.1386.

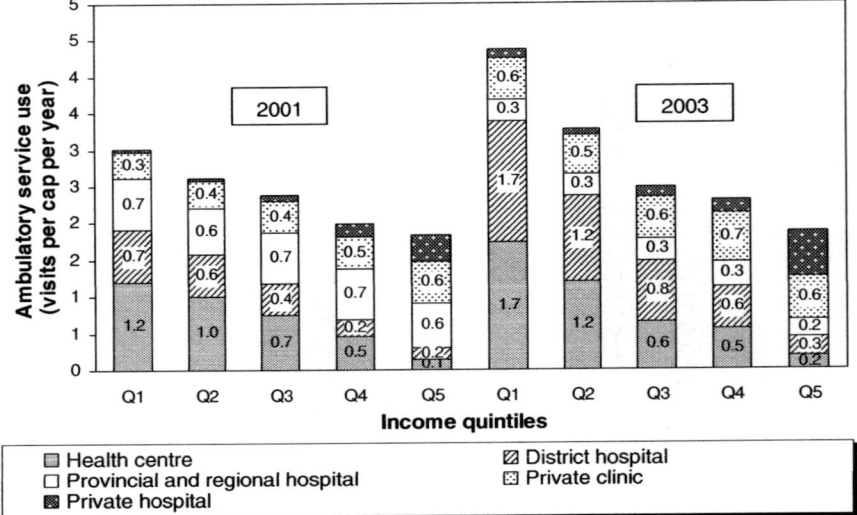

Fig. 3.   Distribution of Ambulatory Service Use Among Different Income Quintiles
in 2001 and 2003 (by Types of Health Facilities).

Table 4.   Concentration Index of Ambulatory Service and
Hospitalization by Types of Health Facilities (2001 and 2003).

Type of Health Facilities	Ambulatory Services		Hospitalization	
	2001	2003	2001	2003
Health centers	−0.2944	−0.3650	NA	NA
District hospitals	−0.2698	−0.3200	−0.3157	−0.2934
Provincial and regional hospitals	−0.0366	−0.0802	−0.0691	−0.1375
Private hospitals	0.4313	0.3484	0.3199	0.3094
Overall Concentration Index	−0.0898	−0.1386	−0.0794	−0.1208

Source: Authors analyzed from the data of 2001 and 2003 Health and Welfare Survey (HWS).

The CI for hospitalization in Table 4 indicates an increased pro-poor
outcome of UC in 2003, notably at the provincial and regional hospitals.
This finding refutes the criticism that UC members were not able to access
more sophisticated tertiary care at provincial and regional hospitals when
needed.

Despite the pro-rich nature of private hospital admission, the CI for overall admission was pro-poor before UC, CI -0.0794 in 2001, and more pro-poor, CI -0.1208 in 2003. This is because private hospitals made up a small portion of total hospital admissions.

Equity in Government Subsidies

Benefit incidence analysis was applied to assess the socioeconomic distribution of the public subsidy. At the time the UC scheme was being developed, some argued that the better-off should pay for their own services and that public funds should not be used to subsidize those who could afford to pay. In contrast, advocates of universalism who were convinced that the rich have made their contributions through a progressive tax system, argued that it is the right of all citizens to health and healthcare, and that it is the legitimate responsibility of government to finance healthcare for all. Another important argument was that collecting insurance premiums and enforcing the payment of contributions, especially among informal sector members, would be technically difficult and costly to implement.

Fig. 4 shows that even before UC (in 2001) public subsidies favoured the poor. Before UC, the 20% poorest population benefited from 28% of total government spending on health. This share increased to 31% after UC, in

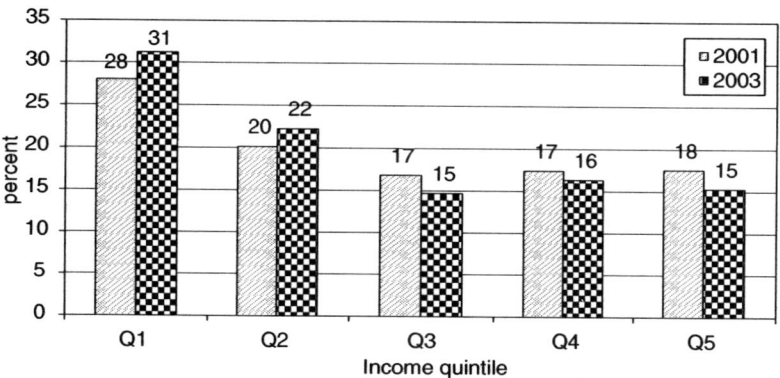

Fig. 4. Percent Distribution of Net Government Health Subsidies by Income Quintiles (Compare Pre-UC 2001 with Post-UC 2003). *Note:* The Overall Net Government Health Subsidies in 2001 were Approximately 58,733 million baht, and in 2003 were 80,678 million baht (in constant 2001 baht).

2003. The CI for the government health subsidy in 2001 was −0.044 and increased markedly to −0.123 in 2003. This finding reinforces a stronger political commitment to adequately finance the UC scheme in view of the pro-poor subsidies.

The Thai experience is in stark contrast to a range of other low- and middle-income countries, where it has been demonstrated that the benefits of public spending are highly skewed in favour of the richer quintiles (World Bank, 2005). The way governments allocate resources among levels of care, whether the poor can or cannot exercise effective use of these public health services, and the level of payment incurred by households are all factors which influence the incidence of public expenditure on health, and determine whether it favours the rich or the poor.

DISCUSSION

The experience of Thailand with a pro-poor incidence of government subsidies is shared by a small number of other countries (Malaysia and Sri Lanka) in the Asia-Pacific region (O'Donnell et al., 2007). Other developing countries in Asia including Bangladesh, China, India, Nepal and Vietnam rely mostly on OOP financing, which has resulted in a relatively high incidence of catastrophic health payment in these countries (Van Doorslaer et al., 2007). Another analysis of 59 countries confirmed that OOP payment was an independent determinant of the proportion of households with catastrophic expenditures (Xu et al., 2003).

This chapter draws several lessons from Thailand's experience with health systems development with implicit equity goals, until it reached UC in 2002. It has indeed been a long march: it took 27 years from the official launch of the Low Income Scheme for the poor in 1975 to achievement of UC in 2002. Successive policy interventions in the past decades were stepping stones for today's health equity achievements. At a later phase of reform in 2002, the design of the UC scheme accelerated and fostered health equity achievements.

Pre-requisite for Success: Functioning PHC Services

The expansion of health service infrastructure in rural areas took almost two decades, receiving particular emphasis in the fifth (1982–1986) and sixth (1987–1991) five-year national health development plans. By the 1990s, every district was covered by a district hospital of 30 beds with well-qualified staff, adequate supplies of medical equipment, medicines and other logistics. Each sub-district was covered by one health centre with four-year degree nurses or trained paramedics with a two-year diploma in public health.

Mandatory rural service by all medical graduates was introduced in 1971. Provision of rural services by medical graduates (and later extended to nurses, pharmacists and dentists) was the most significant enabling factor for a functioning PHC system. These graduates are mandated to serve at least three to four years in rural district hospitals. All other paramedics, such as public health workers, sanitarians, dental nurses and midwives are also required to serve in the rural health centres upon their graduation. This was a strong pro-poor policy intervention taken by the health sector. Such compulsory rural service did not apply to any other professions, for example engineering or agriculture graduates.

In addition to this measure, the MOPH applied a self-reliance policy regarding the production of nursing personnel. The MOPH nursing colleges produced nurses and midwives for deployment in the public sector, as the production capacity in the universities was not adequate to fulfil the demands of rapid scaling up of health infrastructure. By 2006, there were almost 8,000 nurse graduates annually, of which more than 70% were produced by the MOPH nursing colleges.

Together, these policies minimized geographic barriers to use of health services, and facilitated the functioning of the PHC system. Physical expansion required careful human resource planning, production and deployment for which long-term political commitments were needed. This prerequisite is fundamental to ensure that UC is delivered "in action", and not only reflected in political rhetoric or a paper commitment.

Determinants of Success: Right Decision on Financing UC and Design of Provider Payment Method

A piecemeal approach (Tangcharoensathien et al., 2005b) was adopted in the history of health reforms in Thailand. Population groups were classified by their employment characteristics. Public employees and their dependants are covered by CSMBS, a non-contributory health welfare scheme, aiming to compensate the low salary of public sector employees in relation to the market rate. Formal private sector employees are covered by the tripartite payroll tax contributory scheme. Efforts have been made to cover even the smallest firms of at least one employee. The poor were initially covered by the Low Income Scheme. The scheme gradually expanded to include the elderly, children aged under 12 years, the disabled and other socially disadvantaged groups. The near poor were covered initially by the Community-Based Health Insurance Scheme, which gradually developed into a voluntary public-subsidized insurance scheme.

By 2001, around 29% of the population was uninsured, despite the efforts at coverage expansion. This gap was pragmatically covered by a tax-financed insurance scheme, instead of a contributory scheme. This was a major turning point in Thai health financing policy. There was convincing evidence of why the UC scheme should not apply the contributory system to the rest of population who are engaged in the informal sector. First, in 2002 there were neither technical nor administrative capacity to collect insurance premiums from the informal sector. Second, a flat rate premium is easy to collect but it is the most regressive option (Patcharanarumol, 2003). Third, contribution as percentage of income or wealth is progressive, but measurement of income and wealth has proven to be extremely difficult. Fourth, it is difficult to enforce a contributory scheme for the informal sector. Finally, retrospective evidence after UC scheme launched, in Fig. 5, indicates that 25% of UC members belong to the bottom quintile, and 25% to the next poorest quintile. It is therefore the legitimate responsibility of the government to subsidize these groups from general tax revenue, not through contributions.

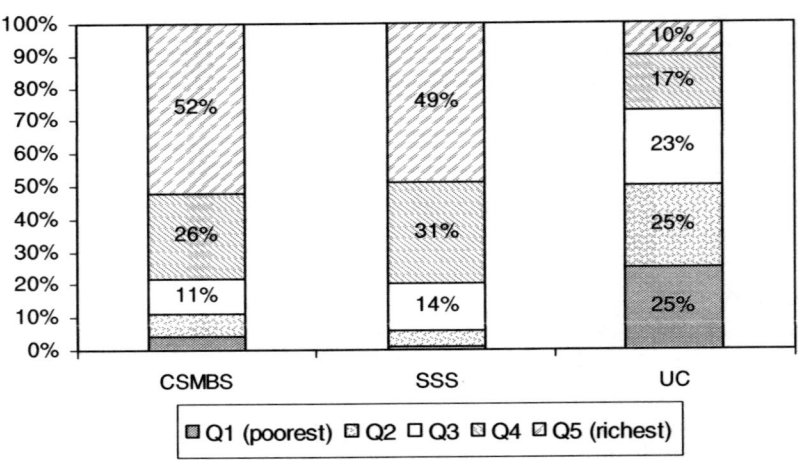

Fig. 5.   Scheme Beneficiaries by Income Quintiles (2004).

Thailand has demonstrated that it is feasible, and equitable, to use tax-financing to cover the majority of population. UC members make up 75% of the population. Half of them belong to the poorest and the second poorest quintiles, whereas 49% of SHI members and 52% of CSMBS members belong to the richest quintile.

The tax-financed scheme is also sustainable in the long term. It links with providers through a contracting model with closed-ended provider payment methods (capitation for outpatient services and global budget with the application of DRG for inpatient services). The capitation contract model has been shown in SHI to be an effective means of cost-containment, and to support adequate quality of care. In contrast, the fee-for-service reimbursement model used by CSMBS has been shown to be associated with cost escalation and inefficiency (Mills, Bennett, Siriwanarangsun, & Tangchar-oensathien, 2000; Tangcharoensathien et al., 1999).

Finally, there were also historical precedents for the comprehensive benefit package. Both the Low Income Scheme and the Voluntary Health Card Scheme provided a comprehensive package. Given this comprehensive service package, which includes outpatient and inpatient care, disease prevention and health promotion, application of a fee for service payment mechanism would have resulted in cost escalation and was clearly beyond the government's fiscal capacity.

Determinants of Success: The Use of PHC to Achieve Equity and Efficiency

The PHC system plays a pivotal role in health achievements and equity in Thailand (Rohde et al., 2008). Contracting district-level health providers to provide close-to-client services for UC beneficiaries is an important means of ensuring efficient and rational use of services while ensuring proper referral systems. On the technical efficiency dimension, the cost of services provided by primary care providers in the district health system is much lower than through provincial hospital-based services. The transport costs incurred by households to use these close-to-client services are also much lower. When the majority of UC members who are poor rural residents can actually exercise their rights in using a comprehensive range of services provided by the PHC network, it results in equity in utilization and a pro-poor public subsidy on health. Together with the provision of a comprehensive benefit package, the system has resulted in minimal catastrophic health expenditure and impoverishment.

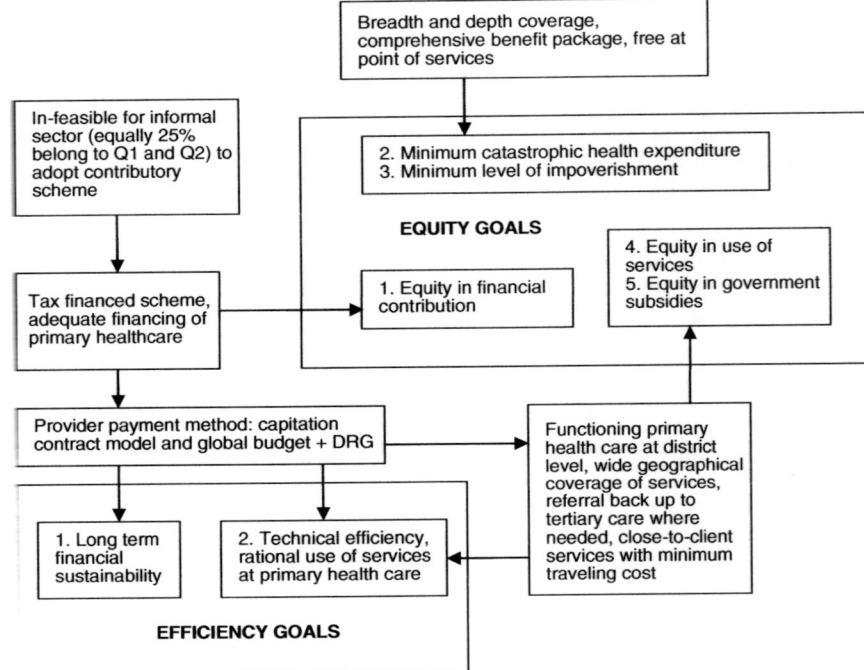

Fig. 6. How Health Equity and Health Systems Efficiency were Achieved.

Having discussed the prerequisites and determinants of success in achieving health equity, a conceptual flow of determinants is summarized in Fig. 6. By adopting a contracting model for primary care and introducing provider payment reforms, the design of the system was able to achieve not only health equity goals, but efficiency goals as well. This figure conveys the most important message to international audiences that a thoughtful systems design is fundamental to achieve the health systems goals of equity and efficiency.

National Institutional Capacity

National institutional capacity to generate evidence from health policy and systems research (Tangcharoensathien & Pitayarangsarit, 2007b) is as important as the capacity to effectively translate the evidence into policy decisions, program design, monitoring and evaluation (Towse, Mills, & Tangcharoensathien, 2004; Tangcharoensathien et al., 2004). The UC reform experienced by Thailand was free from donor influence and advice; but was driven by local evidence and national capacity to effectively scale up the program implementation in a relatively short period.

In this light, the routine collection of nationally representative household data for monitoring health equity and changes over time has been shown to be critical. In the past decade, the IHPP has built up a genuine partnership with NSO in the common effort to maximize the usefulness and quality of nationally representative household survey data, in particular the SES and the HWS. An institutional agreement between the MOPH and NSO was reached in 2006 to ensure that equity stratifiers such as income, expenditure and asset ownership (to generate wealth index) are integrated into all social and health surveys by NSO. A recent review (Tangcharoensathien, Limwattananon, & Prakongsai, 2007a) indicates that national household survey datasets in Thailand are sufficient to undertake equity analysis, monitoring and evaluation of policies, though further efforts should be given to measuring equity in health outcomes, such as disparities in under-five and maternal mortality.

CONCLUSION

A number of policy messages emerge from this analysis. Whether or not reform or UC is part of national policy, governments are obliged to improve service coverage and strengthen PHC, paying particular attention to the needs of the poor rural population. The Thai experience demonstrates the value in equity terms of ensuring a functioning PHC system, through the operation of the district health system. This provides the major pro-poor hub in translating equity policy into practice. Inadequate physical access to care is a result of geographical barriers in most developing countries. Minimizing financial barriers by introducing universal free services where physical barriers are not addressed will eventually favour the rich over the poor.

General tax revenue is the most equitable and feasible (in terms of collection compared to social heath insurance contribution) financing source for providing financial protection for the population, either targeting the poor or adopting a UC approach. The Thai path towards UC incorporated phases of targeting, but reformists kept in mind the ultimate objective of universality. However, the pace in the move towards universality is highly dependent on political will and fiscal space. The piecemeal approach to coverage extension reflected Thai pragmatism.

The way in which systems are designed to support universality is an essential factor influencing whether or not the health system goals of equity and efficiency are obtained. Though it is not the focus of this chapter to address the two other goals of responsiveness and equity in the distribution of health status, future efforts will be addressed to these issues.

Finally, the institutional capacity to generate evidence and translate evidence into policy decision is as important as the capacity to design programs, scale up interventions and regular monitoring and evaluation to inform policies.

NOTES

1. The health card project was initiated in 1983 with a focus on community-based health insurance (CBHI) for maternal and child health (MCH) services managed by village committees. Later in 1984, CBHI was extended to cover healthcare services for other family members. In 1991, the scheme was transformed to a formal voluntary health insurance scheme and finally in 1994, the government decided to subsidize half of the annual cost, with households contributing the other half. The authors view CBHI as a transitional measure towards UC. The voluntary nature of CBHI, with adverse selection and problems of financial sustainability, were major barriers to coverage expansion and reaching universal coverage.

2. Renal replacement therapy (peritoneal dialysis and kidney transplantation) was included in the UC benefit package at the end of 2007.

ACKNOWLEDGMENTS

We wish to acknowledge our national partners for their contributions to the development, implementation, M&E of UC in Thailand especially, NSO for national household surveys to monitor achievement of policy goals, NHSO and other partners who initiate, design and steer the UC scheme, Health Systems Research Institute (HSRI) for support for NHA development and institutionalization, the MOPH healthcare providers which steer the implementation of the UC scheme, and the Thailand Research Fund (TRF) for institutional grants to IHPP.

REFERENCES

Deaton, A. (1997). *The analysis of household surveys: A micro-econometric approach to development policies.* Baltimore: Johns Hopkins University Press.

Frenk, J. (2006). Bridging the divide: Global lessons from evidence-based health policy in Mexico. *Lancet, 368,* 954–961.

Gottret, P., & Schieber, G. (2006). *Health financing revisited: A practitioner's guide.* Washington, DC: World Bank.

Hill, K., Vapattanawong, P., Prasartkul, P., Porapakkham, Y., Lim, S. S., & Lopez, A. D. (2007). Epidemiologic transition interrupted: A reassessment of mortality trends in Thailand, 1980–2000. *International Journal of Epidemiology, 36,* 374–384.

Jongudoumsuk, P. (2002). Achieving universal coverage of health care in Thailand through the 30 Baht Scheme. *SEAMIC Conference, Chiang Mai, Thailand, 2001,* Health Care Reform Office, Ministry of Public Health.

Kutzin, J. (2000). *Towards universal health care coverage: A goal-oriented framework for policy analysis.* Washington, DC: World Bank.

Limwattananon, S., Tangcharoensathien, V., & Prakongsai, P. (2007). Catastrophic and poverty impacts of health payments: Results from national household surveys in Thailand. *Bulletin of the World Health Organization, 85,* 600–606.

Mills, A. (2007). Strategies to achieve universal coverage: Are there lessons from middle income countries? *Publications commissioned by the Health Systems Knowledge Network,* Commission on Social Determinants of Health, World Health Organization, Geneva.

Mills, A., Bennett, S., Siriwanarangsun, P., & Tangcharoensathien, V. (2000). The response of providers to capitation payment: A case-study from Thailand. *Health Policy, 51,* 163–180.

National Statistical Office. (2007). *Household socio-economic survey.* Bangkok: Office of the Prime Minister.

Nitayarumphong, S. (1998). Universal coverage of health care: Challenges for the developing countries. In: S. Nitayarumphong & A. Mills (Eds), *Achieving universal coverage of health care, office of health care reform* (pp. 3–24). Nonthaburi: Ministry of Public Health.

O'Donnell, O., van Doorslaer, E., Rannan-Eliya, R. P., Somanathan, A., Adhikari, S. R., Akkazieva, B., Harbianto, D., Garg, C. C., Hanvoravongchai, P., Herrin, A. N., Huq, M. N., Ibragimova, S., Karan, A., Kwon, S., Leung, G. M., Lu, J. R., Ohkusa, Y., Pande, B. R., Racelis, R., Tin, K., Tisayaticom, K., Trisnantoro, L., Wan, Q., Yang, B., & Zhao, Y. (2008a). Who pays for health care in Asia? *Journal of Health Economics, 27,* 460–475.

O'Donnell, O., van Doorslaer, E., Rannan-Eliya, R. P., Somanathan, A., Adhikari, S. R., Harbianto, D., Garg, C. C., Hanvoravongchai, P., Huq, M. N., Karan, A., Leung, G. M., Ng, C. W., Pande, B. R., Tin, K., Tisayaticom, K., Trisnantoro, L., Zhang, Y., & Zhao, Y. (2007). The incidence of public spending on healthcare: Comparative evidence from Asia. *The World Bank Economic Review, 21,* 93–123.

O'Donnell, O., van Doorslaer, E., & Wagstaff, A. (2008b). *Analyzing health equity using household survey data: A guide to techniques and their implementation.* Washington, DC: World Bank Institute.

Patcharanarumol, W. (2003). *Financial feasibility for introducing contribution to universal healthcare coverage scheme in Thailand.* Master thesis, Maastritch University, The Netherlands.

Rohde, J., Cousens, S., Chopra, M., Tangcharoensathien, V., Black, R., Bhutta, Z., & Lawn, J. E. (2008). Alma-Ata: Rebirth and revision 4, 30 years after Alma-Ata. Has primary health care worked in countries? *Lancet, 372,* 950–961.

Russell, S. (1996). Ability to pay for health care: Concepts and evidence. *Health Policy and Planning, 11,* 219–237.

Srithamrongsawat, S. (2002). The health card scheme: A subsidized voluntary health insurance scheme. In: P. Pramualratana & S. Wibulpolprasert (Eds), *Health insurance system in Thailand* (pp. 79–93). Nonthaburi: Health System Research Institute.

Tangcharoensathien, V., Kasemsup, V., Teerawattananon, Y., Supaporn, T., Vasavid, C., & Prakongsai, P. (2005a). *Universal access to renal replacement therapy in Thailand: A policy analysis.* Nonthaburi: International Health Policy Program.

Tangcharoensathien, V., Limwattananon, S., & Prakongsai, P. (2007a). Improving health-related information systems to monitor equity in health: Lessons from Thailand. In: D. McIntyre & G. Mooney (Eds), *The economics of health equity* (pp. 222–246). New York: Cambridge University Press.

Tangcharoensathien, V., & Pitayarangsarit, S. (2007b). Capacity development for health policy and systems research: Experience and lessons from Thailand. In: A. Green & S. Bennett (Eds), *Sound choices: Enhancing capacity for evidence-informed health policy.* Geneva: World Health Organization.

Tangcharoensathien, V., Prakongsai, P., Limwattananon, S., Patcharanarumol, W., & Jongudomsuk, P. (2007c). Achieving universal coverage in Thailand: What lessons do we learn? In: *A case study commissioned by the health systems knowledge network.* Geneva: WHO Commission on Social Determinants of Health, World Health Organization.

Tangcharoensathien, V., Supachutikul, A., & Lertiendumrong, J. (1999). The social security scheme in Thailand: What lessons can be drawn? *Social Science and Medicine, 48,* 913–923.

Tangcharoensathien, V., Teokul, W., & Chanwongpaisarn, L. (2005b). Challenges of implementing universal health care in Thailand. *Social Policy in a Development Context Series: Transforming the Developmental Welfare State in East Asia,* UNRISD.

Tangcharoensathien, V., Wibulpolprasert, S., & Nitayarampong, S. (2004). Knowledge-based changes to health systems: The Thai experience in policy development. *Bulletin of the World Health Organization, 82*(10), 750–756.

Towse, A., Mills, A., & Tangcharoensathien, V. (2004). Learning from Thailand's health reforms. *British Medical Journal, 328,* 103–105.

Van Doorslaer, E., O'Donnell, O., Rannan-Eliya, R. P., Somanathan, A., Adhikari, S. R., Garg, C. C., Harbianto, D., Herrin, A. N., Huq, M. N., Ibragimova, S., Karan, A., Lee, T., Leung, G. M., Lu, J. R., Ng, C. W., Pande, B. R., Racelis, R., Toa, S., Tin, K., Tisayaticom, K., Trisnantoro, L., Vasavid, C., & Zhao, Y. (2007). Catastrophic payments for health care in Asia. *Health Economics, 16,* 1159–1184.

Van Doorslaer, E., O'Donnell, O., Rannan-Eliya, R. P., Somanathan, A., Adhikari, S. R., Garg, C. C., Harbianto, D., Herrin, A. N., Huq, M. N., Ibragimova, S., Karan, A., Ng, C. W., Pande, B. R., Racelis, R., Toa, S., Tin, K., Tisayaticom, K., Trisnantoro, L., Vasavid, C., & Zhao, Y. (2006). Effect of payments for health care on poverty estimates in 11 countries in Asia: An analysis of household survey data. *Lancet, 368,* 1357–1364.

Vapattanawong, P., Hogan, M. C., Hanvoravongchai, P., Gakidou, E., Vos, T., Lopez, A., & Lim, S. S. (2007). Reductions in child mortality levels and inequalities in Thailand: Analysis of two censuses. *Lancet, 369*, 850–855.

Vasavid, C., Tisayatikom, K., Patcharanarumol, W., & Tangcharoensathien, V. (2004). Impact of universal health care coverage on the Thai households. In: V. Tangcharoensathien & P. Jongudoumsuk (Eds), *From policy to implementation: Historical events during 2001–2004 of universal coverage in Thailand* (pp. 129–149). Nonthaburi: National Health Security Office.

Wagstaff, A. (2007). *Social health insurance re-examined.* World Bank Policy Research Paper 4111. World Bank, Washington, DC.

Wagstaff, A., & van Doorslaer, E. (2003). Catastrophe and impoverishment in paying for health care: With applications to Vietnam 1993–98. *Health Economics, 12*, 921–934.

Wibulpolprasert, S. (2005). *Thailand health profile 2001–2004.* Nonthaburi: Bureau of Policy and Strategy, Ministry of Public Health.

World Bank. (2005). *World development report 2004: Making services work for poor people.* Washington, DC: World Bank.

Xu, K., Evans, D. B., Kawabata, K., Zeramdini, R., Klavus, J., & Murray, C. J. L. (2003). Household catastrophic health expenditure: A multi-country analysis. *Lancet, 362*, 111–117.

SOCIAL HEALTH INSURANCE AND LABOR MARKET OUTCOMES: EVIDENCE FROM CENTRAL AND EASTERN EUROPE, AND CENTRAL ASIA [☆]

Adam Wagstaff and Rodrigo Moreno-Serra

ABSTRACT

Objective – *The implications of social health insurance (SHI) for labor markets have featured prominently in recent debates over the merits of SHI and general revenue financing. It has been argued that by raising the nonwage component of labor costs, SHI reduces firms' demand for labor, lowers employment levels and net wages, and encourages self-employment and informal working arrangements. At the national level, SHI has been claimed to reduce a country's competitiveness in international markets and to discourage foreign direct investment (FDI). The transition from general revenue finance to SHI that occurred during the 1990s in many of*

[☆]The findings, interpretations, and conclusions expressed in this chapter are entirely those of the authors and do not necessarily represent the views of the World Bank, its Executive Directors, or the countries they represent.

Innovations in Health System Finance in Developing and Transitional Economies
Advances in Health Economics and Health Services Research, Volume 21, 83–106

ISSN: 0731-2199/doi:10.1108/S0731-2199(2009)0000021007

the central and eastern European and central Asian countries provides a unique opportunity to investigate empirically these claims.

Methodology/approach – *We employ regression-based generalizations of difference-in-differences (DID) and instrumental variables (IV) on country-level panel data from 28 countries for the period 1990–2004.*

Findings – *We find that, controlling for gross domestic product (GDP) per capita, SHI increases (gross) wages by 20%, reduces employment (as a share of the population) by 10%, and increases self-employment by 17%. However, we find no significant effects of SHI on unemployment (registered or self-reported), agricultural employment, a widely used measure of the size of the informal economy, or FDI.*

Implications for policy – *We do not claim that our results imply that SHI adoption everywhere must necessarily reduce employment and increase self-employment. Nonetheless, our results ought to serve as a warning to those contemplating shifting the financing of health care from general revenues to a SHI system.*

1. INTRODUCTION

Social health insurance (SHI) – a model of health financing where a person's entitlements to health care derive from earnings-related payroll contributions – is enjoying something of a revival in parts of the developing world.[1] Many countries that have in the past used general revenues (and out-of-pocket payments) to finance health care have introduced SHI, or are thinking about doing so.[2] And countries with SHI already in place are making vigorous efforts to extend coverage, especially to informal sector workers and their families.[3]

Ironically, this revival is occurring at a time when three of the oldest SHI countries – France, Germany, and the Netherlands – are all in the process of reducing their reliance on payroll contributions.[4] The implications of SHI for labor markets have featured prominently in the debates over the merits of SHI and general revenue financing in these countries. It has been argued that by raising the nonwage component of labor costs, SHI reduces firms' demand for labor, lowers employment levels and net wages, and encourages self-employment and informal working arrangements. At the national level, SHI has been claimed to reduce a country's competitiveness in international markets and to discourage foreign direct investment (FDI). It was primarily these perceived negative consequences of SHI that prompted one German health minister to call the exclusive linking of health care finance to earnings rather than income more generally "the Achilles heel" of Germany's social insurance system (Schmidt, 2006).

Despite their importance, and the vibrancy of the debate surrounding them, there is comparatively little hard evidence on these issues. There are, of course, studies that look at the effects of higher payroll taxes on employment; interestingly, one recent study of the issue in Germany (Bauer & Riphahn 2002) actually found only very limited employment effects of higher payroll taxes. There are also a few studies that look at health financing reforms and their effects on payroll tax rates and the knock-on effects on wages and employment; Kugler and Kugler (2003), for example, conclude that the Colombian health reforms of the 1990s raised the payroll tax rate by five percentage points, and this in turn reduced (net) wages by 0.7–1.1% and employment by 2–2.5%.

These studies, while useful, do not, however, shed light on the effects on labor market outcomes of a policy shift from SHI to general revenue financing (or vice versa). This is what this chapter attempts to accomplish. One might be tempted to get at these effects through a cross-country econometric analysis of a sample of countries where some finance their health care through SHI and others through general revenues. But this would be problematic because there are likely to be unobservable variables that would be correlated with the type of financing system in place and the outcomes of interest (i.e., SHI is likely to be endogenous). A more promising strategy would be to look for *changes* in the way countries finance their health care, exploiting the variations in changes across countries to eliminate (time-invariant) unobservable variables. This is the approach Gruber and Hanratty (1995) adopt in their analysis of the employment effects of Canada's switch during the 1960s from US-style private health insurance to a system financed largely through general revenues; they exploit the fact that the reform was phased by province, with Saskatchewan making the change as early as 1962 and New Brunswick making the shift as late as 1971. Adopting such an approach to shed light on the effects of shifting from SHI to general revenues (or vice versa) requires the use of country-level data, since no federal country has ever phased in a switch from SHI to general revenue finance. However, among the group of countries that are traditionally thought of as having the best data (the Organisation for Economic Co-operation and Development (OECD) countries), there have been very few switches between the SHI and tax-financed camps; moreover, the transitions occurred some time ago, so the available data are very limited.[5]

This chapter looks instead to a (mostly) different group of countries where transitions have occurred with greater frequency and more recently, namely, the countries of (central and eastern) Europe and Central Asia (ECA).[6] Of the 28 ECA countries, 14 abandoned tax finance and adopted SHI at some stage between 1990 and 2004 (and 4 other countries had adopted SHI before 1990). These countries are also data-rich countries, having inherited and largely maintained the Communist tradition of extensive data gathering. The ECA health financing experiment thus affords a valuable "laboratory" to try to shed light on the question of how SHI systems fare vis-à-vis tax-financed systems. In this chapter, we report the results of analysis of the effects of SHI transitions on labor market outcomes; elsewhere (Wagstaff & Moreno-Serra, 2009) we have reported the results of an analysis of SHI adoption on health sector outcomes, namely, health spending, health sector throughputs, and health status. The models we use in this chapter are regression-based generalizations of difference-in-differences (DID) and instrumental variables (IV). We pay particular attention to the issue of the possible endogeneity of SHI, since it seems likely that there may be events that occurred around the time SHI was introduced that we implicitly lump into our error term but which may affect outcomes.

The organization of the chapter is as follows. Section 2 provides a brief history of the SHI reforms in the post-Communist ECA region and discusses the hypothesized effects of SHI adoption on labor market outcomes. Section 3 outlines our methods, Section 4 our data, and Section 5 our empirical results. Section 6 presents our conclusions.

2. ECA'S SHI REFORMS AND HYPOTHESIZED LABOR MARKET CONSEQUENCES

Under communism, health care in almost all of the ECA countries (the former Yugoslavia was the exception) was financed out of general revenues and out-of-pocket payments.[7] In the early 1990s, as most countries shifted away from communism, several looked to SHI to solve a number of emerging problems and improve the performance of the health sector.

2.1. Transitions to SHI

Of the 28 ECA countries, 14 introduced payroll taxes earmarked for health care at some stage between 1990 and 2004, and 4 others had already done so before 1990 (Bosnia and Herzegovina, Croatia, Serbia and Montenegro, and Turkey). Early SHI adopters in the 1990s included Estonia, Hungary, Lithuania, Macedonia, and Slovenia; all adopted SHI in the period 1990–1992. Some countries adopted much later: Bulgaria, for example, adopted SHI as late as 1999. Often, both the employee and the employer are liable, though of course there may be a wide difference between who is legally liable for what and who ends up bearing the incidence of the payroll tax, the latter depending on conditions in the labor and product markets. Contributions are mandatory, and in exchange for them, the contributing employee is entitled to receive health services under the terms of the SHI scheme. Groups other than formal sector workers usually have some coverage. Contributions are required from the self-employed in all SHI countries and from pensioners in some. Other groups are financed out of general revenues, but often the contributions are not specified and insufficient funds are provided in respect of these groups, who sometimes have inferior de facto coverage. Two countries (Latvia and Poland) introduced earmarked taxes for health care, but the tax base is income not earnings; therefore from a financing perspective, these are not "pure" SHI systems. The precise timing of the transitions is shown and discussed further in the work by Wagstaff and Moreno-Serra (2009).

2.2. Hypothesized Labor Market Consequences of the Transition to SHI

The idea that a heavy emphasis on payroll taxes in financing of health care might have negative consequences for employment is consistent with the OECD's recommendations in its Jobs Strategy that its members ought to lower their payroll taxes (OECD, 1999). Fig. 1 shows the textbook analysis of the imposition of a payroll tax. The wage is initially w_0 and employment is initially E_0. A payroll tax drives a wedge between the gross and net wage and causes the demand curve for labor to shift leftward from D_0 to D_1. The gross wage rises to w_1, and the net wage falls to w_1–tax. Employment falls from E_0 to E_1. However, as Summers (1989) has argued, this ignores the fact that the payroll tax induces not only a leftward shift of the labor demand curve but also a rightward shift in the labor supply curve (workers value the benefits financed through the tax and are willing to supply more labor at a given money wage). Depending where the new labor supply curve, S_1, is in Fig. 1, the naive analysis might substantially overstate the disemployment effect of a payroll tax and understate the reduction in the net wage.

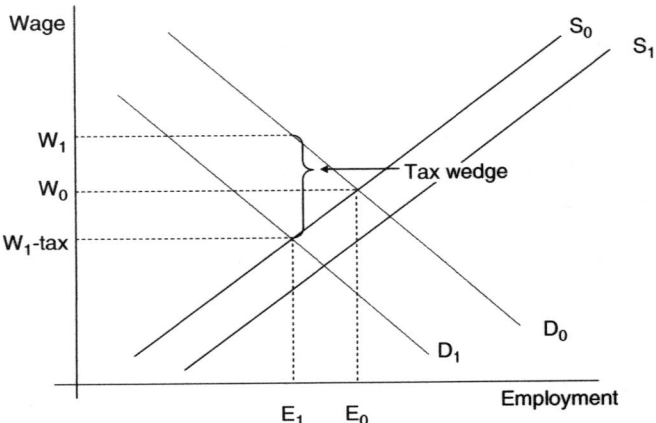

Fig. 1.   Textbook Treatment of Payroll Taxes and Employment.

The textbook analysis ignores another important dimension to the problem, namely, that if payroll taxes were used less, other taxes would have to be used more, and these would also have effects on employment and wages. Raising the income tax would reduce the returns to work and would hence shift the labor supply curve leftward, also causing a reduction in employment. A rise in indirect taxes would reduce real wages, reducing people's willingness to work at a given nominal wage, again potentially reducing employment. In both cases, one could argue that insofar as revenues are used to finance programs that benefit the payers of the taxes, the labor supply curve might shift rightward, along the lines argued by Summers for the payroll tax; this would moderate the disemployment effect. However, it seems likely that because the linkage between taxes paid and the benefits of the health insurance program are likely to be perceived as less close in the case where revenues are raised through the income tax and indirect taxes than in the case where they are raised through a payroll tax, the rightward shift in the labor supply curve is likely to be much smaller in the former case than the latter case and may be imperceptible. It is not inconceivable, therefore, that the disemployment effect of a payroll tax may actually be *less* than that associated with income taxes and indirect taxes.

In practice, it seems that, at least as far as the OECD countries are concerned, payroll, income, and consumption taxes all have broadly similar effects on employment (cf. Nickell, 2004; Nickell, Nunziata, & Ochel, 2005). As Nickell (1997) puts it, "Broadly speaking, the key tax rate for the labor market is the sum of the payroll tax rate, the personal income tax rate and the consumption tax rate. Switching between these taxes will not have an important impact, so payroll taxes, per se, are of little consequence" (p.68). How far this argument applies when other forms of government revenue are taken into account is less clear. It seems likely that some other taxes – such as import duties – may have much smaller effects on employment, in which case, shifting from payroll taxes to general revenues more broadly may help lower unemployment. Ultimately, then, the effects on employment and net wages of shifting between payroll taxation and general revenues to finance health care are unclear a priori.

In contrast, there seems to be less ambiguity about the relative effects of the two systems on levels of self-employment and informal working arrangements. SHI can provide a disincentive for people to join and stay in formal employment, while the same is not true of general revenue financing (cf., e.g., Belev, 2003; Baeza & Packard, 2006; Datta, 2006; Levy, 2007). The incentive is likely to be especially large in the case where among informal sector workers, SHI enrollment is voluntary (as in Germany) or is only weakly enforced (as is the case in many developing countries). In such a setting, people can rely on private insurance (in some countries, they are required by law to have it if they do not join the SHI scheme), or they may opt for informal employment arrangements and resort to using the health ministry's public health care system, albeit facing higher out-of-pocket payments than they would have done under the SHI system and probably ending up with worse quality care. These incentives become even more of an issue if being in formal employment means being drawn into the tax system and having to contribute to a pension scheme that because of limited life expectancy may only pay out for a few years if any. The belief is, then, that SHI encourages self-employment and informal working arrangements, something that may be undesirable; for example, the government's scope to raise taxes is reduced. This is one of the reasons why a recent World Bank book on health systems in Latin America (Baeza & Packard, 2006) recommended a gradual move from payroll financing to general revenue financing.

The final issue we investigate is the link between SHI and FDI. There is plenty of evidence (refer Bellak, Leibrecht, & Riedl (2008) for a recent review) suggesting that high labor costs in a country (gross of social insurance contributions) reduce FDI. This is consistent with theory in that firms can be expected to locate where costs are relatively low, though as Bellak et al. (2008) note, there are clearly mitigating factors. For example, if social insurance contributions result in better preventive and curative health care than would otherwise have been the case, investors may end up with a healthier workforce that may partially or fully compensate foreign investors for the higher labor costs. However, if the comparison is between two equally generous and well-functioning health systems, one financed through payroll contributions and the other through general revenues, the expectation is that the latter will attract more FDI unless the tax system is heavily skewed toward corporate income taxes.

3. METHODS

Let y_{it} be the outcome of interest in country i at time t. In the empirical analysis below, the outcomes studied include gross wages, employment, unemployment, self-employment, informality and FDI. Let X_{it} be a vector of covariates thought to potentially influence both outcomes and the SHI adoption decision, and SHI_{it} be a dummy variable taking on a value of 1 if country i has a SHI health financing system at time t. Consider the model:

$$y_{it} = X_{it}\gamma + \delta SHI_{it} + e_{it}, \tag{1}$$

where the e_{it} capture unobservable variables and noise. Our interest is in the coefficient δ that gives the impact of SHI on the outcome y_{it}. Estimating Eq. (1) by pooled ordinary least squares (OLS) would run the risk that the estimate of δ would be biased because of a correlation between SHI_{it} and e_{it}, that is, SHI status might be endogenous. It could be that countries with unobserved characteristics that led to higher-than-expected levels of, say, self-employment may deliberately choose not to adopt SHI because of the difficulty of having a contribution-based financing system with large numbers of self-employed. Or it might be that certain changes or events occurred broadly around the same time that SHI was introduced; if we do not capture these in our model but instead lump them in the error term, and if they affect the outcomes of interest, our estimate of δ will be biased.

3.1. Difference-In-Differences Models[8]

The simplest way to allow for such a correlation is to let:

$$e_{it} = \alpha_i + \theta_t + \varepsilon_{it}, \tag{2}$$

where θ_t is a period-specific intercept, α_i is a country-specific effect that captures time-invariant unobservables that are potentially correlated with

SHI status, and ε_{it} is an idiosyncratic error term (iid over i and t). Substituting Eq. (2) in Eq. (1) gives

$$y_{it} = \mathbf{X}_{it}\gamma + \delta SHI_{it} + \alpha_i + \theta_t + \varepsilon_{it}. \tag{3}$$

In the special case where the $\mathbf{X}_{it}$ are omitted, Eq. (3) collapses to the standard DID estimator (cf., e.g., Wooldridge, 2002, p. 284). Taking first differences of Eq. (3) gives

$$\Delta y_{it} = \Delta\mathbf{X}_{it}\gamma + \delta\Delta SHI_{it} + \xi_t + \Delta\varepsilon_{it}, \tag{4}$$

which can be consistently estimated by pooled OLS if the endogeneity of SHI adoption is adequately captured by the error term specified in Eq. (2).[9]

This generalized DID estimator assumes a parallel or common trend: the θ_t do not depend on the value of SHI_{it}, and therefore, the "treated" health systems (i.e., those that switch to SHI) and the "untreated" ones exhibit the same trend. In reality, there may be time-varying unobservables that are correlated with both y_{it} and SHI status. One model that allows this parallel trend assumption (PTA) to be relaxed is the somewhat misleadingly named "random trend" (RT) model (cf., e.g., Wooldridge, 2002, p. 316). Eq. (2) is replaced by the assumption

$$e_{it} = \alpha_i + \theta_t + k_i t + \varepsilon_{it}. \tag{5}$$

This allows for the possibility that different countries have different trends, as reflected in different values of k_i. Substituting Eq. (5) in Eq. (1) gives

$$y_{it} = \mathbf{X}_{it}\gamma + \delta SHI_{it} + \alpha_i + \theta_t + k_i t + \varepsilon_{it}, \tag{6}$$

which can be estimated by differencing Eq. (6) and using a fixed effects estimator on the resultant equation:

$$\Delta y_{it} = \Delta\mathbf{X}_{it}\gamma + \delta\Delta SHI_{it} + \xi_t + k_i + \Delta\varepsilon_{it}. \tag{7}$$

If the k_i are jointly insignificant, Eq. (7) collapses to Eq. (4), which would provide some evidence in support of the PTA. Yet even if the k_i were jointly significant, the PTA would still be a reasonable assumption if the k_i are uncorrelated with SHI_{it}. The latter can be tested through a single-variable, generalized version of the Hausman test of fixed versus random effects, which takes into account the clustered nature of our data and is implemented by estimating an auxiliary quasi-demeaned regression (cf. Wooldridge, 2002, p. 290). For each outcome, we implement this test by

estimating an augmented version of Eq. (7) using a random effects estimator – adding the within-country panel means of the original covariates
that vary over i and t as regressors – and testing the null hypothesis of
insignificance of the additional SHI term (with cluster-robust standard
errors). Non-rejection of this hypothesis would suggest that the k_i are
uncorrelated with SHI_{it} and thus provide evidence in favor of the PTA.

The RT model is less restrictive than the standard DID model (the latter is
nested in the former), but nonetheless suffers potentially from two
problems: the assumed trend is linear, and the trend is specific to the
country and assumed not to be modified by the treatment (i.e., the
introduction of SHI). Another model that allows the PTA to be relaxed is
the "differential trend" (DT) model of Bell, Blundell, and Reenen (1999).
They assume:

$$e_{it} = \begin{cases} \alpha_i + k_s m_t + \varepsilon_{it} & if \quad SHI_{it} = 1 \\ \alpha_i + k_n m_t + \varepsilon_{it} & if \quad SHI_{it} = 0 \end{cases} \tag{8}$$

where m_t is an unobserved trend, the influence of which on y_{it} is allowed to
differ between SHI and non-SHI systems. Incorporating this assumption
into Eq. (1) gives:

$$y_{it} = \mathbf{X}_{it}\gamma + \delta SHI_{it} + \alpha_i + k_n m_t + (k_s - k_n)m_t SHI_{it} + \varepsilon_{it}, \tag{9}$$

from which we can get a first differenced estimating equation:

$$\Delta y_{it} = \Delta \mathbf{X}_{it}\gamma + \delta \Delta SHI_{it} + k_n \Delta m_t + (k_s - k_n)\Delta(m_t SHI_{it}) + \Delta\varepsilon_{it}. \tag{10}$$

In the estimation, the Δm_t would be replaced by first differences of year
dummies and the $\Delta(m_t SHI_{it})$ would be replaced by first differences of
interactions between year dummies and the SHI status dummy:

$$\Delta y_{it} = \Delta \mathbf{X}_{it}\gamma + \delta \Delta SHI_{it} + \sum_{\tau=2}^{T} \beta_\tau \Delta YEAR_\tau + \sum_{\tau=2}^{T} \varphi_\tau \Delta(YEAR_\tau SHI_{it}) + \Delta\varepsilon_{it},$$

$$\tag{11}$$

which can be estimated by pooled OLS. In this model, the impact of SHI
varies over time, but one can estimate the average impact of SHI over time:

$$MEAN \ SHI \ IMPACT = \hat{\delta} + \sum_{\tau=2}^{T} \hat{\varphi}_\tau / T - 1. \tag{12}$$

The PTA assumption in this model implies $k_s = k_n$. This can be tested indirectly by testing the nonlinear restriction:

$$\frac{\sum_t m_t(k_s - k_n)}{\sum_t m_t k_n} = \frac{(k_s - k_n)\sum_t m_t}{k_n \sum_t m_t} = \frac{\sum_{\tau=2}^{T} \varphi_\tau}{\sum_{\tau=2}^{T} \beta_\tau} = 0. \tag{13}$$

3.2. Testing for and Dealing with Reverse Causality

Although our DID, RT, and DT models all allow for some correlation between SHI and the original error term e_{it}, they entail specific assumptions that may not adequately capture the endogeneity of SHI. An informal yet intuitive test of reverse causality based on that proposed by Gruber and Hanratty (1995) in a similar modeling exercise is to include in each of our three models a lead dummy variable indicating whether SHI will be adopted the following year. If causality goes from SHI to the outcome variable, the coefficient on the lead dummy will be zero. A nonzero coefficient would point toward causality running the other way or some other type of endogeneity that cannot be captured by the model in question.

For outcomes where none of the DID models mentioned earlier is able to address the endogeneity of SHI_{it}, we resort to IV. Suppose we have a set of instruments Z_{it}. If the Z_{it} are weakly exogenous or predetermined, that is, $E[Z_{is}\, e_{it}] = 0$, $s < t$, $t = 1, \ldots T$, with T representing the number of time periods in the data, it is possible to use lags of the potentially endogenous SHI variable as instruments, in addition to "traditional" instruments obtained outside the model (Anderson & Hsiao, 1981). If these instruments are valid (i.e., exogenous and strong in the sense of being highly correlated with our instrumented SHI dummy – assumptions that can be tested), they should control for any kind of endogeneity *including that arising from country-specific effects and trends*. Eq. (1) can then be consistently estimated by two-stage least squares (IV-2SLS) or using the more efficient two-step generalized method-of-moments (IV-GMM) estimator (cf., e.g., Cameron & Trivedi, 2005).[10]

We use as instruments for SHI_{it} the first lag of the SHI dummy ($SHI_{i,t-1}$) and an indicator for whether the country in question had a SHI system before the communist takeover in the mid-late-1940s. Although under weak exogeneity we could theoretically use more lags of the SHI variable as instruments, we include only its first lag in the instrument set due to the lack of variation over time in our SHI dummy,[11] leading to the redundancy of additional lags and loss of degrees of freedom for overidentifying restrictions tests. The rationale for using the pre-communist presence of SHI arrangements as an instrument is that the tradition of health systems based on the Bismarck model in some ECA countries before communism may have increased the likelihood of SHI re-adoption in these countries after the transition to market economies, but that pre-communist characteristics could reasonably be thought to be uncorrelated with our labor outcomes (measured about 45 years later) except by affecting the probability of SHI adoption.[12] The relevance of our two instruments is assessed through lagrange multiplier (LM) and Wald versions of under-identification and weak identification tests based on the rk statistic recently proposed by Kleibergen and Paap (2006), which account for non-iid structures of the error terms in the estimated equations. Cluster-robust versions of Hansen's J-statistic tests are used to check the exogeneity of the instruments in the estimated models.

4. DATA

We use annual data on SHI status and labor market outcomes for the 28 ECA countries, from 1990 to 2004.[13] Our dataset has been constructed using a variety of sources; the description in this section begins with our independent variable of interest, SHI status, and then continues for our other variables.[14]

4.1. Social Health Insurance Status

We define our SHI dummy SHI_{it} as taking a value of 1 if in country i at time t earmarked payroll taxes for health care were collected from formal sector workers and there was a SHI agency in place.[15] Our strict definition means that we end up classifying as non-SHI some country – year combinations that are often – we believe, erroneously – classified as SHI (such as Latvia and Poland). Furthermore, we classify Romania as SHI only after 1998; despite the fact that payroll taxes were used somewhat before then, it was not until 1998 that SHI was fully set up with a SHI agency and with payroll contributions making up the majority of health care revenues. Our SHI status dummy is equal to 1 in about half (218 observations) of the 442 country – year combinations for which we have non-missing values of the indicator.

4.2. Outcome Variables

Our dependent variables include gross wages, employment, unemployment, registered unemployment, self-employment, informality and FDI.

Total annual gross wages and salaries in local currency units were drawn from the World Bank's World Development Indicators (WDI) ECA regional database and transformed into yearly constant purchasing power parity (PPP) averages for the employed population aged 15–59 years using PPP conversion factors and the US deflator, both available at the WDI database as well. Employment-to-population ratios for individuals aged 15–59 years were obtained from the TransMONEE 2006 Database. We use annual data on total unemployment and registered unemployment rates obtained from the Key Indicators of the Labor Market database, published by the International Labor Organization (ILO). The same database is used for gathering data on agricultural employment and self-employment as shares of total employment; these work categories serve as proxies for informal employment, as they have been argued to be closely associated with last resort, low-productivity jobs in the region, thus masking a situation of worsening underemployment and predominant subsistence farming (Svejnar, 1999; Alam et al., 2005).

Data on informal employment or the size of the informal economy are not readily available for transition countries. Although there are rough estimates provided by ILO and some national statistical offices, their reliability and comparability across countries is not guaranteed and they are available for only a few countries in our sample. However, there have been some attempts in the literature to estimate at least the size of the informal economy using indirect approaches, focusing on various macroeconomic and institutional indicators that are argued to be linked with the evolution of the informal sector. We follow the approach proposed by Kaufmann and Kaliberda (1996) and Johnson, Kaufmann, and Shleifer (1997) and measure the size of the informal economy by comparing official measures of annual gross domestic product (GDP) growth with total electricity consumption growth. The basic assumption is that electricity consumption is closely related to overall economic activity, with a short-run electricity-to-GDP usually close to 1; hence, the annual growth in electricity consumption represents a good proxy for the total (formal plus informal) GDP growth in a given year. If this is the case, rough estimates of the informal GDP can be obtained simply by calculating the difference between the estimated total GDP and the official GDP measure. This simple calculation method avoids important endogeneity problems likely to be found in estimates coming from modeling approaches that derive the size of the informal economy from economic and institutional variables.

The method is not free from criticisms, of course. The assumption of unitary electricity-GDP elasticity has been criticized mainly on the grounds that (i) technical progress over time has made electricity use more efficient than in the past, (ii) higher electricity prices reduce electricity consumption per unit of output, and (iii) many informal activities are not electricity-intensive, such as in the services sector. For these reasons, we also follow Kaufmann and Kaliberda and Johnson et al. and depart from the unitary elasticity assumption, considering three different groups of transition countries identified in previous related research: "energy-efficient" economies (Central and Eastern European countries) that are assumed to have an electricity-GDP elasticity of 0.9 with a growing economy; "energy-neutral economies" (the Baltic countries), assumed to have unitary elasticity; and "energy-inefficient" economies (the rest of the former Soviet republics), assumed to have an elasticity of 1.15 when GDP is growing. We use WDI data on electricity output and official GDP for 17 ECA countries to obtain annual estimates of the size of the informal economy as a share of the total (formal plus informal) GDP for the period 1990–2003. As baseline data, we use the same values as Johnson et al. (1997) for the initial (i.e., 1989) shares of the informal sector in those countries.

Our final outcome variable is FDI, defined in terms of net inflows as a percentage of GDP. The data are taken from the World Bank's WDI database. FDI is defined there as "net inflows of investment to acquire a lasting management interest (10 percent or more of voting stock) in an enterprise operating in an economy other than that of the investor. It is the sum of equity capital, reinvestment of earnings, other long-term capital, and short-term capital as shown in the balance of payments."

Descriptive statistics are summarized in Table 1, which summarizes the averages across the period as a whole and across all countries. Also shown are the averages for the countries and years when SHI was being used to finance health care and the averages for the countries and years when general revenues were being used. In our sample, average gross wages tended to be higher in SHI countries than in non-SHI countries; Armenia and Tajikistan exhibited the lowest averages in 2004 (less than US$150 PPP) while Croatia and Lithuania presented the highest averages in the same year (more than US$2,500 PPP). Average total unemployment rates seem to have been very similar for SHI and non-SHI countries, with Hungary and Slovenia presenting rates around 6% in 2004, and Macedonia and Poland reaching at least 19% in the same year. Registered unemployment rates and

Table 1. Labor Market Outcome Variables: Descriptive Statistics.

	Full Sample			SHI = 1			SHI = 0		
	Mean	SD	Obs	Mean	SD	Obs	Mean	SD	Obs
Gross wage	1115.49	876.72	257	1555.22	921.52	119	736.31	626.16	138
Employment as % population	67.31	9.00	360	64.54	9.12	158	69.47	8.30	202
Unemployment	11.68	5.91	229	11.66	6.16	162	11.73	5.29	67
Registered unemployment	9.27	8.26	295	12.98	9.11	141	5.87	5.56	154
Self-employment	17.24	9.26	190	16.13	8.85	132	19.77	9.73	58
Employment in agriculture	25.26	16.64	268	23.07	18.93	162	28.61	11.64	106
Informal economy	27.66	16.22	203	26.03	15.52	84	28.81	16.66	119
FDI	5.13	20.18	357	3.66	3.15	181	6.65	28.52	176

Note: Mean, standard deviation (SD), and number of observations (Obs) for the full sample and for the sub-samples of observations with the SHI dummy equals to one (SHI = 1) and zero (SHI = 0).

employment-to-population ratios for individuals aged 15–59 years indicate a somewhat worse employment situation for SHI adopters in such period. Self-employment, agricultural employment, and the estimated size of the informal economy were lower on average for SHI countries over the study period: the estimates of the share of the informal GDP for the Czech Republic and Slovakia were lower than 17% in 2003, in contrast to estimates higher than 35% for Azerbaijan, Georgia, and Ukraine in that year. Finally, FDI was a good deal lower, on average, in SHI countries.

4.3. Covariates in the Estimating Equation

Although evidence on the determinants of SHI adoption is scarce, it has been indicated that SHI schemes emerged first in countries with higher initial (i.e., pre-transition) per capita income levels, whilst tax-based funding prevailed in countries with lower initial per capita income (Preker, Jakab, & Schneider, 2002). This positive correlation between income levels and SHI status is also present in our data; thus, we include GDP per capita – measured in constant 2000 dollars adjusted for PPP – in our X_{it} vector. This is, in fact, the only variable we include among the X_{it}; our specification is thus similar to that of Gruber and Hanratty (1995) in their study of the employment and wage effects of the introduction of tax-financed health insurance in Canada.

5. RESULTS

We begin this section with the results of our specification tests and then present the estimates of the models.

5.1. Specification Tests

Table 2 reports the results of our PTA tests for our RT and DT models, that is, Eqs. (7) and (11). The PTA is not rejected in any of the RT models, but is rejected in two of the DT models at the 1% level, namely, for unemployment and FDI, and is rejected at the 12% level for self-employment. To be on the safe side, we focus on the DT model results for these three outcomes.

Table 3 reports the results of our reverse causality tests. For the unemployment, self-employment, and FDI variables, the relevant test statistic is that for the DT model; for the others, the relevant statistic is for the DID model. The only two outcomes where the preferred generalized DID model does not appear to account adequately for the potential endogeneity of SHI are the share of the population in employment and the informality variable. For outcomes other than these two, we use either the basic DID model or the DT model, depending on the PTA test results in Table 2.

For the employment–population share and the informality variable, we employ IV. Table 4 summarizes the relevant IV diagnostic test statistics for these two outcomes; all lend support to our IV specification. The two

Table 2. Tests of the Parallel Trend Assumption.

Dependent Variable	Random Trend Model Generalized Hausman Test on Eq. (7)		Differential Trend Model Non-linear Restriction Test on Eq. (13)	
	Chi-square	p-value	F	p-value
Gross wage	1.84	0.175	0.01	0.929
Employment as % population	0.00	0.988	0.08	0.779
Unemployment	1.19	0.276	57.34*	0.000*
Registered unemployment	0.11	0.746	0.01	0.915
Self-employment	0.39	0.530	2.77*	0.114*
Employment in agriculture	0.89	0.345	0.01	0.933
Informal economy	0.37	0.544	0.20	0.665
FDI	0.05	0.821	24.65*	0.000*

*$p < 0.1$

Table 3. Tests of Reverse Causality.

Dependent Variable	DID Model Lead SHI Dummy Test on Eq. (4)		Random Trend Model Lead SHI Dummy Test on Eq. (7)		Differential Trend Model Lead SHI Dummy Test on Eq. (10)	
	Coefficient	p-value	Coefficient	p-value	Coefficient	p-value
Gross wage	−0.038	0.772	0.005	0.973	−0.022	0.859
Employment as % population	0.029*	0.019*	0.032*	0.018*	0.024*	0.039*
Unemployment	0.093	0.404	0.071	0.463	0.031	0.776
Registered unemployment	0.202	0.154	0.236*	0.044*	0.208	0.139
Self-employment	0.172	0.250	0.140	0.150	0.083	0.607
Employment in agriculture	−0.002	0.925	−0.002	0.931	−0.007	0.768
Informal economy	0.282*	0.098*	0.283*	0.078*	0.267	0.195
FDI	−0.399	0.569	0.108	0.914	−1.184	0.369

*$p < 0.1$

Table 4. Estimates of SHI Effects on Labor Outcomes.

	Preferred Model	Coefficient	p-Value	Kleibergen–Paap LM Tests H_0: Under-Identified	Kleibergen–Paap Wald tests H_0: Weakly Identified	Hansen J-tests H_0: Over-Identified
Gross wage	DID	0.199*	0.02*			
Employment as % population	IV	−0.097*	0.09	0.000*	435.32*	0.436
Unemployment	DT	−0.008	0.91			
Registered unemployment	DID	0.182	0.37			
Self-employment	DT	0.173*	0.02*			
Employment in agriculture	DID	−0.021	0.22			
Informal economy	IV	−0.168	0.61	0.006*	236.17*	0.577
FDI	DT	−0.154	0.95			

Notes: In all models except FDI, the natural logarithm of the dependent variable is used. The reported IV point estimates are from 2SLS estimation, where the excluded instruments are the first lag of the SHI dummy and an indicator for whether SHI existed in the country before communism. p-Values are reported for the Kleibergen–Paap LM and Hansen tests, whereas the values reported for the Kleibergen–Paap Wald tests of weak identification correspond to the estimated rk Wald F statistics; in our case, the critical value for the weak identification tests (tabulated by Stock & Yogo, 2002, 10% maximal IV size) is 19.93. In the last column, the joint null hypothesis of the over-identification tests is that the instruments are uncorrelated with the error term and that the excluded instruments are correctly excluded from the main equation. *$p < 0.1$

instruments are highly relevant in both models, with high partial F statistics (not shown in Table 4). Kleibergen–Paap LM and Wald tests strongly reject the null hypotheses of model under-identification and weak instruments, respectively (Stock & Yogo, 2002). The Hansen tests for overidentifying restrictions are consistent with our excluded instruments being exogenous.

5.2. Estimates of SHI Impacts

Table 4 reports the coefficient estimates (and associated p-value for the null hypothesis of a zero SHI impact) for our preferred model.[16] Our preferred model points to SHI significantly increasing average (gross) wages and salaries by 20% and significantly reducing employment (as a share of the population) by 10%. However, we find no significant effect of SHI on unemployment, whether self-reported unemployment in the labor-force survey or registered unemployment; the coefficient on registered unemployment (which is closer to being significant) is, however, the expected sign. Our preferred model points to SHI significantly increasing self-employment by 17%. By contrast, we find no significant effects of SHI on either agricultural employment or the indicator of informality; moreover, both coefficients are the "wrong" sign. Finally, while the coefficient on FDI has the hypothesized negative sign, it is nowhere near being statistically significant.[17]

6. SUMMARY AND DISCUSSION

The transition that occurred during the 1990s in many of the central and eastern ECA countries from financing health care through general revenues to a SHI system provides a unique opportunity to test hypotheses about SHI on labor market outcomes. We use panel data from the 28 ECA countries for the period 1990–2004. We employ both regression-based generalizations of DID and IV to estimate the effects of SHI (versus general revenues) on various labor market outcomes. We find that, compared to tax-funded systems and controlling for GDP per capita, SHI increases (gross) wages by 20%, reduces employment (as a share of the population) by 10%, and increases self-employment by 17%. In contrast, we find no significant effects of SHI on unemployment (both registered and self-reported), agricultural employment, a widely used measure of the size of the informal economy, or FDI.

Our results thus lend some support to the view that SHI has a negative effect on employment. They also provide some evidence – albeit less clear-cut – that SHI encourages informalization of the economy: our results on self-employment are consistent with this view, although our results on agricultural employment and the informal economy measure are not. Our results do not lend support to the view that SHI diminishes a country's international competitiveness as measured by a reduction of FDI.

How plausible are our results? A skeptic might claim that we have omitted variables other than GDP that influence labor market outcomes and that are correlated with SHI status. These might include dummy variables capturing the timing of other reforms, as well as dummy variables capturing key events in the region and in specific countries in it. Doubtless, there are other important determinants of our labor market outcome variables than GDP per capita. Just to give one example, we know that FDI decisions in a subset of the ECA countries are influenced not just by whether firms have to pay social security contributions (which, in effect, we are capturing through our SHI dummy) but also by labor costs more generally, labor productivity, and corporate income taxes (cf. Bellak et al., 2008). The relevant question, though, is whether the variables we have omitted are correlated with SHI status. It is certainly possible. Whether *changes* in these variables are also correlated with *changes* in SHI status is less clear. Some obvious candidates do not appear to be. For example, as far as we can establish, reforms to unemployment benefits did not occur in the year when countries switched from general revenues to SHI.

Suppose, though, for the sake of argument, that omitted variables are correlated with SHI status and with outcomes, either in levels or differences. A least squares regression of Eq. (1) in levels or first differences would, in such circumstances, produce a biased estimate of δ, our parameter of interest. But this is why we do not estimate Eq. (1) in levels or first differences, but rather employ a variety of models that allow for a correlation between the error term and the SHI status. These include generalized DID models and where these seem to allow inadequately for such a correlation, IV; we check that our IV models pass the relevant identification tests. We therefore believe that our estimates of the impact of SHI are robust to the exclusion of variables other than GDP and represent reliable parameter estimates for the causal effect of SHI adoption on our labor market outcomes.

The textbook analysis of the imposition of a payroll tax, which predicts an increase in the gross wage accompanying the fall in the employment level, is thus supported by our data. Higher gross wages are consistent with the fact that, in the SHI countries of the ECA region, usually both the employee and the employer have been legally required to pay SHI contributions since the switch from tax financing (with employers normally required to pay higher percentages than employees). It is likely, then, that the introduction of a SHI system has created a wedge between gross and net wages in the countries of the region – or, at least, increased this gap relatively to the situation under general tax financing – which has been responsible for the estimated disemployment effect. Yet, due to lack of data, we are unable to further investigate the effect of SHI adoption on *net* wages and therefore the remaining incidence characteristics of the payroll tax.

The mixed evidence we find on the impacts of SHI adoption on informal employment reflect the limits imposed on our analysis by the available data. Although we employ the best available proxies, neither agricultural employment nor self-employment rates are perfect substitutes for the actual share of informal employment in the economy; moreover, our measure of the size of the informal economy is not free from criticism, as we have discussed earlier. As a consequence, it is possible that we are not capturing the actual extent to which workers have moved into informal job arrangements after SHI adoption, despite the lack of estimated effects on our indicators of agricultural employment and the size of the informal economy. By the same token, the sizeable positive impact we find on self-employment rates after SHI introduction is worrying in that it may indicate a situation where firms have started to offer informal job contracts to many workers to minimize or avoid the payment of payroll taxes by both parties, thus eroding the government's tax base. And even if the measured increase in self-employment after SHI implementation does reflect a jump in the number of "truly" self-employed individuals (as an alternative to the more difficult task of finding a formal job in a labor market under strain), tax evasion is still likely to have become more of a problem in those countries in view of the typically more challenging conditions for enforcing the payment of SHI contributions among the self-employed. This negative feature adds, of course, to the higher likelihood of workers falling through the unemployment safety net in countries with a higher relative prevalence of self-employment and informality.

The generalization of our results for other countries is not automatically warranted, of course. We do not claim that our results imply that SHI adoption everywhere must necessarily reduce employment and increase self-employment. The latter pair of results could differ in other countries if SHI is introduced along with other institutional reforms (e.g., unemployment benefits, corporate tax, or pensions reforms) able to stimulate the demand

and supply of labor. Nonetheless, the largely negative employment results in this chapter ought to serve as a warning to those contemplating shifting the financing of health care from general revenues to a SHI system.

NOTES

1. Two quite recent conferences focused on SHI in developing and transition economies, one in Berlin in November 2005 and the other in Manila in October 2006. Details are to be found in the website http://www.shi-conference.de/.
2. Examples include Vietnam (1993), Nigeria (1997), Tanzania (2001), and Ghana (2005). Discussions are under way in South Africa, Zimbabwe, Cambodia, and Laos. Malaysia also recently began debating a shift to SHI.
3. Examples include Colombia, Mexico, the Philippines, and Vietnam.
4. France widened the tax base from earnings to include nonwage income, Germany has decided that from 2009 onward, it will reduce the emphasis on payroll taxes, while the Netherlands introduced a reform in 2005 where insurers receive only half their income from payroll revenues (albeit channeled through a central fund), the rest coming from flat rate direct contributions from members (with offsetting income supplements for low-income groups). For further details, refer, for example, Gottret and Schieber (2006) and the Health Policy Monitor website http://www.hpm.org/en/index.html. In addition to these changes, it is worth noting that both Iceland and Spain shifted wholesale from SHI to tax finance in the late 1980s.
5. Six "old" OECD countries abandoned SHI in the 1970s and 1980s, notably Denmark, Greece, Iceland, Italy, Portugal, and Spain.
6. The countries treated in this chapter as being located in central and eastern ECA (the countries in the World Bank's ECA region) are Albania, Armenia, Azerbaijan, Belarus, Bosnia and Herzegovina, Bulgaria, Croatia, Czech Republic, Estonia, Georgia, Hungary, Kazakhstan, Kyrgyz Republic, Latvia, Lithuania, Macedonia FYR, Moldova, Poland, Romania, Russian Federation, Serbia and Montenegro, Slovak Republic, Slovenia, Tajikistan, Turkey, Turkmenistan, Ukraine, and Uzbekistan.
7. This section draws heavily on Langenbrunner, Sheiman, and Kehler (2008) and the Health Systems in Transition (HiT) series, downloadable from http://www.euro.who.int/observatory/Hits/TopPage.
8. This subsection draws heavily on Wagstaff and Moreno-Serra (2009), which provides a more detailed description of the DID models used.
9. Standard errors need to be adjusted for clustering at the country level to allow for serial correlation (cf. Bertrand, Duflo, & Mullainathan, 2004; Cameron & Trivedi, 2005, p.705).
10. In other words, for our IV estimations with lagged instruments, SHI_{it} is required to be weakly exogenous aside from being contemporaneously correlated with the error term in Eq. (1). This is analogous to the approach used by Ziliak (1997) in his labor supply analysis, except that we do not assume a priori the presence of a fixed effect in our original Eq. (1), and therefore, our IV models are estimated in levels. We formally test for the plausibility of the weak exogeneity assumption in the

context of our models as we describe in the text; if the instruments are found to be exogenous and strongly correlated with SHI status according to the appropriate statistical tests, we can argue with more confidence that such instruments affect outcomes in the current period only indirectly through their effect on current SHI status, not directly. Since we are not primarily interested in the estimated coefficients of the remaining regressors used in the models, these are considered weakly exogenous in the sense above and also contemporaneously uncorrelated with the error term, being instrumented by themselves in the IV regressions.

11. Transitions between tax-funded health and SHI systems occur only once (if at all) in all but one of the countries in our sample, the only exception being Kazakhstan.

12. The countries that had a Bismarckian model before communism in our sample are Bosnia and Herzegovina, Bulgaria, Croatia, Czech Republic, Estonia, Hungary, Latvia, Lithuania, Moldova, Poland, Romania, Russian Federation, Serbia and Montenegro, Slovak Republic, Slovenia, and Ukraine. Of these, four countries – namely, Latvia, Moldova, Poland, and Ukraine – did not adopt a SHI system during 1990–2004 according to the definition used in this chapter (see Section 4.1). Moreover, six countries that did not have a Bismarckian health system before 1945 (Albania, Georgia, Kazakhstan, Kyrgyz Republic, Macedonia, and Turkey) had a SHI system in place at some point between 1990 and 2004. The historical information on health systems in the ECA region comes from the World Health Organization's *Health Systems in Transition* series.

13. In the case of Bosnia-Herzegovina, the period between 1992 and 1996 has been excluded from the analysis due to the lack of data for some variables and the complete disorganization of the health system – which obviously included the SHI scheme – during the war period.

14. For more information on our variables and data sources, refer Wagstaff and Moreno-Serra (2007).

15. Our classification is consistent with that of Langenbrunner et al. (2008). For more information, refer Wagstaff and Moreno-Serra (2007).

16. The models are estimated using the natural logarithm of the dependent variable, except in the case of FDI (which can be negative).

17. The reported IV point estimates are those from the (simpler) 2SLS estimations. We have also estimated the same models using a more efficient two-step GMM procedure; although the estimated standard errors are usually slightly smaller for the latter method, the estimated GMM coefficients (not shown) are remarkably similar to the reported 2SLS ones.

ACKNOWLEDGMENTS

Our thanks to the World Bank's Research Support Budget for financial support; Armin Fidler, Ana Djordjevic, Peyvand Khaleghian, Jack Langenbrunner, Silvia Mauri, and Pia Schneider for information on social health insurance transitions in Europe and Central Asia; and the participants of seminars at Erasmus University, the Nordic Health

Economists Study Group, the University of Oxford, the University of York, and the World Bank for helpful suggestions and comments on earlier versions of this chapter.

REFERENCES

Alam, A., Murthi, M., Yemtsov, R., Murrugarra, E., Dudwick, N., Hamilton, E., & Tiongson, E. (2005). *Growth, poverty, and inequality: Eastern Europe and the former Soviet Union.* Washington, DC: World Bank.

Anderson, T. W., & Hsiao, C. (1981). Estimation of dynamic models with error components. *Journal of American Statistical Association, 76,* 598–606.

Baeza, C., & Packard, T. (2006). *Beyond survival: Protecting households from health shocks in Latin America.* Washington, DC: World Bank.

Bauer, T., & Riphahn, R. T. (2002). Employment effects of payroll taxes – An empirical test for Germany. *Applied Economics, 34*(7), 865–876.

Belev, B. (Ed.) (2003). *The informal economy in the EU accession countries: Size, scope, trends and challenges o the process of EU enlargement.* Sofia: Center for the Study of Democracy.

Bell, B., Blundell, R., & Reenen, J. (1999). Getting the unemployed back to work: The role of targeted wage subsidies. *International Tax and Public Finance, 6*(3), 339–360.

Bellak, C., Leibrecht, M., & Riedl, A. (2008). Labour costs and FDI flows into Central and Eastern European countries: A survey of the literature and empirical evidence. *Structural Change and Economic Dynamics, 19*(1), 17–37.

Bertrand, M., Duflo, E., & Mullainathan, S. (2004). How much should we trust differences-in-differences estimates? *Quarterly Journal of Economics, 119*(1), 249–275.

Cameron, A., & Trivedi, R. (2005). *Microeconometrics: Methods and applications.* Cambridge, MA: Cambridge University Press.

Datta, S. (2006). Is Germany gearing up for health care reform? Available at http://www.frost.com/prod/servlet/cif-econ-insight.pag?docid = 77082735. Retrieved on 10/31/06.

Gottret, P. E., & Schieber, G. (2006). *Health financing revisited: A practitioner's guide.* Washington, DC: World Bank.

Gruber, J., & Hanratty, M. (1995). The labor-market effects of introducing national health insurance: Evidence from Canada. *Journal of Business and Economic Statistics, 13*(2), 163–173.

Johnson, S., Kaufmann, D., & Shleifer, A. (1997). The unofficial economy in transition. *Brookings Papers on Economic Activity, 2,* 159–221.

Kaufmann, D., & Kaliberda, A. (1996). Integrating the unofficial economy into the dynamics of post-socialist economies: A framework of analysis and evidence. In: B. Kaminsky (Ed.), *Economic transition in the newly independent states.* New York: ME Sharpe Press.

Kleibergen, F., & Paap, R. (2006). Generalized reduced rank tests using the singular value decomposition. *Journal of Econometrics, 133*(1), 97–126.

Kugler, A., & Kugler, M. (2003). *The labour market effects of payroll taxes in a middle-income country: Evidence from Colombia* (CEPR Discussion Paper 4046). London: C.E.P.R.

Langenbrunner, J. C., Sheiman, I. M., & Kehler, J. C. (2008). Sources of health financing and revenue collection: Reforms, lessons, and challenges. In: J. Kutzin, et al. (Eds), *Lessons of health reforms in Eastern Europe and Central Asia*. Brussels: European Observatory.

Levy, S. (2007). Pueden los programas sociales disminuir la productividad y el crecimiento economico? Una hipotesis para Mexico. (With English summary). *El Trimestre Economico, 74*(3), 491–540.

Nickell, S. (1997). Unemployment and labor market rigidities: Europe versus North America. *Journal of Economic Perspectives, 11*(3), 55–74.

Nickell, S. (2004). *Employment and taxes, centre for economic performance*. CEP Discussion Papers. London School of Economics, Centre for Economic Performance, Paper No. CEPDP0634, May 2004.

Nickell, S., Nunziata, L., & Ochel, W. (2005). Unemployment in the OECD since the 1960s: What do we know? *Economic Journal, 115*(500), 1–27.

OECD. (1999). *The OECD jobs strategy implementing the OECD jobs strategy: Assessing performance and policy*. Paris: OECD.

Preker, A., Jakab, M., & Schneider, M. (2002). Health financing reforms in central and Eastern Europe and the former Soviet Union. In: A. D. E. Mossialos, J. Figueras & J. Kutzin (Eds), *Funding health care: Options for Europe*. Buckingham: Open University Press.

Schmidt, U. (2006). *Health policy and health economics in Germany* (Speech). Washington, DC: Friedrich Ebert Foundation.

Stock, J. H., & M. Yogo (2002). *Testing for weak instruments in linear IV regression*. NBER, Technical Working Paper # T 0284. National Bureau of Economic Research, Cambridge, MA.

Summers, L. H. (1989). Some simple economics of mandated benefits. *American Economic Review, 79*(2), 177–183.

Svejnar, J. (1999). Labor markets in the transitional Central and East European economies. In: O. Ashenfelter & D. Card (Eds), *Handbook of labor economics, Vol. 3*. Amsterdam: Elsevier.

Wagstaff, A., & Moreno-Serra, R. (2007). *Europe and Central Asia's great post-communist social health insurance experiment: Impacts on health sector and labor market outcomes*. Policy Research Working Paper #4371. World Bank, Washington, DC.

Wagstaff, A., & Moreno-Serra, R. (2009). Europe and Central Asia's great post-communist social health insurance experiment: Impacts on health sector outcomes. *Journal of Health Economics, 28*(2), 322–340.

Wooldridge, J. M. (2002). *Econometric analysis of cross section and panel data*. Cambridge, MA: MIT Press.

Zilak, J. P. (1997). Efficient estimation with panel data when instruments are predetermined: An empirical comparison of moment-condition estimators. *Journal of Business and Economic Statistics, 15*(4), 419–431.

TRUST IN THE CONTEXT OF COMMUNITY-BASED HEALTH INSURANCE SCHEMES IN CAMBODIA: VILLAGERS' TRUST IN HEALTH INSURERS

Sachiko Ozawa and Damian G. Walker

ABSTRACT

Objective – *To understand the role and influence of villagers' trust for the health insurer on enrollment in a community-based health insurance (CBHI) scheme in Cambodia.*

Methodology/approach – *This study was conducted in northwest Cambodia where a CBHI scheme operates with the highest enrollment rates in the country. A mixed method approach was employed to gauge how individuals in the community trust the health insurer, and whether this plays a role in their decisions to enroll in CBHI schemes. Focus groups and household surveys were carried out to identify and measure trust levels, and to explore the association between insurer trust and enrollment in CBHI schemes.*

Findings – *Although villagers generally trusted the health insurance organization, villagers with poor experiences with other organizations in*

Innovations in Health System Finance in Developing and Transitional Economies
Advances in Health Economics and Health Services Research, Volume 21, 107–132
Copyright © 2009 by Emerald Group Publishing Limited
ISSN: 0731-2199/doi:10.1108/S0731-2199(2009)0000021008

the past were less willing to trust the insurer. Insurer trust represented a combination of interpersonal and impersonal trust. After controlling for demographic factors, health care utilization, and household socio-economic status, insurer trust levels for villagers who newly enrolled (RRR = 1.07, p<0.001) and renewed insurance (RRR = 1.15, p<0.001) were significantly higher than those who never enrolled in CBHI schemes.

Implications for policy – *This study illustrates the relationship between CBHI enrollment and villagers' trust for the health insurer in a low-income, post-conflict country. It highlights the need for staff of health insurance organizations to place greater emphasis on building trusting interpersonal relationships with villagers. Understanding the nature of trust for the health insurer is essential to improve health insurance enroll-ment and protect people in poor rural communities against the impact of health-related shocks.*

1. INTRODUCTION

Cambodia is a small, poor, and sparsely populated country between Vietnam and Thailand, making a slow recovery from a long history of conflict. With a quarter of the population killed by execution, starvation, and disease in the Khmer Rouge era (1975–1979) and in the war with Vietnam (1979–1991), reconstruction efforts only began in the past 15 years. Against this backdrop, a number of health financing initiatives have been initiated in Cambodia. These include official user fees with exemp-tions for the poor, contracting of government health service delivery to non-government providers, health equity funds to remove financial barriers to access for the poor, and community-based health insurance (CBHI) schemes (Ekman, 2004; Hardeman et al., 2004; Jacobs, Price, & Sam, 2007; Schwartz & Bhushan, 2005; Van Damme, Van Leemput, Por, Hardeman, & Meessen, 2004).

   Lack of financial protection is one of the main barriers to accessing health care in Cambodia (Annear, Wilkinson, Chean, & Van Pelt, 2006). Households frequently choose not to access health care because it results in catastrophic health expenditure that prevents households from obtaining basic necessities such as food, education, and shelter (WHO, 2000). For example, health care expenditures represent 22 percent of household income in Cambodia, which is one of the highest in the world (GRET, 2005). The economic burden can be so large that according to one study, 46 percent of households that lost their land in Cambodia in 2000 reported selling it to pay for health care (Biddulph, 2000).

CBHI schemes, also known as health insurance for the informal sector or microinsurance, are "voluntary health insurance schemes organized at the level of the community" (Carrin, Waelkens, & Criel, 2005). As Cambodia does not have any formal social security schemes run by the government, CBHI schemes are the only insurance schemes operating in the country. The first CBHI scheme in Cambodia started in 1998 (MOH, 2007). The longest standing scheme is called the SKY Health Insurance scheme operated by a French non-governmental organization (NGO), Groupe de Recherche et d'Échanges Technologiques (GRET). This scheme has had the greatest geographical reach, operating in multiple operational districts. However, the enrollment rate for this scheme remains to be low at 5–10 percent (GRET, 2005). Increasing enrollment in CBHI schemes has been one of the key challenges to finance the Cambodian health system.

The CBHI scheme with the highest enrollment rate to date is operated by a local Cambodian NGO called the Cambodian Association for Assistance to Families and Widows (CAAFW). This scheme started in February 2005 in Thmar Pouk operational district of Banteay Meanchey province. This province is located in northwest Cambodia near the border with Thailand, an area which used to be a stronghold of the Khmer Rouge. Table 1 presents the key health indicators in Banteay Meanchey province as compared to the national average in Cambodia.

As a community-led initiative to provide financial protection for health care, CAAFW initiated the CBHI scheme by building on its reputation as a

Table 1. Key Indicators for Cambodia vs. Banteay Meanchey Province.

	Cambodia	Banteay Meanchey Province
Population	14 Million	650,000
Area	$181,035 \, km^2$	$6,679 \, km^2$
Number of Villages	13,505 villages	614 villages
Percentage of population living in urban areas	15.6%	17.2%
Infant mortality rate	66/1000 live births	76/1000 live births
Under 5 mortality rate	83/1000 live births	96/1000 live births
Percentage of illiterate adults	30.3% females	35.1% females

Source: Cambodia Demographic and Health Survey, 2005

microcredit organization. By the end of 2005, the CBHI scheme covered 25,000 insured individuals and 6,000 insured families, achieving an enrollment rate as high as 25–30 percent (CAAFW, 2007). Enrollment is family-based, with a premium of US$2.00 (8000 Riels as of 2008) per person per year and up to US$12.00 per family per year (Por & Hardeman, 2006). In most cases, insured families can go to any of the 10 health centers and two referral hospitals for no charge, as insurance covers almost all primary health care and hospital costs at public facilities with no user fees. This study hypothesized that one of the factors influencing households' decisions to enroll in CAAFW's CBHI scheme may be the level of trust people have for CAAFW as the insurance provider.

The main characteristic that distinguishes CBHI from national or social health insurance is that enrollment is voluntary, which gives credence to the hypothesis that trust for health insurers may matter when people decide whether to enroll in a CBHI scheme. Health insurance is based on the fundamental idea that there is a level of uncertainty about a future health outcome, and that this risk could be transferred to another party in advance. Prepayment is made to transfer this risk to the insurer, in exchange for an agreement that the insurer will reimburse the insured for covered losses in the future. Trust plays a critical role in this process, due to the nature of the uncertainty of this interaction. With a long history of deception and mistrust in Cambodia (Chandler, 2007; Dubois et al., 2004), trust may play a critical factor in the local demand for CBHI schemes.

Trust is defined as "the *optimistic* acceptance of a *vulnerable* situation in which the truster believes the trustee will *care* for the truster's interests" (Hall, Dugan, Zheng, & Mishra, 2001; italics in original). There are two main forms of trust: interpersonal and impersonal trust. Interpersonal trust is what we commonly think of as trust, where we trust in people we know. The established relationships between two individuals serve as the basis of interpersonal trust. The other form of trust is called impersonal trust, also known as institutional or organizational trust, where we trust in strangers, social systems or organizations. When interacting with strangers, there may be various forms of impersonal trust in effect, where we decide to trust strangers after receiving recommendations from close acquaintances, hearing of the stranger's reputation, or identifying shared norms with the stranger such as belonging to the same group or community (Gilson, 2003). Trust in strangers may also be rooted in institutions that lower the risks individuals face in trusting them, thereby allowing the development of delegated or fiduciary trust for the individual (Lane, 1998). Monitoring and disciplinary procedures embedded in many institutions make it possible for individuals to trust employees of organizations even when individuals have never had contact or share no relevant communal allegiance (Newman, 1998; Offe, 1999).

Recent work has begun to highlight the potential value of trust in understanding the performance of health care organizations and health systems (Gilson, 2003, 2006; Mechanic, 1998). Although various studies have examined trust in patient–provider relationships (Hall, Camacho, Dugan, & Balkrishnan, 2002; Kao, Green, Davis, Koplan, & Cleary, 1998; Thom & Stanford Trust Study Physicians, 2001), trust in patient–insurer relationships is only starting to be explored (Balkrishnan, Dugan, Camacho, & Hall, 2003; Jowett, 2003). The literature on how to measure trust in health care settings is also in its early years (Dugan, Trachtenberg, & Hall, 2005; Goold, Fessler, & Moyer, 2006; Goudge & Gilson, 2005; Zheng, Hall, Dugan, Kidd, & Levine, 2002). This study is the first to examine and measure trust for the health insurer in the context of a CBHI scheme and to assess whether trust for the health insurer appears to matter in people's decisions to enroll in CBHI schemes.

2. METHODOLOGY

This research employed a mixed method approach using both qualitative and quantitative research techniques. The study population included community members in Thmar Pouk operational district in Banteay Meanchey province above 18 years of age, without a health care provider or an employee of the health insurance organization in the family. These screening criteria were applied to capture insurer trust by a typical villager without occupational ties to health care.

Qualitative methods were first used to understand how villagers view and trust the health insurer. Focus group discussions were organized to learn about villagers' interactions with the health insurer as well as their thoughts and expectations about the insurance organization. The study also asked about villagers' knowledge and opinions about CBHI, as well as the social norms around the decision to enroll in CBHI schemes. A standard interview guide was used with various probes to stimulate discussion and elicit villagers' responses.

Focus groups were conducted among villagers who were currently, formerly or never enrolled in the CBHI scheme. These groups were selected based on the hypothesis that individuals who have, no longer have, or never had insurance have distinct experiences with CBHI schemes and different levels of trust for the insurer. A total of seven focus groups were formed: one group with mixed insurance status, and two groups each from the three enrollment groups. Focus groups were held in seven villages spread out across the district. A snowball sample was used to find individuals who fit the screening criteria. Each focus group consisted of between 7 and 13 individuals. Table 2 presents the characteristics of individuals who participated in the focus groups. Those who joined the focus groups tended to be females, married, in their 40s and 50s.

Table 2. Characteristics of Focus Group Participants.

	Number	Percentage
CBHI status		
Currently enrolled	27	36.5
Drop out	20	27.0
Never enrolled	27	36.5
Gender		
Male	9	12.2
Female	65	87.8
Age		
18–29	14	18.9
30–39	7	9.5
40–49	26	35.1
50–59	25	33.8
60+	2	2.7
Marital status		
Single	1	1.4
Married	63	85.1
Widowed	7	9.5
Separated or divorced	3	4.1
Education		
No formal schooling	42	56.8
Primary incomplete	27	36.5
Primary complete	2	2.7
Secondary incomplete	3	4.1
Job/profession		
Farmer	60	81.1
Agricultural wage labor	7	9.5
Self-business	2	2.7
Housewife	5	6.8
Average number of children	2.34	–
Total	74	100.0%

All focus group discussions were tape recorded, transcribed, and translated. Transcripts from these focus groups were analyzed using the framework approach, an applied qualitative research method which evolved from grounded-theory (Pope, Ziebland, & Mays, 2000). Both inductive and deductive methods were used in the analysis, where pre-set aims and objectives were reflected on and themes were brought out of the data. The analysis involved line-by-line coding, writing of memos, indexing, charting, and mapping the data, as well as reflexivity by the researcher. A conceptual framework of insurer trust was developed to reflect the results. Analysis was conducted using the latest version of the Atlas.ti software.

Findings from focus group discussions were incorporated into questions measuring insurer trust in the subsequent questionnaire. Based on a literature review of existing constructs and measures of trust, a trust scale developed to measure patients' trust in health insurers in the United States (Zheng et al., 2002) was culturally adapted to fit the Cambodian context. A technique using qualitative research to inform survey development was applied (Nichter, Nichter, Thompson, Shiffman, & Moscicki, 2002), where words and phrases in the questionnaire were modified and new questions were added. Since meanings of trust are known to be highly context-dependent (Goudge & Gilson, 2005), this process ensured that the trust questions were locally appropriate, clear, and comprehensive.

Quantitative methods were then applied to measure insurer trust levels. A cluster random household survey was carried out with a 28-cluster, 20-persons per cluster sample ($n = 560$). Stratified sampling on insurance status ($n = 360$) was combined with population-proportional-to-size sampling ($n = 200$) to ensure both the statistical power and generalizability of findings. Stratified sampling allowed the sample to have a relatively even representation of four insurance status groups: renew, new, drop out, and never. Households who have had CBHI for more than one year and were enrolled at the time of the survey were classified as "renew," whereas households who joined CBHI for the first time in the past 12 months were categorized as "new." Households who used to have CBHI but were not enrolled at the time of the survey were classified as "drop out," whereas those who had never had CBHI were grouped as "never." The questionnaire included insurer trust questions along with questions on background demographics, social factors, household assets, and health care utilization. Questions were translated, back-translated, and piloted prior to data collection.

Statistical analyses were conducted to develop an insurer trust scale and assess the relationship between people's trust for the insurer and their enrollment in CBHI schemes. Trust questions were measured using a five-point Likert scale, where responses ranged between: strongly agree, agree, neutral, disagree, strongly disagree, and don't know. Twenty-five individuals who responded "don't know" to all insurer trust questions who were demographically similar to the rest of the sample were removed from the analysis ($n = 535$). The "don't know" answers were converted to values on the trust scales using multiple imputations from a uniform distribution, resulting in conservative estimates. Factor analysis was used to uncover the underlying dimensions of the scale. The resulting trust scale was assessed for validity and reliability. Test–retest and inter-rater reliability of the 12-item trust scale was also assessed. Test–retest reliability was measured where respondents were asked the same questions by the same interviewers, 6 to 7 days apart. A combination of test–retest and inter-rater reliability was also captured where respondents were asked the same questions by different interviewers, 6 to 7 days apart. Multinomial logistic regression models were used to ascertain associations between the insurer trust scale and enrollment in CBHI schemes. Multivariate regression models controlled for demographic factors, health care utilization, as well as socio-economic status.

This study was approved by the Cambodia National Ethics Committee for Health Research (NECHR) as well as the ethics committee at the Johns Hopkins School of Public Health. Informed consent was sought from all study participants.

3. RESULTS

3.1. Qualitative Analysis

3.1.1. Trust for the Health Insurer
When focus group participants were asked about the organization managing the CBHI scheme, many villagers said they did not know much about the organization, even if they had health insurance. Most respondents were not able to name CAAFW, calling it "the organization," "health organization," "Mr. (promoter/founder's name) organization," or "widow organization." However, the image people had of the health insurance organization appeared to be positive: "I think the organization is good;" "[organization] staff have good reputation;" "reason for dropping out is not because of the staff." Villagers suggested that "staff are good and friendly," "staff say

good words to us" and that they were happy when the staff came to visit them at the referral hospital when they were sick.

The health insurance organization appeared to have earned some trust in the community: "what the organization told us is true;" "[I] believe in the organization because they encourage us to go to the hospital." Some tactics appeared to be particularly effective for the insurer to gain people's trust. Many villagers mentioned how the insurer told the truth about them not having to pay when they go to the health center: "the organization is good. We see with our own eyes that they pay everything for us;" "before we just followed what the organization said, but we see that we really don't need to pay when we go to the hospital." In addition, villagers spoke well of the insurer's timing to collect money: "the organization only takes money after they give the [CBHI] card to us;" "when the organization staff take a photograph, [they do] not yet take money;" "[we] joined because the organization staff gives [the CBHI] card before they collect money." Allowing people to owe money to the insurer was also an important factor in facilitating insurer trust and enrollment: "we can owe [the health insurer] some money after getting [the CBHI] card;" "if we can owe the organization, [we] can join." Some villagers noted that the ways in which the organization staff came to their village to explain about CBHI mattered: "staff came to give information before they took photograph;" "the organization contacted health center staff, commune chief, and village chief to inform people about health insurance."

In deciding whether to trust the insurance organization, villagers appeared to consider both their beliefs about the organization, as well as their personal interactions with organization staff. Many participants noted their belief in the organization as a whole, exhibiting impersonal trust: "the organization is good [because] it helps people;" "I trust the organization and want to take a photograph [and join CBHI] in order to protect my health, [because] one day I can be sick." However, interpersonal trust with organizational staff also appeared to matter in their decisions to trust the organization: "[The staff] talk to us softly and do not say any bad words;" "[The staff] are good [and] they call us Uncle, Brother ... and if we need to take a photograph we just call [them over] when we see them coming [to the village]."

Yet some villagers also revealed some misgivings about the health insurance organization: "[the organization] never asks us about our experience or relationship between us and the doctor. They just come and ask us to pay fees at the end of the year." Some respondents complained about the lack of visibility of the organization: "staff come only to take photo and collect money. They rarely come to the village;" "When there is no NGO staff to stand by [for us] at the hospital, [we feel that] they do not care about us." Other respondents noted how little knowledge they have about the organization: "we have no information about the organization;" "[We] want staff of organization to come to our village and explain clearly to villagers about the goal of the organization." Villagers who already have CBHI were worried that the insurance organization may stop offering CBHI: "We might pay more if [the organization] stop[s] [and] our [CBHI] cards cannot be used at the hospital. We would like the organization to continue [offering the CBHI scheme]." Villagers also revealed how some people were apprehensive about the service the insurer provides:

> "Some family did not join [CBHI] because they don't trust it. They think that they might not get sick, the [health insurance] organization might not care for them carefully when [they become] sick, and they might [have] to go [see] private [providers] again."

Most focus group participants were not worried that this particular health insurance organization might be dishonest: "[We are] not worried that the organization cheats, because we just pay them when they give us the card." However, trust in the insurer was especially poor in one village which had had a poor experience trusting another organization in the past:

> "[We] don't believe in organizations. Before, there was an organization that came, took a photo and asked for 50 Baht[1] (US$1.25) each but they cheated us. They said they will come again but never came back. All the villagers [in this village] gave him 50 Baht each. [We] do not know what they took the money for. We do not trust organizations because of this cheating."

The study team then asked whether the national identity of the health insurance organization made a difference in people's decisions to trust or not trust the organization. Most villagers said that they trust foreign organizations and Cambodian organizations equally: "[I] believe in organizations, both Khmer and foreign;" "Organizations are good. Both Khmer and foreign [organizations] are the same." Yet some noted that they trust foreign organizations more than Cambodian ones: "Between foreign and local NGOs, [I] believe foreign NGOs because [they are] honest, not corrupt, and have lots of money. Some local NGOs cheat the people." Others noted their worry about the difficulty of communicating with foreign organizations: "Khmer or foreigner, [our trust is] the same if they both help us. But foreign NGO is difficult to understand because we don't know how to speak with them."

3.1.2. Conceptual Framework of Insurer Trust

Based on these findings and a review of the limited theoretical literature, a conceptual model was developed to describe villagers' trust for the health insurer in Cambodia (Fig. 1). The model postulates that insurer trust has five components. First, there is organizational trust, which is people's belief in the health insurance organization as an institution, a form of impersonal trust. Secondly, there is financial trust, which is having confidence in financial transactions with the health insurer. The third domain is honesty, which is the perception that the health insurer is telling the truth. The fourth domain is competence, which is to receive service from staff of the health insurance organization at a level that meets their basic expectations. The last domain is personal interactions, which is having a positive rapport with employees of the health insurance organization.

This conceptual framework complements the existing model of health insurer trust developed in the United States (Zheng et al., 2002). The domain of personal interaction encompasses the idea of fidelity discussed by Zheng et al. (2002), which is to care for villagers' interests or welfare. Honesty and competence were included in both models. Confidentiality, a domain included in the original model, was not a critical component of insurer trust in Cambodia. Focus group participants were not worried about disclosure of sensitive information by the insurance organization. Organizational trust and financial trust were separated out from the domain of global trust in the model by Zheng et al. (2002), as important separate domains of

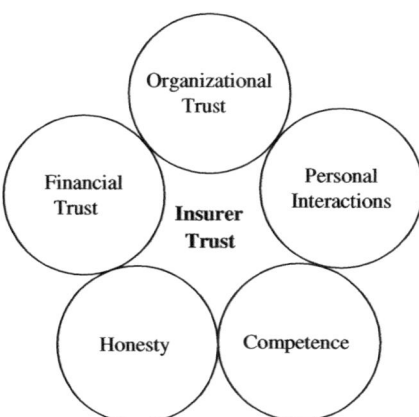

Fig. 1. Conceptual Framework for Insurer Trust.

insurer trust. This conceptual framework was subsequently used in culturally adapting the trust questions and selecting the items on the insurer
trust scale.

3.2. Quantitative Analysis

3.2.1. Development of the Insurer Trust Scale

A household survey resulted in 535 households being interviewed from 28
randomly selected villages in Banteay Meanchey province. Table 3
summarizes the demographic characteristics of survey respondents by
insurance status. The majority of individuals in the sample were female
(69%) and married (85%), with an average age of 41.3 years (SD = 13.17),
average years of education of 2.9 years (SD = 2.98), and average family size
of 4.8 individuals (SD = 1.59). Core demographic characteristics such as
gender, age, marital status, and number of family members were not
statistically significantly different across insurance status groups. However, individuals who were never insured tended to have more years of
education (3.83 years, $p = 0.002$), not be from Banteay Meanchey province
originally ($p < 0.001$), and have spent time in a refugee camp ($p = 0.002$).
The CBHI scheme appears to have attracted individuals of all wealth
quintiles, with recent success in recruiting new households from the lowest
quintile.

Twenty-four candidate questions were included in the household survey
to measure villagers' trust for the health insurer. Table 4 presents the initial
24 items with the sources, means, standard deviations, and item-to-total
correlations from the household survey. The source of the item describes
whether the question was taken directly from the scale developed in the
United States (Zheng et al., 2002), modified to fit the Cambodian context, or
added by the study team to reflect the findings from focus group discussions.
Asterisks denote items which were incorporated in the final insurer trust
scale. The final insurer trust scale consist of 12 questions: six developed by
the study team, three from the original scale, and three which were culturally
adapted to fit the Cambodian context. The means of selected items range
from 3.66 to 4.23, with standard deviations between 0.89 and 1.26. The
response categories range from strongly agree (coded as 5), agree, neutral,
disagree, to strongly disagree (coded as 1), with reverse scoring for
negatively worded items.

The final 12-item insurer trust scale was chosen based on a number of
considerations: response distribution, factor structure, internal consistency,

Table 3. Characteristics of Household Survey Participants by CBHI Enrollment.

CBHI Enrollment	Renew		New		Drop out		Never		p-value
	Number	Percentage	Number	Percentage	Number	Percentage	Number	Percentage	
Gender									
Male	45	32%	33	27%	50	34%	37	30%	0.565
Female	95	68%	91	73%	96	66%	88	70%	
Age									
18–29	25	18%	37	30%	31	21%	35	28%	0.319
30–39	39	28%	26	21%	29	20%	21	17%	
40–49	36	26%	34	27%	38	26%	38	30%	
50–59	27	19%	17	14%	33	23%	21	17%	
60+	13	9%	10	8%	15	10%	10	8%	
Mean (SD)	41.88	(12.24)	39.56	(13.46)	42.87	(13.80)	40.41	(13.01)	0.167
Marital status									
Single	2	1%	11	9%	8	5%	4	3%	0.055
Married	126	90%	103	83%	119	82%	106	85%	
Widowed	12	9%	10	8%	15	10%	12	10%	
Separated or divorced	0	0%	0	0%	4	3%	3	2%	
Years of schooling									
Mean (SD)	2.83	(2.90)	2.52	(2.90)	2.68	(2.74)	3.83	(3.26)	0.002

Table 3. (*Continued*)

CBHI Enrollment	Renew		New		Drop out		Never		p-value
	Number	Percentage	Number	Percentage	Number	Percentage	Number	Percentage	
Number of family members									
Mean (SD)	4.98	(1.66)	4.77	(1.67)	4.55	(1.47)	4.78	(1.56)	0.152
Province of origin									<0.001
Banteay Meanchey	128	91%	86	69%	133	91%	96	77%	
Other provinces	12	9%	38	31%	13	9%	29	23%	
Ever in refugee camp									0.002
Yes	41	29%	44	35%	26	18%	45	36%	
No	99	71%	80	65%	120	82%	80	64%	
Wealth quintile									<0.001
Lowest	17	12%	43	35%	26	18%	21	17%	0.009
Second	25	18%	15	12%	32	22%	36	29%	0.151
Middle	33	24%	21	17%	34	23%	18	14%	0.284
Fourth	31	22%	20	16%	35	24%	21	17%	0.076
Highest	34	24%	25	20%	19	13%	29	23%	
Total (*n* = 535)	140	100%	124	100%	146	100%	125	100%	

Table 4. Insurer Trust Questions: Means, Standard Deviations and Item-to-Total Correlations.

Items	Source	Mean	Standard Deviation	Item-to-Total Correlation
1. Organization staff are very friendly and approachable	Study team	4.49	0.75	0.54
2. Organization staff are easy to make contact with*	Study team	3.99	1.20	0.61
3. Organization staff care about your health just as much or more than you do*	Study team	3.88	1.13	0.62
4. Sometimes organization staff allow you to owe money*	Study team	3.92	1.26	0.43
5. Organization staff only collects money after distributing card	Study team	4.49	0.81	0.33
6. Organization staff comes to village to explain what health insurance is	Study team	4.33	1.00	0.36
7. If you have a question, you think organization staff will give you a straight answer*	Zheng	4.01	1.06	0.58
8. Organization staff visit people at the health center or referral hospital when they are sick	Study team	3.70	1.26	0.51
9. You believe organization staff will help you if you had problems at the health center or referral hospital*	Study team	3.96	1.13	0.60
10. You think the organization staff are completely honest and reliable*	Zheng (modified)	3.97	1.00	0.67
11. As far as you know, the organization staff are very good at what they do*	Zheng	4.15	0.95	0.67
12. Sometimes organization staff do not pay full attention to what you are trying to tell them	Study team	3.43	1.34	0.38
13. Sometimes you wait a long time before organization staff reach you	Study team	2.76	1.26	0.28
14. You worry that organization staff might share embarrassing information about you with others	Zheng (modified)	3.83	1.34	0.34
15. If someone at the organization made a serious mistake, you think they would try to hide it	Zheng	2.57	1.42	0.40
16. You feel like you have to check everything the organization staff say	Zheng (modified)	1.75	0.92	0.22
17. As far as you know, the quality of service by the organization is very good*	Study team	4.15	0.93	0.67

Table 4. *(Continued)*

Items	Source	Mean	Standard Deviation	Item-to-Total Correlation
18. You feel that the organization cares more about poor people than rich people	Study team	3.02	1.48	0.17
19. You believe the organization will pay for everything it is supposed to, even really expensive treatments*	Zheng	3.84	1.25	0.53
20. You believe organization does good for the community*	Study team	4.23	0.89	0.63
21. You worry there are a lot of expenses that the organization does not pay for	Zheng (modified)	2.71	1.35	0.29
22. The organization cares more about making money than about getting you the treatment you need*	Zheng (modified)	3.66	1.26	0.56
23. If you got seriously sick, you're afraid the organization might try to stop paying for you altogether	Zheng (modified)	3.28	1.49	0.29
24. All in all, you have complete trust in the organization*	Zheng	4.11	0.98	0.71

*Items in the final insurer trust scale.

face validity, content validity, external construct validity, test–retest reliability, and inter-rater reliability.

First, the response distributions of each trust item was examined. No items had responses concentrated in one or two categories, suggesting that all items had acceptable response patterns and adequate discriminatory power. Two questions (items 8 and 15) were dropped from the analysis due to high percentages of "don't know" responses of 32 percent and 22 percent, respectively. An iterated principal factor analysis was conducted to examine the latent dimensions underlying the items. The first factor with an eigenvalue of 5.49 explained 74 percent of the variance in the data, whereas the second factor with an eigenvalue of 1.13 explained 17 percent of the variance. The scree plot showed a large break between the first factor and the second factor. Based on these results, one factor was selected to model insurer trust. This supported the findings of the original scale for insurer trust, which also modeled insurer trust as a unidimensional construct.

The trust scale was then developed by deleting items with low factor loadings, high uniqueness, and low item-to-total correlations. Under these criteria, 10 questions (items 1, 5, 6, 12, 13, 14, 16, 18, 21, and 23 shown in Table 4) were deleted. The remaining 12 items exhibited high internal consistency (Cronbach's alpha of 0.87), with an eigenvalue of 4.43 for the first factor explaining 96 percent of the estimated common variance. Scores from these 12 items were summed, displaying good response variability (range = 20–60, mean = 47.87, SD = 8.28).

Face and content validity was also considered in the item selection. The final 12 items selected represents all 5 domains of insurer trust in the conceptual model: organizational trust (items 17, 20, and 24), financial trust (items 4, 19, and 22), honesty (items 7 and 10), competence (items 9 and 11), and personal interaction (items 2 and 3). External construct validity was also assessed by examining the relationship between the trust scale and two general trust questions in the household survey. The first trust question asked: Which of the following best fits how you trust others? (1) I tend not to trust anyone, (2) I trust a few people, (3) I trust some people, (4) I trust most people, and (5) I tend to trust everyone. Association between the developed trust scale and this question was examined using simple linear regression, where a statistically significant positive association was found (1.67, 95% CI: 0.94 to 2.41, $p < 0.001$). A separate question captured villagers' trust for their neighbors in a binary response (yes/no): Do you believe your neighbors will be kind to you if you are kind to them? Villagers who responded yes to this question were likely to have a 2.64 point higher score for insurer trust compared to those who responded no, with a statistically significant difference (95% CI: 0.31 to 4.16, $p = 0.026$). These relationships affirmed that the insurer trust scale has good construct validity. The test–retest reliability of the scale ($r = 0.65$) and the combined test retest reliability and inter-rater reliability score ($r = 0.48$) suggest that the 12-item scale is reliable.

3.2.2. Insurer Trust and CBHI Enrollment

Both univariate and multivariate analyses were conducted to examine the relationship between insurer trust levels and CBHI enrollment. Multinomial logistic regression models were used for this analysis, where differences in household insurance status were examined by levels of insurer trust. Table 5 presents the results.

With univariate analysis, significant associations were found when assessing the relationship between insurer trust levels and CBHI enroll-ment. People who dropped out (RRR = 1.06, $p < 0.001$), newly enrolled

Table 5.   Multinomial Logistic Regression: Insurer Trust and
CBHI Enrollment.

	Univariate Analysis			Multivariate Analysis[a]		
CBHI enrollment	RRR[b]	95%CI	p-value	RRR[b]	95%CI	p-value
Never	1.00	–	–	1.00	–	–
Drop out	1.06	(1.033–1.096)	<0.001	1.06	(1.025–1.093)	<0.001
New	1.07	(1.039–1.106)	<0.001	1.08	(1.041–1.122)	<0.001
Renew	1.15	(1.108–1.190)	<0.001	1.15	(1.102–1.196)	<0.001

[a] Controlled for demographic factors, health care utilization and socio-economic status
[b] Relative risk ratio – the ratio of two relative risks, comparing each of the drop out, new and renew categories to those who never enrolled in CBHI.

(RRR = 1.07, $p < 0.001$) and renewed the insurance scheme (RRR = 1.15, $p < 0.001$) had significantly higher insurer trust scores than those who had never had insurance. Villagers who renewed the insurance scheme were found to have statistically significantly higher trust levels compared to those who were new to the scheme (RRR = 1.07, $p < 0.001$) and those who dropped out of the scheme (RRR = 1.08, $p < 0.001$).

With multivariate analysis, this association between insurer trust levels and CBHI enrollment changed little after controlling for demographic factors, health care utilization, and socio-economic status. Insurer trust levels for those who never enrolled in CBHI remained statistically significantly different from other CBHI enrollment groups after adjusting for measured confounders. The multivariate analysis presented in Table 5 controlled for the following demographic variables: age (in 10-year categories), gender, marital status, years of schooling, number of household members, province of origin, and having ever been in a refugee camp. Villagers' level of worry about paying for health care (4-point scale) was also added to the model. The following health care utilization variables were included: having had a household member (1) be admitted to a hospital in the past 12 months, (2) deliver a baby in the past 12 months, or (3) be ill or injured in the past 30 days. A household asset index was also incorporated in the model to control for differences in socio-economic status.

Fig. 2 displays the relative risk ratios (also known as conditional odds ratios) comparing the drop out, new, and renew group to those who never enrolled in CBHI. Comparing villagers who renewed CBHI to those who never had insurance, the ratio of relative risks for one unit increase in insurer trust levels was 1.15 (95% CI: 1.102–1.196, $p < 0.001$) holding other covariates fixed. Conditional on being in renew or drop out category, the ratio of the

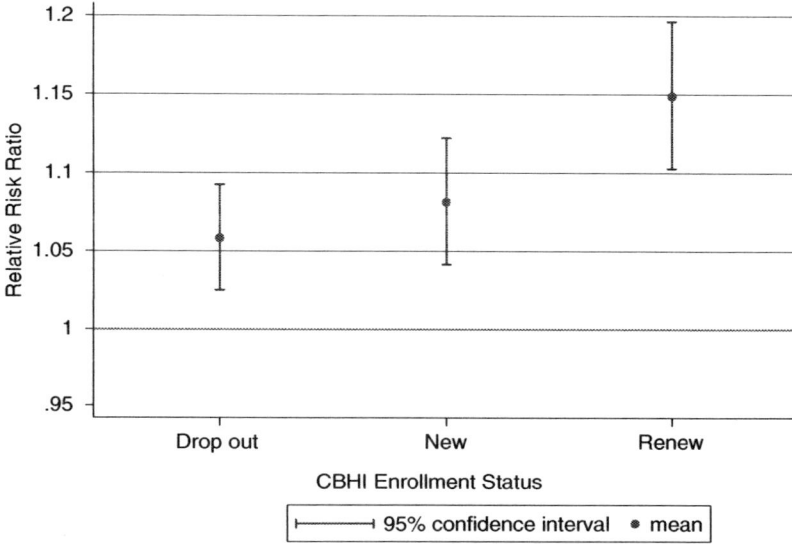

Fig. 2. Relative Risk Ratios by CBHI Enrollment. The Comparison Group is Never Insured Individuals.

odds of renewed individuals for one unit increase in trust levels was also statistically significant (1.08, 95% CI: 1.04–1.13, $p < 0.001$) holding other covariates fixed.

4. DISCUSSION

4.1. Community-Based Health Insurance and Trust

This study examined villagers' trust for health insurers and the association between insurer trust and CBHI enrollment. Trust for the health insurance organization was generally high, though villages with unfavorable experiences with other organizations in the past were less willing to put their faith in the insurer. Insurer trust was found to be based on a combination of impersonal and interpersonal trust. Five domains of insurer trust were identified: organizational trust, financial trust, honesty, competence, and personal interactions. Some villagers suggested that perceived honesty, timing of fund collection, ability to owe money to the insurer and the method of recruitment had a bearing on their trust for the insurer.

A statistically significant association was found between villagers' trust levels for the health insurer and CBHI enrollment after controlling for demographic factors, health care utilization, and socio-economic status. Individuals who continue to purchase insurance have higher levels of trust for the health insurer compared to those who had just enrolled, dropped out or never enrolled in CBHI. Individuals who never enrolled in CBHI also had statistically significantly lower trust levels compared to those who renewed or newly enrolled in CBHI. This supports the original hypothesis that trust for the health insurer varies across villagers with different CBHI enrollment status, and that health insurer trust is associated with CBHI enrollment. The result confirms that health insurer trust is an important consideration in villagers' decision to participate in CBHI schemes.

These findings complement and contribute to what has already been found in the literature about the link between trust and CBHI enrollment in other countries. Schneider (2005) conducted an exploratory study using focus groups, and found that trust for the CBHI scheme appeared to influence the enrollment in micro-health insurance schemes in Rwanda. In China, Zhang, Wang, Wang, and Hsiao (2006) attempted to capture individual level social capital as measured by a trust index and found that individuals' general trust for others was positively associated with the probability of farmers' willingness to join CBHI schemes in rural China. Trust in the integrity and competence of people managing CBHI schemes and access to choice of physicians have also been described to have an effect on enrollment (Balkrishnan, Hall, Blackwelder, & Bradley, 2004). Insurers who had existing entry points into the community and insurers who were more responsive to the community's preferences tended to have an easier time attracting villagers to enroll in CBHI schemes (Carrin et al., 2005).

Some limitations must be noted about the generalizability of this study. This study was conducted in one area in northwest Cambodia, where CAAFW operates a CBHI scheme. Since no comparisons are presented between CAAFW's scheme and other CBHI schemes in the country, this study may provide limited insight into trust relationships in other CBHI schemes. It is also important to note the historical background of the research area, which was a Khmer Rouge stronghold until the late 1990s. The trauma brought about by the Khmer Rouge and the mental health issues that continue to persist in the population may affect the trust relationships today. Given the context-specific nature of trust, this cultural and historical setting may limit the generalizability of results about the meaning of trust in this study. This study also focused only on the community's perceptions. Focus groups were conducted among villagers and not among staff of the health insurance organization. Since trust is a two-way road, understanding the trust mechanisms by health insurers to trust villagers is also an important area for future research.

Despite these limitations, parallels can be drawn among operational aspects of CBHI schemes on how villagers in low-income, post-conflict settings may decide whether to trust a health insurance provider. Although specific reasons to trust health insurance organizations may differ across regions or CBHI schemes, the idea that the relationships built between villagers and insurers matter in their decisions to enroll in CBHI is likely to be transferable. The finding that health insurer trust consists of both impersonal trust with the organization and interpersonal trust with organization staff is also likely to be transferable to other settings, which merits further research to strengthen the research base.

4.2. Factors Influencing CBHI Enrollment

Beyond the issue of trust, the literature also offers some guidance in identifying factors that are associated with enrollment in CBHI schemes. An extensive review of CBHI schemes was conducted in 1998 by the World Health Organization, examining 82 non-profit health insurance schemes for people outside the formal sector employment in developing countries (Bennett, Creese, & Monasch, 1998). This review identified affordability of premiums or contributions as one of the main determinants of membership. Other factors contributing to enrollment included units of enrollment (e.g., individual versus family-based membership) and timing of collecting the contributions (e.g., monthly, quarterly, annually) to fit the seasonality of income (Bennett et al., 1998). Income was also found to be a significant factor in explaining enrollment in CBHI based on application of econometric models to investigate the extent to which specific individual and household characteristics influence the decision to enroll in health insurance (Drechsler & Jutting, 2007; Jutting, 2004).

These factors were also identified in our study. The premium was discussed as a deciding factor, where many villagers who never enrolled or dropped out of CBHI noted their lack of ability to pay the premium. The borrowing practices for CBHI also appeared to be a hurdle for enrollment, where villagers mentioned the ability to owe money to the insurer as playing a role in their decision to trust the insurer and enroll in the CBHI scheme.

The timing to collect premiums was also noted in this study, where it was important for villagers to receive the CBHI card before being asked to pay for premiums. However, income did not appear to play a significant role in explaining enrollment in the CBHI scheme in this study. Households that renewed or newly enrolled in the CBHI scheme represented all five wealth quintiles in socio-economic status, suggesting an equitable provision of CBHI coverage.

In addition to the abovementioned factors supported by the literature, knowledge about health insurance also appeared to influence CBHI enrollment to a great extent. In communities where literacy is low and information is scarce, enrollment in CBHI may be closely related to people's understanding about CBHI. This was endorsed by villagers' requests for the health insurance organization to provide more information and explanations about the CBHI scheme. Some villagers also requested information about exactly when the staff would come back to take the photo or collect money, and when the card expires.

To better understand and appreciate the reasons villagers choose to enroll or not enroll in CBHI schemes, further research is called for to study the appropriate rankings and weights that villagers place among possible considerations including trust. A conjoint analysis can offer important insight into villagers' health financing decisions, and allow health insurers to prioritize their efforts in attracting enrollment in CBHI schemes.

4.3. Trust in Health Financing Systems

This study highlights that trust plays a vital role in health financing systems where the entire arrangement is largely relational. Interactions among patients, providers, insurers, suppliers, regulators, and other health care agents are critical to financing a health system. As Gilson notes, "trust is important to health systems because it underpins the co-operation throughout the system that is required for health production" (Gilson, 2003).

Study findings revealed that both impersonal and interpersonal trust matter in villagers' trust for the health insurer. This is an essential finding in building a functioning Cambodian health system as the system relies on interactions among many individuals. Unlike in Western cultures where trust between patients and health insurers only exemplifies impersonal trust, interpersonal relationships are given greater weight in villagers' health financing decisions in Cambodia. This highlights the dependence of organizations on individual workers' personal traits and social networks.

It also points to an opportunity for staff of organizations to place greater weight on building trusting interpersonal relationships with villagers. Improving the trust relationships between villagers and staff of the health insurance organizations may not only increase enrollment in CBHI schemes, but also have positive spillover effects.

The results of this study support the need for further research on trust in health systems, as it can inform many of the fundamental aspects of health systems. In human resource management, trust in health systems points to the need to consider the institutions and behaviors that shape performance, relationships that must be managed to deliver outcomes and the importance of developing shared meanings to sustain delivery (Gilson, Palmer, & Schneider, 2005). In health financing, health systems face many pressures to provide financial incentives that undermine trustworthy behavior. Since individual behavior is largely understood to be influenced by financial incentives (Gottret & Schieber, 2006), many governments and international organizations are increasingly adopting financial incentives to generate performance gains (Akashi, Yamada, Huot, Kanal, & Sugimoto, 2004; Noirhomme et al., 2007; Schwartz & Bhushan, 2005). Yet without careful design, such incentives may reinforce self-interested rather than altruistic trust-building behavior. Further research is needed to understand the role and assess the impact of trust in other health financing arrangements such as contracting, health equity funds and conditional cash transfer programs.

Funding arrangements influence the trust between the patient and the insurer. These arrangements can serve as direct incentives for the insurer, which may "support or undermine the fiduciary relationship between the provider and patient" (Gilson, 2003). It could also reveal norms and values in the health system such as solidarity, fairness, and procedural justice that promote trust in the system (Braithwaite, 1998; Brockner, Siegel, Kramer, & Tyler, 1996; Mladovsky & Mossialos, 2008). The relationships insurers have with their staff and the management practices of the health insurance organization are also found to strongly shape insurer attitudes and practices. Building trusting relationships is imperative to having a well-functioning health system. Having a trusting and trusted health system can then contribute to fostering wider social value and social order (Gilson, 2003).

In conclusion, this study has illustrated the importance of insurer trust in the CBHI context in Cambodia. Further research is essential to understand and measure levels of insurer trust in similar settings, as well as to identify and evaluate some interventions to develop trusting relationships in health systems in similar low-income, post-conflict settings.

NOTE

1. The Thai currency (Baht) is commonly used in this region near the Thai border.

ACKNOWLEDGMENTS

We thank the Center for Advanced Study (CAS) in Cambodia for the data collection efforts, especially Sovuthikar Inuong, Mealea KeKantha, Hun Thirith, Chean Rithy Men, and Hean Sokhom. We also thank Roger Hay, Katherine Fritz, Karen Bandeen-Roche and Adrijana Corluka for their advice, as well as the Cambodian Association for Assistance to Families and Widows (CAAFW), especially Sour Iyong for local support. The authors express their appreciation for the financial support (Grant No. H050474) provided by the UK Department for International Development (DFID) for the Future Health Systems research program consortium. This document is an output from a project funded by DFID for the benefit of developing countries. The views expressed are not necessarily those of DFID.

REFERENCES

Akashi, H., Yamada, T., Huot, E., Kanal, K., & Sugimoto, T. (2004). User fees at a public hospital in Cambodia: Effects on hospital performance and provider attitudes. *Social Science & Medicine, 58*(3), 553–564.

Annear, P., Wilkinson, D., Chean, M., & Van Pelt, M. (2006). *Study of financial access to health services for the poor in Cambodia. Phase I: Scope, design and data analysis.* Phnom Penh: Research Report for the Ministry of Health Cambodia, World Health Organization, AusAID and RMIT University.

Balkrishnan, R., Dugan, E., Camacho, F. T., & Hall, M. A. (2003). Trust and satisfaction with physicians, insurers, and the medical profession. *Medical Care, 41*(9), 1058–1064.

Balkrishnan, R., Hall, M. A., Blackwelder, S., & Bradley, D. (2004). Trust in insurers and access to physicians: Associated enrollee behaviors and changes over time. *Health Services Research, 39*(4 Part 1), 813–824.

Bennett, S., Creese, A., & Monasch, R. (1998). *Health insurance schemes for people outside formal sector employment.* WHO/ARA/CC/98.1, Division of Analysis, Research and Assessment, Paper No. 16. World Health Organization, Geneva.

Biddulph, R. (2000). *Making the poor more visible: Landlessness and development research report.* Cambodia Land Study Project, Oxfam, Phnom Penh.

Braithwaite, V. (1998). Communal and exchange trust norms: Their value base and relevance to institutional trust. In: V. Braithwaite & M. Levi (Eds), *Trust and governance.* New York: Russell Sage Foundation.

Brockner, J., Siegel, P., Kramer, R. M., & Tyler, T. R. (1996). Understanding the interaction between procedural and distributive justice: The role of trust. In: R. M. Kramer &

T. R. Tyler (Eds), *Trust in organizations: Frontiers of theory and research.* Thousand Oaks, CA: Sage.

CAAFW. (2007). *Community health insurance in Thmar Pouk – A presentation.* Phnom Penh: Cambodian Organization for Assistance to Families and Widows.

Carrin, G., Waelkens, M. P., & Criel, B. (2005). Community-based health insurance in developing countries: A study of its contribution to the performance of health financing systems. *Tropical Medicine & International Health, 10*(8), 799–811.

Chandler, D. (2007). *A history of Cambodia* (4th ed.). Boulder, CO: Westview Press.

Drechsler, D., & Jutting, J. (2007). Different countries, different needs: The role of private health insurance in developing countries. *Journal of Health Politics, Policy and Law, 32*(3), 497–534.

Dubois, V., Tonglet, R., Hoyois, P., Sunbaunat, K., Roussaux, J. P., & Hauff, E. (2004). Household survey of psychiatric morbidity in Cambodia. *International Journal of Social Psychiatry, 50*(2), 174–185.

Dugan, E., Trachtenberg, F., & Hall, M. A. (2005). Development of abbreviated measures to assess patient trust in a physician, a health insurer, and the medical profession. *BMC Health Services Research, 5*, 64.

Ekman, B. (2004). Community-based health insurance in low-income countries: A systematic review of the evidence. *Health Policy and Planning, 19*(5), 249–270.

Gilson, L. (2003). Trust and the development of health care as a social institution. *Social Science & Medicine, 56*(7), 1453–1468.

Gilson, L. (2006). Trust in health care: Theoretical perspectives and research needs. *Journal of Health Organization and Management, 20*(5), 359–375.

Gilson, L., Palmer, N., & Schneider, H. (2005). Trust and health worker performance: Exploring a conceptual framework using South African evidence. *Social Science & Medicine, 61*(7), 1418–1429.

Goold, S. D., Fessler, D., & Moyer, C. A. (2006). A measure of trust in insurers. *Health Services Research, 41*(1), 58–78.

Gottret, P., & Schieber, G. (2006). *Health financing revisited: A practitioner's guide.* Washington, DC: The World Bank.

Goudge, J., & Gilson, L. (2005). How can trust be investigated? Drawing lessons from past experience. *Social Science & Medicine, 61*(7), 1439–1451.

GRET. (2005). *GRET-SKY Health Insurance Project Cambodia: Briefing note.* Phnom Penh: Groupe de Recherche et d'Échanges, Technologiques.

Hall, M. A., Camacho, F., Dugan, E., & Balkrishnan, R. (2002). Trust in the medical profession: Conceptual and measurement issues. *Health Services Research, 37*(5), 1419–1439.

Hall, M. A., Dugan, E., Zheng, B., & Mishra, A. (2001). Trust in physicians and medical institutions: What is it, can it be measured, and does it matter? *The Milbank Quarterly, 79*(4), 613–639.

Hardeman, W., Van Damme, W., Van Pelt, M., Por, I., Kimvan, H., & Meessen, B. (2004). Access to health care for all? User fees plus a health equity fund in Sotnikum, Cambodia. *Health Policy and Planning, 19*(1), 22–32.

Jacobs, B., Price, N., & Sam, S. O. (2007). A sustainability assessment of a health equity fund initiative in Cambodia. *The International Journal of Health Planning and Management, 22*(3), 183–203.

Jowett, M. (2003). Do informal risk sharing networks crowd out public voluntary health insurance? Evidence from Vietnam. *Applied Economics, 35*(10), 1153–1161.

Jutting, J. (2004). Do community-based health insurance schemes improve poor people's access to health care? Evidence from rural Senegal. *World Development*, *32*(2), 273–288.

Kao, A. C., Green, D. C., Davis, N. A., Koplan, J. P., & Cleary, P. D. (1998). Patients' trust in their physicians: Effects of choice, continuity, and payment method. *Journal of General Internal Medicine*, *13*(10), 681–686.

Lane, C. (1998). Introduction: Theories and issues in the study of trust. In: C. Lane & R. Bachmann (Eds), *Trust within and between organizations: Conceptual issues and empirical applications*. Oxford: Oxford University Press.

Mechanic, D. (1998). The functions and limitations of trust in the provision of medical care. *Journal of Health Politics, Policy and Law*, *23*(4), 661–686.

Mladovsky, P., & Mossialos, E. (2008). A conceptual framework for community-based health insurance in low-income countries: Social capital and economic development. *World Development*, *36*(4), 590–607.

MOH. (2007). *Launching community-based health insurance in Cambodia: Concept note*. Phnom Penh: Ministry of Health, Cambodia.

Newman, J. (1998). The dynamics of trust. In: A. Coulson (Ed.), *Trust and contracts: Relationships in local government, health and public services*. Bristol: The Polity Press.

Nichter, M., Nichter, M., Thompson, P. J., Shiffman, S., & Moscicki, A. B. (2002). Using qualitative research to inform survey development on nicotine dependence among adolescents. *Drug and Alcohol Dependence*, *68*(Suppl. 1), S41–S56.

Noirhomme, M., Meessen, B., Griffiths, F., Por, I., Jacobs, B., Thor, R., Criel, B., & Van Damme, W. (2007). Improving access to hospital care for the poor: Comparative analysis of four health equity funds in Cambodia. *Health Policy and Planning*, *22*(4), 246–262.

Offe, C. (1999). How can we trust our fellow citizens? In: M. E. Warren (Ed.), *Democracy and trust*. Cambridge: Cambridge University Press.

Pope, C., Ziebland, S., & Mays, N. (2000). Qualitative research in health care. Analyzing qualitative data. *BMJ*, *320*(7227), 114–116.

Por I., & Hardeman, W. (2006). *Briefing paper on CAAFW's community health insurance in Thmar Pouk, Cambodia*. Phnom Penh: Cambodian Organization for Assistance to Families and Widows.

Schneider, P. (2005). Trust in micro-health insurance: An exploratory study in Rwanda. *Social Science & Medicine*, *61*(7), 1430–1438.

Schwartz, J. B., & Bhushan, I. (2005). Cambodia: Using contracting to reduce inequity in primary health care delivery. In: D. Gwatkin, A. Wagstaff & A. Yazbeck (Eds), *Reaching the poor with health, nutrition and population services – What works, what doesn't, and why*. Washington, DC: The World Bank.

Thom, D. H., & Stanford Trust Study Physicians. (2001). Physician behaviors that predict patient trust. *The Journal of Family Practice*, *50*(4), 323–328.

Van Damme, W., Van Leemput, L., Por, I., Hardeman, W., & Meessen, B. (2004). Out-of-pocket health expenditure and debt in poor households: Evidence from Cambodia. *Tropical Medicine & International Health*, *9*(2), 273–280.

WHO. (2000). *The World Health Report 2000 Health Systems: Improving performance*. Geneva: World Health Organization.

Zhang, L., Wang, H., Wang, L., & Hsiao, W. (2006). Social capital and farmer's willingness-to-join a newly established community-based health insurance in rural China. *Health Policy*, *76*(2), 233–242.

Zheng, B., Hall, M. A., Dugan, E., Kidd, K. E., & Levine, D. (2002). Development of a scale to measure patients' trust in health insurers. *Health Services Research*, *37*(1), 187–202.

METHODOLOGICAL CHALLENGES IN EVALUATING HEALTH CARE FINANCING EQUITY IN DATA-POOR CONTEXTS: LESSONS FROM GHANA, SOUTH AFRICA AND TANZANIA ☆

Josephine Borghi, John Ataguba, Gemini Mtei, James Akazili, Filip Meheus, Clas Rehnberg and Di McIntyre

☆This chapter draws on the work of SHIELD – Strategies for Health Insurance for Equity in Less Developed Countries. SHIELD is a collaborative research project comprised of researchers from the following institutions: Health Economics Unit, School of Public Health and Family Medicine, University of Cape Town and Centre for Health Policy, University of the Witwatersrand in South Africa; Ifakara Health Institute in Tanzania; Ghana Health Service (including the Ghana Health Research Unit and its field site Navrongo Health Research Centre) in Ghana; Health Economics and Financing Programme, London School of Hygiene and Tropical Medicine in the United Kingdom; Development, Policy & Practice, Royal Tropical Institute (KIT) in the Netherlands; and Medical Management Centre, Karolinska Institute in Sweden.

Innovations in Health System Finance in Developing and Transitional Economies
Advances in Health Economics and Health Services Research, Volume 21, 133–156
Copyright © 2009 by Emerald Group Publishing Limited
All rights of reproduction in any form reserved
ISSN: 0731-2199/doi:10.1108/S0731-2199(2009)0000021009

ABSTRACT

Objective – *Measurement of the incidence of health financing contributions across socio-economic groups has proven valuable in informing health care financing reforms. However, there is little evidence as to how to carry out financing incidence analysis (FIA) in lower income settings. We outline some of the challenges faced when carrying out a FIA in Ghana, Tanzania and South Africa and illustrate how innovative techniques were used to overcome data weaknesses in these settings.*

Methodology – *FIA was carried out for tax, insurance and out-of-pocket (OOP) payments. The primary data sources were Living Standards Measurement Surveys (LSMS) and household surveys conducted in each of the countries; tax authorities and insurance funds also provided information. Consumption expenditure and a composite index of socio-economic status (SES) were used to assess financing equity. Where possible conventional methods of FIA were applied. Numerous challenges were documented and solution strategies devised.*

Results – *LSMS are likely to underestimate financial contributions to health care by individuals. For tax incidence analysis, reported income tax payments from secondary sources were severely under-reported. Income tax payers and shareholders could not be reliably identified. The use of income or consumption expenditure to estimate income tax contributions was found to be a more reliable method of estimating income tax incidence. Assumptions regarding corporate tax incidence had a huge effect on the progressivity of corporate tax and on overall tax progressivity. LSMS consumption categories did not always coincide with tax categories for goods subject to excise tax (e.g. wine and spirits were combined, despite differing tax rates). Tobacco companies, alcohol distributors and advertising agencies were used to provide more detailed information on consumption patterns for goods subject to excise tax by income category. There was little guidance on how to allocate fuel levies associated with 'public transport' use. Hence, calculations of fuel tax on public transport were based on individual expenditure on public transport, the average cost per kilometre and average rates of fuel consumption for each form of transport. For insurance contributions, employees will not report on employer contributions unless specifically requested to and are frequently unsure of their contributions. Therefore, we collected information on total health insurance contributions from individual schemes and regulatory authorities. OOP payments are likely to be under-reported due to long recall periods; linking OOP expenditure and illness incidence questions – omitting preventive care; and focusing on the last service used when people may have used multiple services during an illness episode. To derive more robust estimates of financing incidence, we collected additional primary data on OOP expenditures together with insurance enrolment rates and associated payments. To link primary data to the LSMS, a composite index of SES was used in Ghana and Tanzania and non-durable expenditure was used in South Africa.*

Policy implications – *We show how data constraints can be overcome for FIA in lower income countries and provide recommendations for future studies.*

INTRODUCTION

Health insurance is increasingly being seen as presenting an opportunity to increase the resource base for domestic health sector funding, to expand coverage of health services to a wider proportion of the population and to promote equity within health systems. Health care financing is also once again relatively high on the policy agenda within Africa (e.g., International Labour Organization, 2007). However, little is known about the mechanisms to extend health insurance coverage in the African context or the potential equity implications of such a change. Insurance implies pooling health funds and risks such that citizens can be provided with financial protection against the potentially high costs of health care when in need (World Health Organization, 2005). From an equity perspective, individuals should contribute to the funding of health care according to their ability to pay (ATP), which will promote income cross-subsidies within the overall health system. Therefore, a key element of the information required to inform health care financing reforms relates to the incidence of contributions to different financing mechanisms across socio-economic groups.

Against this background, the SHIELD (Strategies for Health Insurance for Equity in Less Developed countries) research project aims to evaluate existing inequities in health care financing in Ghana, South Africa and Tanzania and the extent to which health insurance mechanisms could address equity challenges. These three African countries were selected because, to varying degrees, they all have existing voluntary insurance and are incorporating elements of mandatory health insurance into their health systems. Ghana has a small private commercial health insurance sector, which covers a limited number of formal sector workers, and also had an extensive network of community-based pre-payment schemes. In 2003, Ghana initiated a National Health Insurance Scheme (NHIS) with the intention of achieving universal coverage in a short space of time. South Africa has a well-established private voluntary health insurance sector covering some formal sector workers and their dependents (less than 15% of the population). Although the possibility of introducing some form of mandatory health insurance system in South Africa has been under discussion since the late 1980s, the ruling party has only recently committed to implementing National Health Insurance (NHI) with universal coverage. Tanzania has very limited commercial health insurance and growing experience of community-based pre-payment schemes in rural areas. There are also two national level compulsory insurance schemes for formal sector workers. The different experiences and approaches to voluntary and mandatory health insurance in these countries provide a basis for useful comparative analyses. SHIELD first provided an overview of existing health financing systems within each country and then, for each source of finance, sought to identify who bears the burden by socio-economic status (SES) and the extent of the health financing burden (financing incidence analysis (FIA)). SHIELD will also evaluate the extent to which alternative health insurance mechanisms could promote a more equitable distribution of the burden of health care financing across socio-economic groups.

Whilst financing incidence analyses have been carried out in a variety of different country contexts relying solely on secondary data sources, no such analysis has yet been conducted in Africa. During the process, the SHIELD research team encountered numerous methodological challenges both in compiling and in analysing the data needed for a comprehensive and accurate FIA. The objective of this chapter is to describe the problems encountered and possible approaches for addressing them to assist other researchers in data-scarce low- and middle-income country contexts in undertaking similar research. The chapter focuses on strategies for overcoming potential methodological constraints and is intended to minimise the need to 're-invent the wheel' and also to encourage other researchers to avoid using 'quick and dirty' methods when they encounter methodological challenges. To be able to inform health care financing policy discussions, researchers have an obligation to produce evidence that is as accurate as possible.

This chapter begins by providing a brief overview of the structure of health care financing within the three countries (refer McIntyre et al., 2008 for greater detail), followed by a description of the main national household surveys used for the FIA and methods for SES measurement. The rest of the chapter is structured in relation to the steps taken to undertake a FIA of the main domestic health care financing mechanisms, namely tax funding, health insurance and out-of-pocket (OOP) payments. In each section, we present the key challenges in relation to data sources and estimation techniques experienced in the SHIELD project and how they were addressed (e.g. through collection of additional primary data, making innovative use of existing datasets, triangulating with data from a range of different sources). The focus is on how we estimated the distribution, *between different socio-economic groups*, of contributions to each health care financing mechanism.

OVERVIEW OF HEALTH CARE FINANCING IN SOUTH AFRICA, GHANA AND TANZANIA

Based on the most recent National Health Accounts data in each country,[1] tax represents around half of total health sector revenue in Ghana and South Africa (56% and 40% respectively) – Table 1. OOP payments represent around 24% in Ghana and only 14% in South Africa. In contrast, Tanzania relies heavily on OOP payments (47%) for health sector funding, with tax representing less than a quarter of total health funding. OOP payments include user fees at public health facilities, payments to informal or formal private health care providers (especially in Ghana and Tanzania) and co-payments by insured groups (South Africa). Private medical schemes make up a large proportion of health sector funds in South Africa (45%). In both Ghana and Tanzania, the breakdown of health financing sources relies

Table 1. Overview of Main Sources of Health Care Financing by Country.

Financing Source (Data Source)	South Africa (McIntyre et al., 2007)	Ghana (MOH, 2006)	Tanzania (MOHSW, 2001)
Donors	–	1	23
Taxes	40	56	22
Private insurance	45	–	–
Firms/NGOs	–	7	8
Out-of-pocket	14	24	47
Other[a]	<1	12	–

[a]Ghana = Parastatals (6.4%); non-profit institutions (5.7%).

Table 2. Overview of the Percentage Contribution of Each Form of Tax
to the General Tax Base by Country.

Tax Category (Data Source)	South Africa (National Treasury, 2005)	Ghana (RAGB, 2005)	Tanzania (TRA,[a] 2005)
Personal income	30	11	14
Corporate income	25	15	10
VAT	27	25	44
Domestic		8	16
Imports		17	28
Fuel	5	18	7
Excise	3.8	3	
Import duty	4	17	17
Export duty	<0.1	<1	<0.1
Other[b]	5	10	9

Note: RAGB, Revenue Agency Governing Board; TRA, Tanzania Revenue Authority.
[a]These data were derived from the following website for the year 2005: http://www.tra.go.tz/
Current_National_Statistics.htm. Accessed on November 1, 2008. A personal communication
from the Tanzania Revenue Authority.
[b]In South Africa, other includes taxes on property (<3%) and unidentified levies, stamp duties
and fines, air departure tax and skills developed levy (<3%). In Ghana, other includes national
health insurance levy (5%); other (stamp, fines, etc.) (3%); self-employed tax (1.5%) and airport
tax (<1%). In Tanzania, other includes other income tax, for example, housing tax, tax on
interest and dividends (7%) and other domestic taxes and charges, for example, stamp duty,
vehicle registration taxes (2%).

on NHA data that precedes the widespread introduction of national health
insurance schemes.

In Tanzania, the main source of tax financing is value-added tax (VAT)
that accounts for just under half of total tax revenue (44%), followed by
revenues from import duty (17%) (Table 2). In Ghana and South Africa,
VAT contributes around a quarter of total tax revenue. Ghana also benefits
from significant contributions from fuel tax (18%) and import duty (17%).
In South Africa, personal income tax is the largest source of tax revenue.
Personal income tax is structured progressively in each country.

In Tanzania, there are two forms of compulsory insurance schemes for the
formal sector. The National Health Insurance Fund (NHIF) covers public
employees and up to five dependants, with premium contributions of 6% of
salary, shared equally between the employer and the employee. The Social
Health Insurance Benefit (SHIB) covers formal sector private and parastatal
employees who are contributing to the National Social Security Fund;
6.25% of their salary goes to health insurance, shared equally between

employer and employee. The NHIF covers around 5% of the total population and the SHIB 4%. For the rural population, the community health fund (CHF) is a voluntary scheme relying on an annual flat rate contribution of around Tsh 5–10,000. The average CHF enrolment within rural districts is estimated to be less than 10%.

In Ghana, the NHIS covers both the formal and the informal sectors and has currently registered around 60% of the population. However, only 32% of the population have the requisite identity cards and are able to access services. The NHIS is implemented through a network of District Mutual Health Insurance Schemes (DMHIS). Formal sector workers contribute a premium equivalent to 2.5% of their salaries through the Social Security and National Insurance Trust (SSNIT). For those outside the formal sector, premiums are officially graduated according to income varying from US$8 to US$53 per annum. However, in practice, premium payment appears to be more of a flat rate of US $8 per annum due to the difficulty of categorising people into different socio-economic groupings.

In South Africa, the main form of insurance is private voluntary health insurance. There is community rating of contributions to schemes, often shared between employers and employees, with the percentage share varying across companies, and contribution rates are differentiated by benefit package rather than income level. Medical schemes cover less than 15% of the population and include high- and middle-income formal sector workers and sometimes their dependents. Private commercial schemes cover less than 5% of the population in both Tanzania and Ghana.

There is no cross subsidisation in Tanzania across schemes, and for the CHF, there is no risk pooling across districts. In Ghana, there is currently no risk pooling between the individual DMHIS. In South Africa, there is risk pooling within individual schemes in relation to the prescribed minimum benefit package, but most schemes have individual 'medical savings accounts' for primary care services. There is no risk pooling between the tax funded pool and insurance schemes.

OVERVIEW OF DATA SOURCES

Before exploring in detail how the data for the financing incidence study were analysed, it is helpful to briefly outline the main household survey datasets that were drawn on in each country.

Each country relied on the most recent national dataset containing information on income and expenditure (Table 3). Income and consumption

Table 3.   Overview of National Household Survey Data Sources Used
for the FIA.

Country/Variables	South Africa	Ghana	Tanzania
Name of survey	Income and Expenditure Survey	Ghana Living Standards Survey	Household budget survey (HBS)
Year	2005/2006	2005/2006	2000/2001
Number of households	21,144	8,687	22,178
Number of individuals	84,978	36,488	108,672
Sample size (individuals in sample as % total population[a])	0.18%	0.17%	0.3%
Organisation that conducted survey	Statistics South Africa	Ghana Statistical Service	National Bureau of Statistics

[a]National population of Tanzania, 36.5 million; Ghana, 22 million; South Africa, 46.9 million (PRB, 2005).

expenditure on durable items was measured as reported income/expenditure in the past 12 months within the main household survey. Consumption expenditure on food and non-durable items was collected by means of monthly household diaries for the same sample of households.

Whilst the national survey data provided detailed information on income and consumption expenditure, they generally lacked detailed information on OOP payments for health services and on contributions to health insurance schemes. OOP payment data were collected in aggregate as expenditure in the past year, with no means of associating expenditure with visits to particular providers or breaking down expenditure by line item (e.g. drugs, tests and travel). Furthermore, in Tanzania, at the time of data collection, individuals were not yet fully benefiting from the NHIF.

Consequently, for the purposes of the study, each country team also carried out their own household survey to compile detailed information on OOP payments associated with health care seeking by type of provider visited and for each category of insured and non-insured groups, as well as information on general household characteristics and socio-demographic characteristics of households, and health status.

In Tanzania and Ghana, the survey was carried out in 6 districts and covered a total of 2,234 and 2,960 households, respectively. In both countries, sampling was stratified according to rural and urban areas and health insurance membership status to ensure that the full range of health insurance schemes (mandatory and voluntary) were represented. These samples were not designed to be nationally representative but rather to allow the calculation, with statistical confidence, of the impact of insurance membership on utilisation of health care and associated OOP expenditures. In South Africa, the survey comprised all nine provinces of South Africa and was nationally representative. It had a sample size of 4,800 households. One of the purposes of this chapter is to illustrate how supplementing secondary with primary household survey data can improve the accuracy of financing incidence analyses.

FINANCING INCIDENCE ANALYSIS

FIA is concerned with the assessment of which socio-economic groups bear the burden of health care financing, in terms of taxes, insurance contributions and OOP expenditures, or the relative progressivity of financing mechanisms relative to living standards. The living standards measure to classify households into socio-economic groups is therefore a key component in the analysis, and we begin by considering how this might be done. We then review the financing incidence methods used for tax incidence, OOP payments and insurance.

MEASURING AND CATEGORISING SOCIO-ECONOMIC STATUS

Living standards are generally defined in terms of reported income, consumption expenditure or a composite index of SES (O'Donnell et al., 2008). Reported income is not usually considered appropriate for SES classification, particularly in low- and middle-income countries with large informal sectors and considerable subsistence agriculture. In these settings, income is frequently under-reported and consumption expenditure, which is smoothed over periods of variable income, is regarded as more indicative of living standards. For example, while there was little difference between per capita income and consumption expenditure (mean $349 and $387) in Tanzania, per capita expenditure was about 35% greater than income in South Africa (mean $4,707 and $3,493 respectively). Given uncertainties about income, our primary method of living standards measurement for the financing incidence analysis was per capita consumption expenditure (including the value of subsistence consumption).

A key challenge faced by the SHIELD team was the need to draw on data from both the secondary household surveys (particularly for the tax incidence analysis) and the primary household surveys conducted specifically for SHIELD (particularly for assessing the incidence of OOP payments). This was undertaken by means of a composite index of SES. In Ghana and Tanzania, both secondary and primary datasets collected detailed information on ownership of assets and housing particulars; the identical questions contained in the secondary household survey on these variables were included in the primary survey questionnaire to ensure consistency. In line with international practice, principal component analysis (PCA) was applied to the secondary household survey data to construct the composite index (Filmer & Pritchett, 2001). We divided households into quintiles, or five groups of equal sizes, based on the absolute size of index value (e.g. Vyas & Kumaranayake, 2006; Mckenzie, 2004; Chuma & Molyneux, 2008; Filmer & Pritchett, 2001; Schellenberg et al., 2003). This index was then applied to the data in the primary household survey to be able to allocate households into one of the five quintiles, and in this way link the data in the primary and secondary household surveys. The average consumption expenditure in each quintile (estimated from the secondary household survey) was used to calculate the percentage of household consumption expenditure devoted to funding health care.

In South Africa, the secondary data source did not include data on assets and housing characteristics, and therefore, information on non-durable consumption expenditure was collected in the SHIELD survey, allowing the linking of the two datasets.

Having established the SES measure to classify households, the next stage is to estimate the amount of health sector funding contributed by each of the socio-economic quintiles in terms of tax, OOP payments and insurance contributions. All our analyses of financial data are presented in 2005 prices (the latest year for which data were available) and adjusted when necessary using the general consumer price index.

EVALUATING FINANCING INCIDENCE

Health care financing incidence studies typically examine how the burden of health financing is distributed across socio-economic groups, and to what extent the burden of health financing affects the underlying distribution of income (Wagstaff, 2002). It is generally believed that health care ought to be financed according to ATP; this is partly to ensure equity in access to health care and also to avoid impoverishment resulting from health care utilisation in case of need. The incidence of health financing is, therefore, considered in terms of the share of income constituted by health care payments and the rate at which this share rises with income. Health care payments are said to be proportional if the payments comprise an equal share of household income across socio-economic groups; they are regressive if the share of income devoted to health care payments decreases as income rises; they are progressive if the share of income rises as income rises. Most commonly, the degree of progressivity of health financing is measured in terms of the Kakwani index (Kakwani, 1977). Health financing is then considered to be progressive if the index is positive, regressive if the index is negative, and proportional if the index is zero.

The first step to analysing financing incidence is to assess the progressivity of each source of financing, and then to establish the overall progressivity of the system. In the current study, we used consumption expenditure as a measure of ATP or income, due to the limitations of income outlined earlier. The average amount of per capita health care payments made (by each source of financing) is then considered for each of five socio-economic groups, in relation to the average consumption expenditure per capita of that group.

In low- and middle-income countries where a large share of health care financing is attributable to OOP payments and voluntary health insurance (whether commercial or community-based pre-payment schemes), there are important caveats in the interpretation of financing incidence. As indicated by O'Donnell et al. (2008, p. 474) 'Interest in the distribution of health financing arises, in part, from its potential redistributive effect ... a redistributive interpretation cannot be placed on payments that are voluntary and made in direct return for health care [i.e. out-of-pocket payments, but also private voluntary insurance] ... With respect to such payments, it is their impact on utilisation of health care ... that is the major equity concern ... ' It is for this reason that the SHIELD project is also undertaking a comprehensive benefit incidence analysis (to be reported on in future publications) to complement the interpretation of the financing incidence findings.

TAX INCIDENCE ANALYSIS

This section reviews the methods used to assess tax incidence, or who bears the burden of tax payments by socio-economic group. Tax incidence incorporates direct (income and corporate tax) and indirect taxes (VAT, excise, fuel taxes and import and export duty). In keeping with published tax incidence analyses, a series of incidence assumptions were made based on our knowledge of the local context. In part, this requires us to make assumptions about the pattern of tax shifting (or who ultimately pays the tax). Where possible, we first review what has been done elsewhere, and then highlight our own methods, indicating how we have dealt with knowledge gaps.

Assessment of Personal Income Tax Incidence

Owing to the unreliability of reported income, a number of studies appear to have based their assessment of income tax incidence on data obtained by tax authorities, using the income classification defined by these authorities (e g. Younger, Sahn, Haggblade, & Dorosh, 1999; Tabi, Urie, & Etoh-Anzah, 2004). However, as the primary method of classifying households by SES in a lower income setting is through consumption expenditure and composite indices, secondary household data sources are the only option for the assessment of income tax incidence.

There are three possible variables reported in Living Standards Measurement Surveys (LSMS) (or equivalent) that could be used to estimate personal income tax:

1. the income variable itself (excluding earnings in kind and interest on dividends), which is an estimate of reported gross income (method 1);
2. average consumption expenditure adjusted to reflect gross income, which relies on the assumption that tax payments do not impact on the tax bracket that individuals fall into (method 2) and[2]
3. reported income tax payments (method 3).

In higher income countries, studies have tended to rely on reported income tax payments derived from income and expenditure surveys (e.g. Wagstaff et al., 1999), but such data is less reliable in lower income settings. In Tanzania, for example, only 0.21% of the sample reported paying income tax, although 47% were identified as earners. In South Africa, the proportion reporting tax payments was higher (23.7%) but remains lower than expected.

When using reported income or consumption expenditure data as a basis for tax calculation, it is difficult to identify who is actually eligible to pay tax As far as we are aware, this issue has not been discussed in the existing literature, because of the reliance upon reported tax payments. In Tanzania, we decided to adopt a fairly inclusive definition of eligibility, where anybody

Table 4. Income Tax Progressivity: A Comparison of Three Methods of Tax Calculation (Tanzania).

Quintiles of Socio-economic Status	Income Tax Payments as a Proportion of Consumption Expenditure		
	Method 1	Method 2	Method 3
1	1%	0.0%	0.0%
2	1%	0.3%	0.1%
3	1%	1%	0.2%
4	5%	5%	0.4%
5	25%	30%	2%
Kakwani index	0.48	0.50	0.36

whose reported main activity was formal sector employment was included as a potential tax payer, and a variable entitled 'earner' used to identify them. Then, the average income per earner was estimated, based on household income data as individual income data were not available. This approach was not required in South Africa where we had individual level data.

We consider the effect of each of the three methods of income tax estimation on the progressivity of income tax payments, drawing from the example of Tanzania (Table 4).

All three methods result in a progressive tax distribution. The most striking difference between the three methods is in terms of the overall burden of tax on consumption expenditure. Reported tax implies virtually no tax payments by the first 4 quintiles, with the highest quintile only contributing 2% of household consumption expenditure. In contrast, the distribution of tax based on either income or consumption expenditure illustrate that the highest quintile are contributing a quarter or more of their income as income tax.

For future surveys, and to increase response rates, it may be helpful to add a question on whether an individual pays income tax, in addition to the amount of tax paid, to facilitate identification of tax payers.

Assessment of Corporate Income Tax Incidence

There is no consensus in the literature as to how to deal with corporate income tax in terms of incidence assumptions (e.g. Nevin, 1963; Bradford, 1981; Kotlikoff & Summers, 1987). It is generally assumed that shareholders, capital owners (typically higher income groups) and consumers (typically lower income groups) bear the burden of the tax through lower profits and higher prices on goods and services, respectively (Martinez-Vazquez, 2001). It has been noted that market conditions and the degree of competition can affect the allocation of the burden, with consumers being more likely to bear the burden as the degree of monopoly power increases (Herberger, 1962). We considered three scenarios and their impact on the progressivity of corporate tax:

1. that consumers bear the full burden of corporate tax (scenario 1);
2. that the tax burden is shared equally between consumers and shareholders (scenario 2) and
3. that shareholders bear the full burden of corporate tax (scenario 3).

Using the secondary data sources, shareholders were identified as those reporting revenue from dividends. They were assumed to lie in the highest wealth groups. Indeed, in South Africa, over 97% of dividends received were amongst those in the top quintile. However, in Tanzania, only 3% of households reported receiving dividends, and they were fairly evenly distributed across socio-economic groups. To estimate the burden of corporate tax on consumers, a list of the products manufactured by the companies responsible for 70% of overall corporate tax payments were also obtained, and the tax allocated to individuals consuming these products (as for VAT).

Assumptions regarding corporate tax calculation have a significant effect on the resulting tax progressivity, as seen in the example of South Africa (Table 5). When assuming the tax is fully passed on to consumers, the result is highly regressive, with the first quintile contributing twice as much of their income as the highest quintile. The second scenario is almost proportional, and the third scenario is highly progressive.

Table 5.   Progressivity of Corporate Tax Using Three Scenarios.

Quintiles of Socio-economic Status	Scenario 1	Scenario 2	Scenario 3
1	24.3%	12.3%	0.3%
2	21.4%	11.6%	1.9%
3	19.2%	10.1%	1.1%
4	17.6%	9.2%	0.8%
5	12.4%	16.4%	20.4%
Kakwani index	−0.12	0.06	0.19

The assumptions used to measure corporate tax also have a significant effect on total tax incidence. For example, using the assumption of scenario 3, total tax incidence appears to be highly progressive, ranging from 18% of consumption expenditure for Q1 to 56% for Q5. Whereas when we use the assumptions of scenario 1, total tax incidence shifts to 42% for Q1 to 48% for Q5. This wipes out the relative progressivity of some of the other taxes so that total tax incidence is nearly proportional.

Assessment of Indirect Tax Incidence

The assessment of VAT followed the standard methods that have been employed in other studies, and we assumed that the tax is shifted to the consumer (Martinez-Vazquez, 2001).

Excise tax is levied on certain locally manufactured goods as well as their imported equivalents and is applied at specific rates (e.g. tobacco, alcohol and fuel) and ad valorem (e.g. for cars and other luxury goods). Ad valorem excise duty revenue can be easily apportioned to households according to their share of consumption of goods that are subject to ad valorem tax, in the same way as VAT.

To estimate taxes paid for those commodities with a tax rate dependent on the quantity consumed, it is possible to use information derived from the LSMS on related expenditure combined with unit retail price information for the respective commodities in 2005. In this way, the quantity (or number of taxable units consumed) could be measured for each household and the tax rate applied and total tax payments estimated.

However, in some cases, the LSMS do not provide adequate disaggregation of commodities to allow for a precise tax calculation. For example, the tax rates on imported/local, filter/non-filter cigarettes were very different; yet, it is not possible to ascertain the type of cigarette consumed from the LSMS. In such cases, national data can be obtained on consumption patterns of cigarettes (from tobacco company advertising agencies) to assess the likelihood of individuals smoking each type of cigarette. Similar issues were faced in the disaggregation of taxes on wines. For spirits and brewed beer in South Africa, the tax is levied per litre of absolute alcohol content. An average of 5% alcohol content was used for beer and 43% for spirits, based on a survey of beer and spirits sold in shops in South Africa.

Fuel levy is a specific excise tax levied on petrol (leaded or unleaded), kerosene and diesel. It is paid by private users, commercial users and businesses. For private users, expenditure on fuel was obtained from the secondary datasets. The number of litres consumed can then be estimated as a function of the price of each fuel type in 2005 and reported consumption expenditure on fuel. The excise tax payments were then based on the number of litres consumed.

For commercial or 'public transport' users, the calculation is more challenging. Previous studies have made the crude assumption that 20% of the cost of transportation is attributed to gasoline tax based on input-output coefficients (Younger et al., 1999). In our case, we assumed that the fuel levy is shifted to consumers reporting expenditure on minibus taxis, buses, bakkies[3] and cabs. We calculated taxes based on a range of parameters including expenditure on transport, the average cost of the form of transport per kilometer (charges per km and average number of passengers) and average rate of fuel consumption for each form of transport.

We assumed that fuel tax accruing to businesses was also passed on to consumers.

It is often assumed that import duties passed on to the consumer have the same incidence as VAT in the absence of information regarding consumption of imported versus local goods (Martinez-Vazquez, 2001). We followed two approaches in our calculations. Firstly, using standard methods, we obtained information from the tax authorities regarding the key import commodities in the country and allocated the total value of import tax generated from these commodities across those individuals reporting expenditure on these items. In a second stage, we identified consumers of those commodities that are both imported and locally produced and made assumptions about the likelihood of the good having been imported or locally produced based on national statistics on domestic production versus imports of given commodities. The tax rate was then applied to the amount apportioned to imports.

Export taxes for goods produced by small farmers may fall on the producer. Taxes on larger companies may effectively be transferred to foreign consumers. However, as export taxes were so small in our countries, they were not included in the calculation of FIA.

Adjustments to Aggregate Tax Estimates

Estimates of total tax payments derived from the above-mentioned analyses of national survey data will inevitably be lower than those reported as received by the tax revenue authority, as the former are based on a series of assumptions (Robilliard & Robinson, 2001). In South Africa, for example, the total estimate for personal income tax was 15.4% lower than that reported by the South African Revenue Service (SARS). To adjust for this underestimation, the difference between the survey-based estimate and the actual revenue collected for each type of tax was allocated across households based on their proportional share of contributions to that particular tax.

HEALTH INSURANCE

Household surveys in many countries (including South Africa and Ghana), which collate data on income and expenditure, include questions on contributions to health insurance organisations. However, these surveys can heavily underestimate the actual contributions to health insurance schemes.

Contribution levels may be underestimated for various reasons. In the formal sector, insurance contributions may be shared between employers and employees. Employees will not report on employer contributions unless specifically requested to and are frequently unsure of the level of employer contributions. They are also typically unaware of the exact value of their own contributions to health insurance, which are deducted directly from payroll. For example, in South Africa, the Income and Expenditure Survey indicated that a total of R23.8 billion was contributed by individuals and R21.1 billion by employers to medical schemes. In reality, based on reporting of all schemes to the regulatory body (the Council for Medical Schemes), total medical scheme contributions were R54.2 billion in 2005.

One approach to addressing this deficiency in household survey data is to secure information on total health insurance contributions either from individual schemes themselves or from a regulatory authority if insurance schemes are required to report to such an agency (in South Africa, schemes report regularly to the Council for Medical Schemes). An assumption could be made that the household surveys at least accurately reflect the distribution of health insurance contributions across socio-economic groups (i.e. that total contributions could be distributed across socio-economic groups according to the respective shares indicated in the household survey). However, it is possible that the proportion of health insurance contributions paid by employers may vary across socio-economic groups (e.g. employers may pay a greater proportion of contributions on behalf of lower income employees). Hence, the extent of the under-reporting of insurance contributions may be greater for some socio-economic groups than for others.

For this reason, it was necessary to triangulate between estimates based on the secondary household survey data and the data secured directly from health insurance schemes. In the South African context, data was obtained from the largest medical schemes and administrators, which were able to provide information on the majority of total medical scheme beneficiaries. Not all schemes were able to provide information on members' income levels (as contributions are only income-related in certain 'closed schemes' – i.e. schemes that are restricted to employees of a specific company, industry or sector). Nevertheless, it was possible to obtain information on contributions for individual benefit options within the largest schemes, and a broad socio-economic profile of those choosing each option. Data from the insurance schemes were used to assess whether the distribution of contributions across socio-economic groups from the household survey was accurate and provided a basis for undertaking sensitivity analyses on the incidence of health insurance contributions.

A key assumption made in the health insurance incidence analysis was that the burden of all insurance contributions is borne by the household, even if employers pay something towards these contributions. The basis for this assumption is that although employers may claim that contributions they make on behalf of their employees are an additional employment benefit, in reality most employers (certainly in South Africa) operate on a total 'cost to company' basis. Thus, they have a total remuneration package ceiling that they are willing to pay. If health insurance contributions increase more rapidly than expected in a particular year, they will offset this cost by agreeing to relatively lower increases in the cash salary component. The same assumption has been made in earlier studies (O'Donnell et al., 2008).

In Tanzania, the 2001 household budget survey (HBS) did not include any questions on contributions to insurance schemes. Our own household survey data gives an indication of the socio-economic levels of insured groups in Tanzania (public insurance, community insurance and private insurance). Private health insurance cover is limited to the highest income groups. Community Health Fund contributions are restricted to the rural population and are regressive as the premiums are community rated and the same for all. Furthermore, the concentration of community health insurance membership is amongst the poor (75% of members earning less than $70 per month), and only 1% earning more than $300 per month. The NHIF membership caters to a larger proportion of higher income earners. Only 4% of NHIF members have household monthly incomes less than $70, and 11% have incomes above $300. The premiums represent a fixed proportion of income, and therefore, the distribution of financing in terms of insurance contributions amongst members is proportional. The government matches these contributions (as the employer) from general tax revenue.

In Ghana, comprehensive data on NHI payments is being collected in the case study and will be used to triangulate with the Ghana Living Standards Survey (GLSS) data on insurance contributions.

OUT-OF-POCKET PAYMENTS

Once again, household surveys frequently under-report OOP expenditure on health services. This is sometimes due to long recall periods in the household survey (typically previous 12 months). Another reason is because sometimes the questions on OOP spending are linked to questions on recent illness and service utilisation for that illness. This means that health service use for other reasons (e.g. for ante-natal care, other preventive services and deliveries), and associated OOP payments, will not be reported. In addition, survey questionnaires generally only ask about the use of one service while many people may have used more than one service during an illness episode.

Given the magnitude of OOP spending in many countries, we undertook our own household surveys to obtain a precise measure of the extent of OOP payments (both formal and informal) and their distribution across socio-economic groups. The surveys ask about outpatient service use by any household member in the previous month, recording all visits to all service providers and OOP payments for the most recent visit. Average OOP payments for each type of service were calculated and applied to each reported visit. Similar data were collected for hospitalisations, using a one-year recall period. These were separated into user fees in government and private facilities and co-payments for the insured population, based on the insurance status of the household member. Whilst OOP payments were found to be largely concentrated amongst the better off in Asia (O'Donnell et al., 2008), in South Africa, OOP payments were found to be regressive with expenditures representing a slightly higher proportion of consumption expenditure in the lowest quintiles (1.8% in quintile 1 compared with 1.6% in quintile 5). In Tanzania, the non-insured incurred significantly higher costs during outpatient visits than the insured.

These estimates were then triangulated against other sources of data on OOP payments. In relation to user fees at government facilities, information on total user fee revenue was obtained from the Department of Health in the case of South Africa and National Health Accounts data in Ghana and

Tanzania. In the case of OOP payments by the insured population, information on the difference between claims submitted to the insurance scheme and the amount paid by the scheme was obtained directly from the insurance organisations. It is recognised that this will be an underestimate as the insured will not submit claims for services that are not covered in the scheme's benefit package or when their benefits for the year have been exhausted. Nevertheless, based on data obtained directly from medical scheme administrators, it was estimated that OOP payments by scheme members was approximately R7 billion. In contrast, household survey data indicated that OOP payments by medical scheme members were well below R2 billion. Where the household survey under-reported OOP payments, the difference was allocated to individual socio-economic groups according to the distribution of total OOP payments across the groups identified through the household survey.

DISCUSSION

Researchers from African countries interested in undertaking finance incidence studies will face considerable challenges. The current literature on financing incidence does not provide clear guidance on tackling these practical challenges. This chapter presented an overview of how we addressed these methodological challenges when undertaking health care financing incidence studies in three sub-Saharan African countries as part of the SHIELD project. It particularly highlights issues arising from problems with access to, and quality of, data used for analysing the distribution of health care financing between socio-economic groups.

The first step was to investigate and use secondary data sources, most commonly large national household surveys of reported income and expenditure. These national datasets have been designed for several purposes and do not provide all the appropriate information needed. Most commonly, these surveys are the main source of data for estimating the incidence of various taxes but lack reliable information about OOP payments and levels of health insurance scheme contributions. In all three countries, new household surveys were undertaken to fill these gaps, albeit with smaller sample sizes than the secondary surveys.

To link data from the secondary and primary household survey datasets, a comparable measure of SES had to be applied. Given the difficulty of collecting comprehensive and accurate data on household income or consumption expenditure in surveys whose primary purpose is to collect information on health care utilisation, expenditure and financing, a composite SES index was used in some countries as the mechanism for linking the two datasets. The major constraint with this approach was that the variables that could be included in constructing the composite index were governed by the indicators contained in the secondary household surveys. In this way, it was possible to assess health care financing contributions drawn from the primary household surveys (particularly OOP payments and health insurance contributions) as a proportion of household consumption expenditure.

While the primary household surveys filled some of the gaps we identified, the other strategy we used was to triangulate our estimates with information from a wide range of secondary sources. Other financing incidence studies (such as those produced by the ECuity Project and Equity in Asia-Pacific Health Systems (EQUITAP)) have triangulated estimates of tax revenue based on household surveys with actual revenue reported by the tax collection authorities, but do not appear to have undertaken extensive triangulation for other health care financing mechanisms. OOP payments are an important financing mechanism in many low- and middle-income countries, yet are often heavily under-reported in household surveys. We sought to triangulate data obtained from the household surveys with other data sources to obtain a more comprehensive and accurate estimate of the extent and distribution of OOP payments. For example, one of the largest components of OOP payments is spending on medicines. Information on total retail sales of medicines is often tracked by market research and related companies (such as IMS, http://www.imshealth.com) and if spending on medicines by health insurance schemes is deducted from this total, an accurate estimate of OOP spending on medicines can be obtained.

This chapter has illustrated how innovative techniques and thinking can be used to overcome data weaknesses in lower income settings. There is also a need to improve data routinely collected by the official statistics organisations. For example, the FIA could have been enhanced if the living standards or income and expenditure surveys in these three countries had included questions on:

- whether members of each household pay income tax (as opposed to only asking about amounts of income tax paid);
- whether household members hold any shares, along with a clear definition of what is meant by shareholding to avoid confusion (as opposed to only asking about dividend receipts, which seems to have unreliable reporting) and

- cigarette and alcohol consumption patterns in greater detail (specifically, consumption of imported versus local cigarettes, filter versus non-filter cigarettes; consumption of wine versus other spirits, and of local versus imported spirits).

Through undertaking primary household surveys and extensive triangulation with a wide range of secondary data sources, we have been able to undertake comprehensive assessments of health care financing incidence within Ghana, South Africa and Tanzania (whose results will be reported in other publications in the near future). We believe that it is important to invest in these additional data collection efforts to minimise the assumptions that are made in financing incidence analyses, so as to provide the most comprehensive and accurate data possible to promote truly evidence-informed health financing policy making.

NOTES

1. In the case of South Africa, these were updated from secondary sources (McIntyre et al., 2007).
2. One potential challenge with this approach is financial transfers to other family members. Consumption expenditure could conceivably be lower than their taxable income as a result of making the transfer, resulting in an underestimation of tax payments or the misclassification of an individual in a lower tax category.
3. A light delivery vehicle (LDV) that is a truck of one ton or less as used in South Africa. They are often used to convey passengers for monetary rewards.

ACKNOWLEDGMENTS

The authors would like to thank SHIELD colleagues who contributed to workshop discussions on the methodological challenges reviewed in this chapter (Moses Aikins, Mariam Ally, Bertha Garshong, Jahangir Khan and Anne Mills).

We also gratefully acknowledge the financial support of the European Commission (Sixth Framework Programme; Specific Targeted Research Project no: 32289), without which this research would not have been possible. DM is supported by the South African Research Chairs Initiative of the Department of Science and Technology and National Research Foundation. The usual disclaimers apply.

REFERENCES

Bradford, D. F. (1981). The incidence and allocation effects of a tax on corporate distributions. *Journal of Public Economics, 15*, 1–22.

Chuma, J., & Molyneux, C. (2008). Estimating inequalities in ownership of insecticide treated nets: Does the choice of socio-economic status measure matter? *Health Policy & Planning, 24*(2), 83–93.

Filmer, D., & Pritchett, L. H. (2001). *Estimating wealth effect with expenditure data – or tears: An application to educational enrollments in states of India, 38*(1), 115–132.

Herberger, A. C. (1962). The incidence of corporation income tax. *Journal of Political Economy, 70*(3), 215–240.

International Labour Organization. (2007). Africa: Community-based micro-insurance for universal health coverage. 11th African Regional Meeting. Addis Ababa, 24–27 April.

Kakwani, N. C. (1977). Measurement of tax progressivity: An international comparison. *Economic Journal, 87*, 71–80.

Kotlikoff, L. J., & Summers, L. H. (1987). Tax incidence. In: A. J. Auerbach & M. Feldstein (Eds), *Handbook of public economics* (Vol. 2, pp. 1043–1092). North-Holland: Amsterdam.

Martinez-Vazquez, J. (2001). *The impact of fiscal policy on the poor: Fiscal incidence analysis* (International Studies Program Working Paper Series 01–10, Georgia State University, Georgia).

McIntyre, D., Garshong, B., Mtei, G., Meheus, F., Thiede, M., Akazili, J., Ally, M., Aikins, M., Mulligan, J., & Goudge, J. (2008). Beyond fragmentation and towards universal coverage: Insights from Ghana, South Africa and Tanzania. *Bulletin of the World Health Organisation, 86*, 871–876.

McIntyre, D., Thiede, M., Nkosi, M., Mutyambizi, V., Castillo-Riquelme, M., Goudge, J., Gilson, L., & Erasmus, E. (2007). *A critical analysis of the current South African health system*. Cape Town: Health Economics Unit, University of Cape Town and Centre for Health Policy, University of the Witwatersrand.

McKenzie, DJ. (2004). *Measuring inequality with asset indicators* (BREAD Working Paper no. 42). Cambridge, MA: Bureau for Research and Economic Analysis of Development.

MOH. (2006). *National Health Accounts Ghana*. Accra: Ministry of Health.

MOHSW. (2001). *National Health Accounts Tanzania*. Dar es Salaam: Ministry of Health and Social Welfare.

National Treasury. (2005). *2005 Budget review*. Pretoria: National Treasury.

Nevin, E. (1963). Taxation for growth-A factor tax. *Westminster Bank Review* (November), 13–25.

O'Donnell, O, Doorslaer, E, Rannan-Eliya, RP, Somanathan, A, Adhikari, SR, Akkazieva, B, Harbianto, D, et al. (2008). Who pays for health care in Asia? *Journal of Health Economics, 27*, 460–475.

Population Reference Bureau – PRB. (2005). *2005 World population data sheet*. Washington, DC: PRB.

RAGB. (2005). *2005 Tax revenue returns of Ghana*. Ghana: Ministry of Finance and Economic Planning.

Robilliard, A. S., & Robinson, S. (2001). *Reconciling household surveys and national accounts data using a cross entropy estimation method* (TMD Discussion paper no. 50. International Food Policy Research Institute, Washington, DC).

Schellenberg, J. A., Victora, C. G., Mushi, A., de Savigny, D., Schellenberg, D., Mshinda, H., & Bryce, J. for the Tanzania IMCI MCE baseline household survey study group. (2003).

Inequities among the very poor: Health care for children in southern Tanzania. *The Lancet, 361,* 561–566.

Tabi, A. J., Urie, E. J., & Etoh-Anzah, P (2004). *The distributive impact of fiscal policy in Cameroon: Tax and Benefit Incidence.*

Vyas, S., & Kumaranayake, L. (2006). How to do (or not to do)... Constructing socioeconomic indices: How to use principal components analysis. *Health Policy and Planning, 21*(6), 459–468.

Wagstaff, A. (2002). Reflections on and alternatives to WHO's fairness of financial contribution index. *Health Economics, 11,* 103–115.

Wagstaff, A., van Doorslaer, E., van der Burg, H., Calonge, S., Christiansen, T., Citoni, G., Gerdtham, U. G., et al. (1999). Equity in the finance of health care: Some further international comparisons. *Journal of Health Economics, 18,* 263–290.

World Health Organization. (2005). *"Sustainable health financing, universal coverage and social health insurance": World Health Assembly resolution WHA58.33.* Geneva: World Health Organization.

Younger, S. D., Sahn, D. E., Haggblade, S., & Dorosh, P. A. (1999). Tax incidence in madagascar: An analysis using household data. *The World Bank Economic Review, 13*(2), 303–331.

SECTION III
SECURING CARE

THE ROLE OF RISK EQUALIZATION IN MOVING FROM VOLUNTARY PRIVATE HEALTH INSURANCE TO MANDATORY COVERAGE: THE EXPERIENCE IN SOUTH AFRICA

Heather McLeod and Pieter Grobler

ABSTRACT

Objective – *The South African health system has long been characterised by extreme inequalities in the allocation of financial and human resources. Voluntary private health insurance, delivered through medical schemes, accounts for some 60% of total expenditure but serves only the 14.8% of the population with higher incomes. A plan was articulated in 1994 to move to a National Health Insurance system with risk-adjusted payments to competing health funds, income cross-subsidies and mandatory membership for all those in employment, leading over time to universal coverage. This chapter describes the core institutional mechanism envisaged for a National Health Insurance system, the Risk Equalisation Fund (REF). A key issue that has emerged is the appropriate sequencing*

Innovations in Health System Finance in Developing and Transitional Economies
Advances in Health Economics and Health Services Research, Volume 21, 159–196
ISSN: 0731-2199/doi:10.1108/S0731-2199(2009)0000021010

of the reforms and the impact on workers of possible trajectories is considered.

Methodology – *The design and functioning of the REF is described and the impact on competing health insurance funds is illustrated. Using a reference family earning at different income levels, the impact on workers of various trajectories of reform is demonstrated.*

Findings – *Risk equalization is a critical institutional component in moving towards a system of social or national health insurance in competitive markets, but the sequence of its implementation needs to be carefully considered. The adverse impact of risk equalization on low-income workers in the absence of income cross-subsidies and mandatory membership is considerable.*

Implications for policy – *The South African experience of risk equalization is of interest as it attempts to introduce more solidarity into a small but highly competitive private insurance market. The methodology for considering the impact of reforms provides policy-makers and politicians with a clearer understanding of the consequences of reform.*

INTRODUCTION

In May 2005, the Fifty-Eighth World Health Assembly endorsed a resolution calling on member states to work towards universal coverage and pre-payment for healthcare services (World Health Organization, 2005). Countries were called on to share experiences on different methods of health financing, including the development of social health insurance schemes, with particular reference to the institutional mechanisms that are established to address the principal functions of the health financing system. A report on the status of healthcare funding in Africa (Kirigia, Preker, Carrin, Mwikisa, & Diarra-Nama, 2006) concluded that countries need a comprehensive health financing strategic plan with a clear roadmap of how to transit to universal coverage.

In South Africa, there was an attempt in 1944 to introduce universal coverage through a National Health System, similar to that of Britain. The attempt failed when the political landscape changed in 1948 and the subsequent decades under *apartheid* saw increasing privatisation of healthcare. The new democratic government in 1994 had prepared a plan for healthcare reform and a system of National Health Insurance (African National Congress, 1994). The plan envisaged that there would be risk-adjusted payments to competing health funds, income cross-subsidies and mandatory membership for all those in employment, leading over time to universal coverage. As work has progressed since 1994 to prepare the detail of the transition, there has been new understanding of the complexities of the reform and the difficulties in sequencing the reforms.

The goal of this chapter is to describe the reforms needed to move from voluntary health insurance to a system of National Health Insurance with a particular focus on the role of risk equalization. A key issue that has emerged is the appropriate sequencing of the reforms, and the impact on workers of possible trajectories is considered to recommend a preferred sequence of reform.

This chapter describes the core institutional mechanism envisaged for a National Health Insurance system, the Risk Equalisation Fund (REF).[1] The chapter begins with an explanation of the existing healthcare system in South Africa and the reforms envisaged for National Health Insurance. The design and functioning of the REF is described and the impact on competing health insurance funds is illustrated. A series of related reforms is described and their impact explored. The problem with sequencing the reforms is demonstrated and suggestions made as to the preferred reform trajectory.

THE CURRENT HEALTH SYSTEM IN SOUTH AFRICA

The South African health system has long been characterised by extreme inequalities in the allocation of financial and human resources. During the *apartheid* years, the inequalities were established on the basis of race, but despite a strong commitment since 1994, progress has been limited and income inequality has worsened. As a result, inequalities in healthcare are increasingly related to socio-economic class rather than race (Harrison, Bhana, & Ntuli, 2007; McIntyre & Thiede, 2007).

The delivery system is a mix of robust private sector, struggling public sector and some non-governmental not-for-profit organisations. The National Health Act of 2003 makes it clear that all of these form part of the National Health System under the stewardship of the Minister of Health. Approximately 60% of the total expenditure on healthcare in the country flows through private intermediaries and only 40% through the

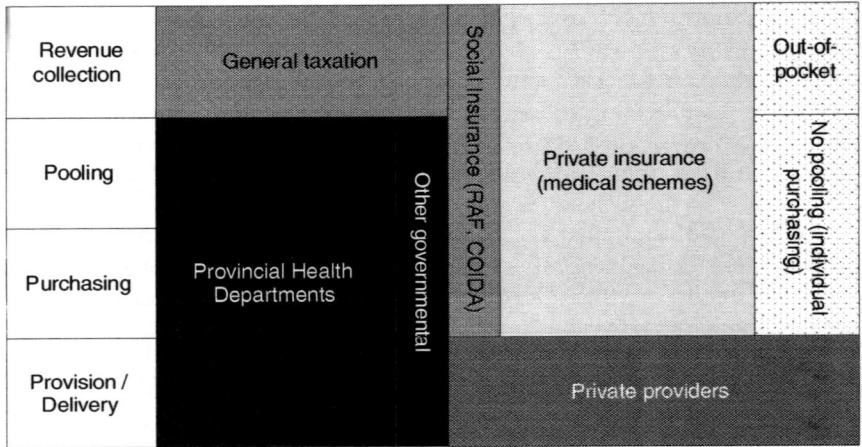

Fg. 1. Current Healthcare Financing in South Africa. *Note:* RAF is the Road Accident Fund. COIDA is the Fund that Provides Compensation for Occupational Injuries and Diseases. Both RAF and COIDA are Funded by Mandatory Levies and use Private Providers to Deliver Care. Out-of-Pocket Payments Include all Amounts Paid Directly by Consumers, Whether as Medical Savings Accounts or as Conventional Out-of-Pocket Payments. *Source:* Ministerial Task Team on Social Health Insurance (2005).

public sector. The Kutzin diagram[2] for South Africa, drawn on the basis of healthcare expenditure, is shown in Fig. 1.

Private health insurance has been in existence since 1889 but remains voluntary. Although it accounts for 60% of total expenditure, it serves only the 14.8% of the population with higher incomes (McIntyre & van den Heever, 2007). The vehicles for private health insurance, known as medical schemes, reimburse their members for actual expenditure on health and are governed under the Medical Schemes Act of 1998. The Council for Medical Schemes[3] is the regulator established under this legislation to protect the interests of beneficiaries. Medical schemes are run on a not-for-profit basis and are essentially mutual societies, owned by their members. They are governed by boards of trustees of which 50% must be elected from the members.

Healthcare is delivered to medical scheme members predominantly in the private sector that is well developed, resource intensive and highly specialised (Harrison et al., 2007). It is estimated (McIntyre & van den Heever, 2007) that 21.0% of the population are not covered by health insurance but prefer to use private primary care doctors and pharmacies on an out-of-pocket basis. This group is almost entirely dependent on the public sector for specialist and hospital care. The remaining 64.2% of the population are dependent on the public sector for all their conventional healthcare services. User fees are charged in the public system and those earning an income of R6,000 per month[4] or more are required to pay in full at a tariff similar to private rates. However, the exemption policy has been liberally applied and bills are not always followed up, perpetuating a public belief that if they run out of medical scheme benefits, they can still obtain care in the public sector.

The major difficulty with the over-resourcing of private health insurance and under-resourcing of the public sector is that healthcare practitioners have been attracted to the more lucrative private system. South Africa has struggled for many years with an inequitable distribution of healthcare personnel. McIntyre and van den Heever (2007) estimate that there are 588 people per primary care practitioner in the private sector (including out-of-pocket usage), but 4,193 people per practitioner for the 64.2% of the population relying on public clinics. The situation with specialists is worse with medical scheme members having one practitioner for every 470 people, while the public sector has 10,811 people per specialist.

There is a tax subsidy for private healthcare that favours the highest income groups but gives no subsidy to those using private insurance that earn below the tax threshold. The tax subsidy for private insurance was estimated for 2005 to be R10.1 billion, 23.7% of the allocation of R42.5 million to the provinces to provide public sector healthcare. (Ministerial Task Team on Social Health Insurance, 2005). The tax break has reduced the sensitivity of higher income groups to the increases in contributions because until 2006 the subsidy escalated at the same rate as contributions. There is generally low awareness amongst individuals of the tax incentive for medical scheme membership.

Out-of-pocket payments account for almost a quarter of private healthcare financing, partly due to the use of personal individual medical savings accounts in many medical schemes.

REFORMS TO ENHANCE RISK POOLING

Free market reforms in private health insurance in the late 1980s and early 1990s had produced adverse results in terms of healthcare equity and access, with the elderly and those with chronic disease being most vulnerable. The new democratic government in 1994 began a process of re-regulation with the completely revised Medical Schemes Act, No. 131 of 1998. This provided for improved governance of medical schemes and for the re-introduction of three key policy issues that enhance the risk pooling function of schemes:

- *Open enrolment*: Open schemes have to accept anyone who wants to become a member at standard rates.
- *Community rating*: Everyone must be charged the same standard rate, regardless of age or state of health (i.e. charging by risk or risk rating is not allowed). However, the current implementation applies to each benefit *option* in each scheme rather than the *scheme* as a whole. Future changes will see community rating applying to the *industry* as a whole.
- *Prescribed minimum benefits (PMBs)*: A minimum package that must be offered by all schemes. Beneficiaries must be covered in full for these conditions[5] with no limits or co-payments.

To manage care for the PMBs, schemes may insist on the use of a contracted network of providers[6] and formularies[7] of medicines. Schemes are in theory able to negotiate fees with healthcare providers but have struggled both against the concentration of power amongst four large private hospital groups and against the complexity of negotiating with thousands of independent practitioners who are not well organised into collective bodies. In practice, most schemes adopt fee schedules that are some percentage of the National Health Reference Price List (NHRPL).

REFORMS FOR A NATIONAL HEALTH INSURANCE SYSTEM

A system of National Health Insurance[8] with income cross-subsidies, risk-adjusted payments and mandatory membership had been envisaged in policy papers from 1994 onwards (African National Congress, 1994; Broomberg & Shisana, 1995; Department of Social Development, 2002; Ministerial Task Team on Social Health Insurance, 2005). In January 2004, the Minister of Health stated there were three issues on the unfinished reform agenda towards implementing mandatory health insurance:

- The introduction of *risk-adjusted cross-subsidies*. This will effectively enforce community rating across all medical schemes so that everyone is charged the same standard rate[9] for the common PMB package, regardless of the benefit option or scheme they choose to join. This will be accomplished through a central REF.

- The introduction of *income-based cross-subsidies.* This de-links the purchase of healthcare from family affordability concerns. It enforces the primary solidarity mechanism under which people receive a common package of benefits according to healthcare needs and contribute to healthcare on the basis of their ability to pay. The REF would accept the income-related payments and in turn pay the amounts on a risk-adjusted basis to medical schemes.
- The creation of a *mandatory environment.* People earning above a certain amount would be required to contribute to mandatory health cover. The level at which contribution would be mandatory and the degree of progressiveness of the contribution has not been publicly debated. It was envisaged that as employment increased and incomes improved, more people would gradually become part of the mandatory system.

The proposals by the Department of Health[10] are expected to impact on the functions of the health system as follows:

- *Revenue collection*: The current role of medical schemes in collecting contributions would be replaced in respect of the minimum benefits by a central collection mechanism. The tax authority, the South African Revenue Service (SARS), has the most complete information on incomes and is thus the logical choice for collecting income-related revenue. Initially, the public sector system would still be tax-funded (also collected by SARS). The tax-funded revenue and an income-related contribution could be combined in a single stream and identified as National Health Insurance contributions.
- *Pooling*: The pooling function of medical schemes would be reduced as the REF and would function as a central pool. Risk-adjusted amounts would flow to each medical scheme and there would be residual pooling within each scheme. In the initial implementation, REF is intended to operate between competing private medical schemes, but it could readily be extended to make risk-adjusted payments to the public sector as well. A good example of the benefits that would flow from having a single risk equalization pool across public and private sectors is that the prevalence of human immunodeficiency virus (HIV)/acquired immune deficiency syndrome (AIDS) in private medical schemes is of the order of one-third of that in the general population. There are also substantial differences between the nine provinces, and risk-adjusted budgeting for the provinces could be done using this mechanism.

- *Purchasing*: The introduction of risk equalization should affect the purchasing function as schemes will be incentivised to compete less on the basis of risk selection and more on the basis of cost effective healthcare delivery. Medical schemes would be encouraged to move away from being passive purchasers to becoming more strategic purchasers of healthcare. A key problem in purchasing is that fee-for-service is still the dominant reimbursement mechanism despite attempts to enter into greater risk sharing with providers.
- *Delivery*: The focus in the reforms has been on changes to the revenue collection and pooling functions in healthcare financing in South Africa, and relatively, little has been written about reform of the delivery function. The National Health Act of 2003 envisages a mixed system of private and public providers. There are plans to improve the governance of the public sector as the quality of delivery remain uneven across the nine provinces.

BENEFIT OPTIONS AND INCENTIVES TO RISK SELECT

South Africa is unusual in having open enrolment, community rating and minimum benefits without risk equalization at present. In the absence of risk equalization, schemes are incentivised to 'risk select' or 'cream-skim' that is, to seek younger and healthier lives and design benefit packages that are not as attractive to those with chronic disease. The design of benefit packages by medical schemes is largely unfettered provided they include the PMBs. Schemes will typically offer several benefit options ranging from a capitated primary care and network option to an option with complete freedom of choice of providers. Benefits may also be designed to move the young and healthy to savings account plans that offer little more than in-hospital care and to move those with chronic disease to so-called comprehensive benefit options.

A fragmentation of risk pools occurs because schemes are required to treat each benefit option as a separate risk pool for community rating. Risk selection can thus effectively occur through benefit design despite open enrolment and community rating.

In 2007, there were 122 medical schemes (Council for Medical Schemes, 2008b), of which 41 were open schemes (open to any member of the public) and 81 were restricted schemes (restricted to an employer, profession, industry or union). These 122 schemes covered 3.179 million members and their families, covering 7.478 million beneficiaries in total. There were 345 benefit options registered in medical schemes in 2007. Consumers in the open fund market were confronted with a choice between 200 different benefit options. However, from 2006, the regulator has been increasingly refusing to register minor variations in benefits as separate benefit options.

In the current South African environment of community rating and open enrolment but with no REF, medical schemes have survived by competing on risk selection on a benefit option level, predominantly through the way that benefits are structured. Examples of benefit structuring to differentiate between the young and healthy and the older and chronic patients are

- differentiated benefits for oncology, organ transplants and dialysis;
- differentiated benefits for internal prosthesis as older patients are more likely to require this benefit;
- differentiated benefits for chronic medication with some benefit options providing just the PMBs, while others cover many more chronic diseases as well as richer formularies;
- older and chronic patients typically require more comprehensive out-of-hospital benefits.

Fig. 2 illustrates the extent to which the chronic disease rate by age can differ across benefit options in a large scheme. The overall scheme has a disease profile very similar to that expected for the industry.[11] Benefit option a has almost no chronic disease across the full range of ages while that for benefit options b and c is less than half of the expected level. In contrast, the rate of chronic disease in benefit option e peaks at a level about 75% higher than the scheme and the industry prevalence.

DESIGN OF THE RISK EQUALISATION FUND

The design of the REF was undertaken in 2003/2004 (McLeod et al., 2004), and the need for risk equalization was found to be urgent (Armstrong et al., 2004). The risk factors in the risk equalization formula are predominantly prospective and are as follows:

- Age last birthday on 1 January, summarised into age bands Under 1, 1–4, 5–9, 10–14, ... , 75–79, 80–84, 85+;
- Gender (recommended for inclusion from 1 January 2007 but not yet implemented);

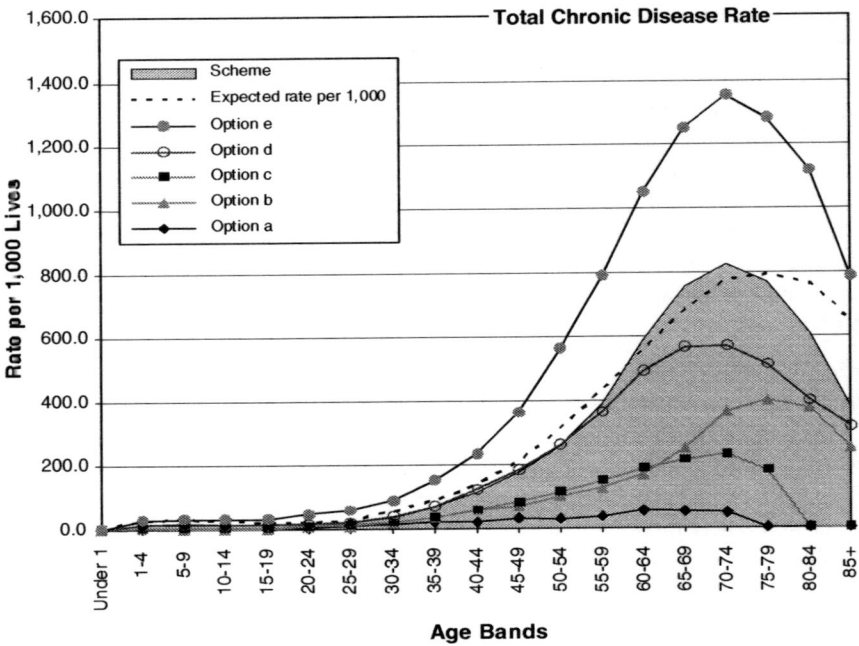

Fig. 2.   Risk Selection through Benefit Design in a Large Medical Scheme in 2007.

- The 25 PMB Chronic Disease List (CDL) conditions. Where a beneficiary has more than one chronic condition, the scheme may select the most expensive of the conditions.
- HIV/AIDS provided the beneficiary is receiving anti-retroviral therapy according to national guidelines;
- An additional factor for multiple chronic conditions with provision for 2, 3 or 4+ simultaneous chronic conditions and
- A retrospective factor for maternity events, defined as the delivery of a single/multiple foetus, either stillborn or alive.

Since 2005, monthly data has been gathered from schemes each quarter to test the functioning of the REF in 'shadow mode', that is, with no money yet changing hands. Concern was expressed in the original design report about the ability to reliably measure the chronic disease factors and about the ability to audit this data. It was seen as critical that there was a trusted and fair way to determine the numbers with chronic disease. In 2005, there were

29 third-party administrators and a further 20 funds were self-administered. Although some administrators used common software and data-switching services, there was a proliferation of different standards for determining eligibility for chronic disease.

Actuarial and clinical teams have collaborated to produce a comprehensive manual of Verification Criteria that is now in its third iteration (Council for Medical Schemes, 2008a, 2008b). The Verification Criteria have been developed with the emphasis on the verifiability of cases and are used to ensure that gaming[12] of the REF is identified and addressed. There are two elements to the criteria:

- the *diagnosis* of a particular disease, which includes specification of applicable ICD-10 codes and limitations on the practitioners that may diagnose certain complex conditions. There may also be certain mandatory tests needed to differentiate between diseases, and these test results must be retained by the fund and
- a *proof of treatment* element, which is based on paid claims data. Claims for at least two of the three calendar months before the month of submission are typically required to demonstrate proof of treatment.

It is conceivable that the REF may initially be implemented with a smaller set of risk factors if the data on each of the 26 chronic diseases is not considered sufficiently reliable at that stage. Accordingly, the actuarial team developing the tables has produced a series of tables ranging from 'Age Only' to the Full Table that includes all risk factors.

The systems for risk equalization have been developed but cannot be fully tested and implemented without the enabling legislation and regulations that will formally allow for the collection of industry data. The draft Bill for an amendment to the Medical Schemes Act to establish the REF was gazetted in November 2006 but not dealt with when submitted to parliament in 2008. The earliest date from which financial transfers could take place is 2011, provided there are no further delays.

IMPACT OF THE RISK EQUALISATION FUND

The effect of risk equalization will be to ensure that everyone across all benefit options and medical schemes pays a similar community rate for the same package of benefits (the PMBs), provided that they are all equally efficient in providing the benefits. If the PMBs can only be delivered for nore than the risk-adjusted amount, the difference to the amount received from REF would need to be charged directly to members. If the PMBs can be delivered more efficiently (less than the risk-adjusted amount), then the scheme can use the balance to fund greater benefits for members. Members would thus be more aware of the efficiency of their scheme and, it is hoped, would choose a scheme more carefully.

The risk profiles of schemes show substantial differences even using only age as a risk factor. Fig. 3 shows the expected impact of REF transfers at scheme level for the whole industry. The net payments to REF are shown as a percentage of the industry community rate for PMBs.

The graph demonstrates the extent of differences in age profile between competing schemes. It is possible for some schemes to attract a much younger profile than others and to maintain this position over a number of years, despite a highly competitive market with members that move freely amongst open schemes. There has been significant movement of members out of restricted schemes and to open schemes in the last decade, leading to some restricted schemes having extreme age profiles. This typically occurs in industries that are shrinking or where brokers have moved younger lives to an open scheme, thus leaving a heavy burden of elderly people on the restricted scheme.

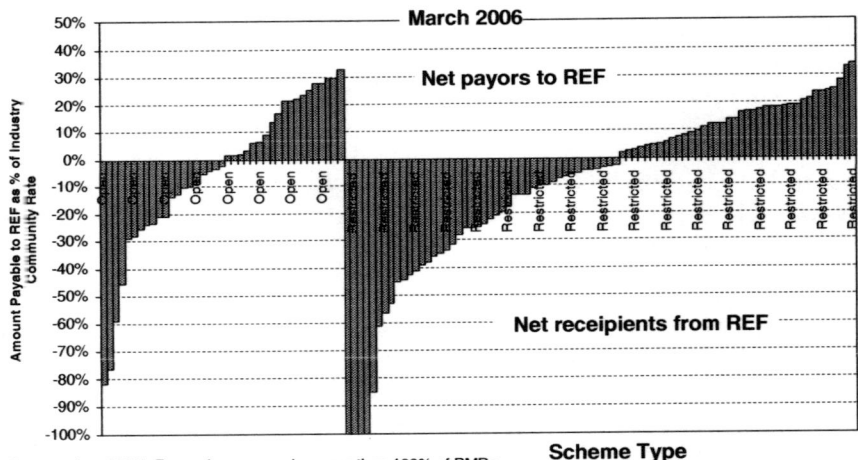

Truncated at -100%. Four schemes receive more than 100% of PMBs, with one extreme scheme receiving 272% of the value of PMBs.

Fig. 3. Net Transfers to REF Using Age Only Tables, March 2006.

Fig. 3 shows that some open schemes might need to increase the price of PMBs by 30% and others would see a reduction of that magnitude. In a highly competitive market where price is published annually and there is significant broker activity, these adjustments are expected to have a significant market impact. In the 'shadow period', the magnitude of adjustments has been kept confidential to prevent gaming in advance of the introduction of REF.

When risk equalization is implemented, the scheme community rate for PMBs should no longer be primarily influenced by age and disease, but rather the efficiency of the medical scheme in purchasing and delivering care to its members. The primary objective of the REF is thus to protect open enrolment and community rating in the highly competitive market.

ADDITIONAL REFORMS TO MINIMUM BENEFITS

The International Review Panel that evaluated the design of the REF and the envisaged mandatory health insurance system expressed concern about the small size of the minimum benefit package relative to the total benefit expenditure by schemes (Armstrong et al., 2004).

A study of the relationship between PMBs and total benefits was conducted in 2007 by the second largest administrator. The study covered 3 open schemes and 15 restricted membership schemes comprising just more than 1 million lives or about 14% of all covered lives in private health insurance. Table 1 summarises the relationship between minimum benefits and total benefits in the study.

Only about 50% of total benefit expenditure is currently part of the PMB package. However, this does seem to vary to a large extent with the

Table 1. PMBs as a Proportion of Total Scheme Benefits.

	Prescribed Minimum Benefits Relative To		
	In-hospital Benefits (%)	Out-of-hospital Benefits (%)	Total Benefits (%)
Open schemes	70.3	22.0	52.7
Restricted schemes	62.6	15.4	39.0
Average	68.8	20.0	49.4
Minimum	60.4	7.7	33.9
Maximum	74.7	34.4	61.6

minimum being 33.9% and the maximum being 61.6% in the 2007 study. The percentage for restricted schemes is also shown to be much lower than for open schemes. Restricted schemes tend to have richer (more generous) benefits than open schemes.

Nearly half of the out-of-hospital PMBs consist of medicine costs for members with chronic diseases. The narrow range of PMBs in-hospital relative to the total in-hospital benefits confirm that the benefit structures for in-hospital benefits have only relatively minor differences. The very wide range of PMBs relative to out-of-hospital benefits is due to a wide range of different benefit structures ranging from only the PMBs covered out-of-hospital to comprehensive out-of-hospital cover.

The current minimum benefit package is orientated towards in-hospital care. At the time of the design of the PMBs, it was envisaged that primary care would be provided free at a system of public clinics (Söderlund & Peprah, 1998). When this did not materialise, the PMBs should have been amended, but this did not occur. The PMBs are also not in line with the benefits in the public sector where there has been a commitment since 1994 to a system based on primary healthcare. The dilution of primary care in medical scheme expenditure in recent years has been dramatic: in 2003, the expenditure on primary care, dental benefits and medicines (out-of-hospital) was 48.2% of total benefit expenditure; by 2006, this had reduced to 32.3%. Medical schemes have increasingly become focussed on providing benefits in hospital with primary care being paid directly by members. Many stakeholders argue that this needs to be reversed by adding more primary care to the minimum benefit package. A comprehensive review of the structure of minimum benefits was initiated by the Council for Medical Schemes in conjunction with the Department of Health in 2008.

Calculations using the findings in Table 1 indicate that a benefit package that includes all hospital cover would increase the minimum cost for an average beneficiary from R257.05 per beneficiary per month in 2007 to R373.79 per beneficiary per month. This is an increase of 45%. An increase in the cost of the minimum benefits provided, without concomitant changes in income cross-subsidies, could force many marginal members out of the system due to them being unable to afford cover. This issue is explored in more detail in the section on the impact on workers and in Tables 3 and 4.

If minimum benefits accounted for almost all expenditure, then a risk equalization system would focus attention away from risk selection and towards cost-efficient delivery of care. However, as minimum benefits in South Africa are only about half of total expenditure, the impact of risk equalization is significantly diluted and there will remain substantial incentives to risk select. There is a clear need to begin to enlarge the pooled benefits that will be subject to risk equalization, but the policy dilemma is that affordability of medical schemes is already problematic (as illustrated in sections A and B of Table 3).

ADDITIONAL REFORMS TO BENEFIT DESIGN

The International Review Panel found that there was a need to simplify and standardise benefit packages to improve competition (Armstrong et al., 2004). Draft legislation that would allow for the simplification of benefits and will require changes in benefit design was published in 2008. The draft legislation tries to correct the incentives to design packages to risk select by introducing a distinction between common benefits and supplementary benefits. Community rating is currently applied at benefit option level but would in future be applied at scheme level with a set of common benefits for all members belonging to the scheme. The common benefits are defined as all the existing PMBs as well as all remaining in-hospital treatment. The common benefits and contributions must be the same for all members of the fund although contributions may vary by income. If only PMBs are risk equalised (as envisaged in draft legislation prepared for parliament in 2008) while community rating is applied to a larger package of benefits, schemes with a younger/healthier profile will still be able to charge less for the same set of benefits than schemes with an older/sicker member profile. Competition based on risk selection would thus be further encouraged.

In a study of three open schemes in 2007, the PMB cost for the benefit option with the best profile was consistently less than 70% of the average PMB cost for the scheme as a whole. While it is widely acknowledged that there is a need to move away from the current environment to one where community rating happens at a scheme level, this would mean that certain members will experience large increases in contributions. If the reform occurs while membership is still voluntary and without additional steps to deal with the affordability problem, this could result in these members electing to opt out of the private health insurance system. The loss of young and healthy members would have a 'death-spiral' effect on the remaining members of medical schemes with healthier lives leaving in each round of price increases.

ANTI-SELECTION BY MEMBERS IN A VOLUNTARY ENVIRONMENT

In considering the price of healthcare for a National Health Insurance system, evidence from the voluntary environment needs to be used with extreme caution. In a voluntary environment, people can move onto medical schemes when they believe they might need cover, despite the existence of waiting periods and late-joiner penalties. This means that the price of healthcare is artificially inflated. It is thus necessary to consider the demographic profile of beneficiaries in the voluntary environment and the proposed mandatory system and to perform all price calculations with regard to at least age and gender.

The age profile of voluntary medical schemes in South Africa, using data submitted to the Council for Medical Schemes, is contrasted with the age profile of the population as a whole in Fig. 4. Medical schemes have a 'twin-peak' age profile, showing that young working age people have remained

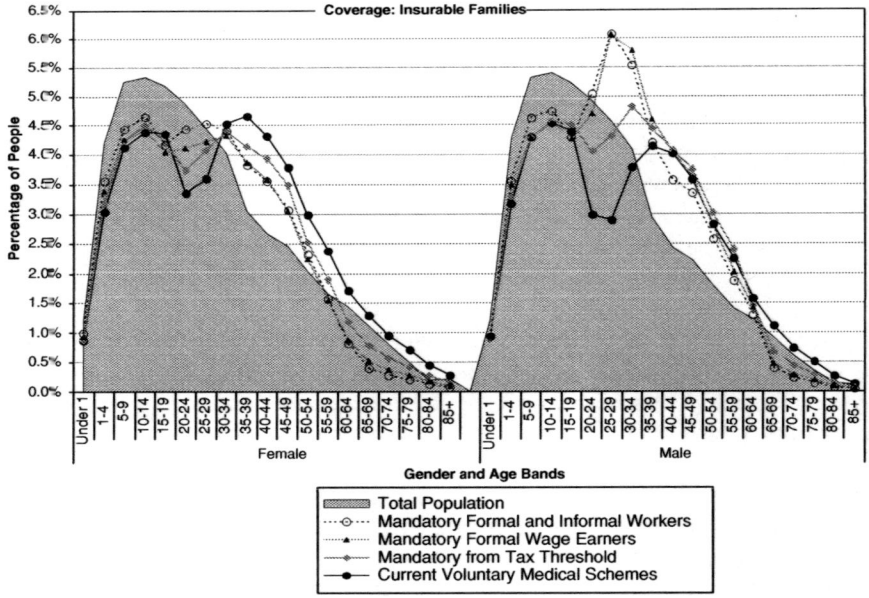

Fig. 4. Standardized Age Profiles for Phased Implementation of Mandatory Insurance.

outside the voluntary health insurance system while older working age people have joined medical schemes in significant numbers.

There is evidence that the proportion of children in medical schemes has reduced substantially in recent years as a response to high contribution increases. The industry has also lost membership in the young adult years with a commensurate increase in membership from age 35 upwards. The impact of the loss of children and young adults on the price of minimum benefits has been an increase of 3.8% between 2002 and 2007.

Fig. 4 shows that the age profile of medical schemes will alter substantially as the reforms to create a mandatory system of National Health Insurance are implemented. The impacts also differ by gender. Fig. 5 shows evidence of anti-selection in the voluntary environment by women in the child-bearing years. The minimum benefit package includes almost all maternity care, and thus, it has become a common phenomenon for women to join a

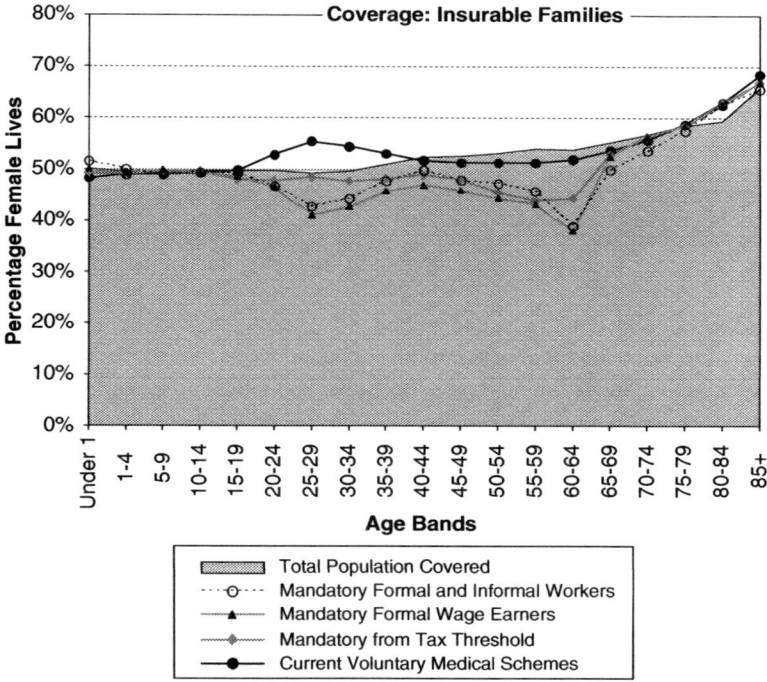

Fig. 5. Proportion of Female Lives during Phased Implementation of Mandatory Insurance.

medical scheme to have their children and to leave if the children are healthy.

Anti-selection by members in the voluntary environment will be eliminated by introducing mandatory membership and this will result in a reduction in the price of healthcare.

IMPACT OF MANDATORY MEMBERSHIP ON THE PRICE OF MINIMUM BENEFITS

It is likely that mandatory membership would need to be implemented in phases. For the purposes of this analysis, five phases in the reform are shown:

- The existing voluntary medical scheme environment;
- All people earning more than the tax threshold[13] become contributors. The insurable families[14] of contributors become members of medical schemes, together with those who were members in the voluntary environment.
- Add as contributors all those earning below the tax threshold but above R1,000 per month. These are typically formal sector workers. There may be a wage subsidy or other support to cover the cost of social security contributions for the group.
- Add as contributors all those earning below R1,000 per month. This group is typically farm and domestic workers and informal traders. They will require almost complete subsidisation.
- Inclusion of all people in the country as members of the National Health Insurance system. This phase will see an extension of beneficiaries but with no added contributors.

The changing age and gender profiles that will occur as South Africa moves from the current voluntary health insurance system to universal coverage can be predicted from census and other national survey data, as shown in Figs 4 and 5.

Table 2 summarises the number of people who would be added and covered in each phase. The impact of the changes in the age and gender profile[15] on the price of minimum benefits are shown using the REF tables.

Considering firstly only the age and gender effects, the price of minimum benefits falls from R257.02 to R210.58 when all those who can be contributors are added with the informal workers. This leaves an unusually

Table 2. Impact of Phased Implementation of National Health Insurance on the Price of Minimum Benefits.

	Current Voluntary Medical Schemes	Mandatory from Tax Threshold	Mandatory Formal Wage Earners	Mandatory Formal and Informal Workers	Total Population Covered
Income level for mandatory membership[a]	Not applicable	R2,917 pm	R1,000 pm	Any earnings	Not applicable
Number currently covered	6,903,683				
Number of additional people covered		5,021,697	6,214,844	5,978,660	23,272,144
Number of people covered	6,903,683	11,925,380	18,140,225	24,118,885	47,391,029
Percentage of population (%)	14.6	25.2	38.3	50.9	100.0
Using age and gender Risk Equalisation Tables					
Community rate for minimum benefits	257.02	232.55	217.73	210.58	221.42
Revised rate as percent of initial rate (%)		90.5	84.7	81.9	86.1
Using age,gender and maternity Risk Equalisation Tables					
Community rate for minimum benefits	257.02	225.33	210.48	203.90	215.98
Revised rate as percent of initial rate (%)		87.7	81.9	79.3	84.0
Using age, gender, maternity and disease Risk Equalisation Tables					
Community rate for minimum benefits	257.02	216.51	203.37	198.55	213.26
Revised rate as percent of initial rate (%)		84.2	79.1	77.3	83.0

[a]2005 data for incomes and coverage.

shaped population in the public sector: a very young group of children, few working age adults and many poor elderly people. The inclusion of this group results in a small increase in the price of minimum benefits from R210.58 to R221.42 per month. In totality, the price of PMBs has fallen to 86.1% of its initial level.

Fig. 5 shows the extent of anti-selection by women of child-bearing age. The total number of children expected to be born in South Africa in 2005 was 22.8 per 1,000 women.[16] In an extensive study covering 63% of the medical scheme beneficiaries (Risk Equalisation Technical Advisory Panel,

2007), the number of children was found to be 26.4 per 1,000 women in medical schemes. This projection for medical schemes has been found to be on the low side compared to actual experience since 2005, suggesting that anti-selection by pregnant women is widespread. The extent of anti-selection by those with chronic disease can only be speculated, but the patterns of disease by age show unusual bulges in the young adult years for some severe diseases such as multiple sclerosis, suggesting that families with someone with an expensive disease would try to join a medical scheme.

Estimates have been made of the possible impact on maternity and chronic disease in the groups that would be added at the various phases of mandatory cover. Table 2 summarises that the price of minimum benefits may be as low as R198.55 pbpm (per beneficiary per month) when informal workers are added or R213.26 for the entire population. Another way to look at this phenomenon is that prices of minimum benefits in the voluntary environment are some 17%–23% more expensive than they could be under this phasing of mandatory cover.

SEQUENCING OF REFORMS

The earlier sections have raised and quantified the impacts of a bewildering number of factors and reforms in moving from the current voluntary medical schemes to a National Health System. While the aim of the reforms is clear to all involved, the trajectory and sequencing of the reforms is not clear and several alternative paths are indicated in Tables 3 and 4. The sequence described here is developed from the Ministerial Task Team on Social Health Insurance (2005), which conceptualised the reforms for the Department of Health.

The key institutional reform is to establish a new statutory body, the REF, as shown in Fig. 6. Although work on the REF and the collection of data during the current 'shadow period' is done on the basis of all schemes contributing the industry community rate to REF and then receiving risk-adjusted payments, this is not the sequence that was envisaged for implementation. The International Review Panel (Armstrong et al., 2004) argued that implementation would be simpler and more acceptable if the flows were organised so that every scheme was a recipient of REF so that there was not the perception of 'winners and losers'. This would occur if the existing unequal tax subsidy was removed and replaced by a direct subsidy per person (the per capita subsidy) between government and REF in Fig. 6. This was adopted in the Ministerial Task Team on Social Health Insurance's (2005) proposals.

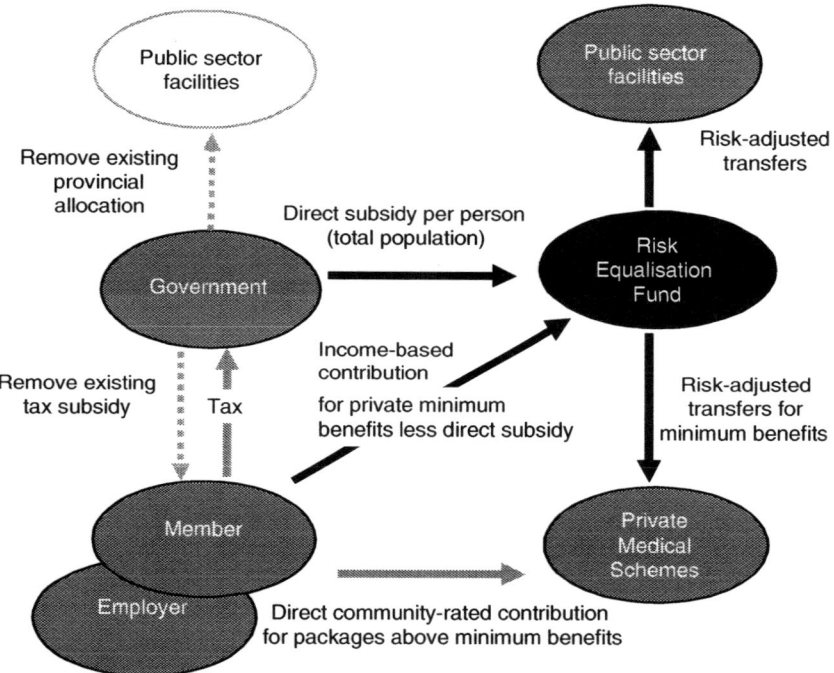

Fig. 6. Envisaged Flow of Funds under Mandatory Health Insurance.

The amount would be the same per person and equivalent to the amount being spent per head in the public sector. This would immediately provide substantial relief for lower income groups and make contributions more affordable for these families as indicated in Table 3. The direct subsidy per person would be sourced from tax revenue and paid from government to the REF. The REF would in turn make monthly risk-adjusted payments of this amount to medical schemes, as shown in Fig. 6.

The next reform would be to raise an income-related contribution for the difference between the price of the minimum benefit package and the public sector subsidy. This amount would be paid to the REF together with the direct subsidy per person, enabling the REF to make monthly risk-adjusted payments to medical schemes in respect of the total minimum benefit package. This income-related contribution would be mandatory for all people earning over a certain amount and would replace about half of the amounts paid directly to medical schemes at present. It is estimated that an income-related contribution of the order of 3.0%–4.1% of income would be needed to cover the current definition of the minimum benefit package, depending on the income level at which contributions become mandatory.[17] Direct payments to medical schemes as a whole would reduce by the amount of the direct subsidy plus the amount raised by the income-related contribution.

The amount needed to be raised to cover PMBs depends on the definition of the minimum package. Every R10 change in the cost of the PMB package for the industry increases the income-related contribution by between 0.32% and 0.53%, depending on the income threshold.[18]

Members would still be allowed to choose packages greater than the minimum benefits, but would pay the additional amounts directly to medical schemes. These are shown in Fig. 6 as being on a community-rated basis, but there could be some limited form of risk rating allowed for standardized benefits above the minimum.

Draft legislation prepared for parliament in 2008 would have seen the creation of the REF and changes to the nature of pooling within medical schemes, as outlined in the section on benefit design. Thus far, there is no sign of the changes to the tax subsidy, the introduction of a per capita subsidy or income cross-subsidies. Stakeholders are deeply concerned that there may be a drive to implement REF, change benefit option design and increase the size of the benefit package before any of the other reforms.

IMPACT ON WORKERS OF THE SEQUENCING OF REFORMS

The greatest challenge facing medical schemes is to make healthcare more affordable to lower income workers (McLeod & Ramjee, 2007). Despite significant attempts to find solutions for so-called low-income medical schemes (Low Income Medical Schemes Process, 2006), there has been little practical progress. Table 3 begins illustrating the problems with the sequencing of reforms by choosing a model worker family of two adults and two children with one income to perform the calculations. A range of illustrative incomes is chosen to reflect the problems.

The first lines of the table show the number of people in insurable families in each income band and the numbers already covered by voluntary medical schemes.[19] There is a strong pattern by income: at the highest income levels, close to 80% are already on medical schemes, but this falls off very rapidly

Table 3. Impact on Workers of the Preferred Sequencing of Reforms.

All Calculations in 2007 on a Monthly Basis for a Family of Four (Two Adults+Two Children) with One Income	Informal Workers	Formal Farm and Domestic Workers	Formal Workers below Tax Threshold	Worker Just above Tax Threshold	Low-Paid Civil Servants	Clerical and Service	Supervisory and Managerial	Professional
Income range for phased National Health Insurance[a]	Under R1,000 pm	R1,000 to R2,000 pm	R2,000 to tax threshold	Above tax threshold to R5,000 pm	R5,000 to R8,000 pm	R8,000 to R12,000 pm	R12,000 to R30,000 pm	Over R30,000 pm
Estimate of number of people[a]	3,143,779	2,177,341	1,306,436	1,834,778	1,550,869	738,607	681,718	114,582
Proportion on voluntary medical schemes (%)[a]	2.9	5.1	12.1	33.2	63.1	72.6	79.8	78.5
Monthly income of contributor	750.00	1,500.00	3,000.00	4,500.00	6,000.00	9,000.00	20,000.00	50,000.00
A: Illustration of affordability problems: lack of affordability of most comprehensive package								
Monthly contributions for family	3,084.00	3,084.00	3,084.00	3,084.00	3,084.00	3,084.00	3,084.00	3,084.00
Contributions as percent of income (%)	411	206	103	69	51	34	15.4	6.2
Employer subsidy of 50% of package	−1,542.00	−1,542.00	−1,542.00	−1,542.00	−1,542.00	−1,542.00	−1,542.00	−1,542.00
Effective contributions by worker	1,542.00	1,542.00	1,542.00	1,542.00	1,542.00	1,542.00	1,542.00	1,542.00
Contributions as percent of income (%)	206	103	51	34	26	17	7.7	3.1

Table 3. (*Continued*)

All Calculations in 2007 on a Monthly Basis for a Family of Four (Two Adults+Two Children) with One Income	Informal Workers	Formal Farm and Domestic Workers	Formal Workers below Tax Threshold	Worker Just above Tax Threshold	Low-Paid Civil Servants	Clerical and Service	Supervisory and Managerial	Professional
B: Current situation: benefit package chosen according to income								
Monthly contributions for family	900.00	900.00	1,324.00	1,960.00	2,008.00	2,444.00	3,084.00	3,084.00
Contributions as percent of income (%)	120	60	44	44	33	27	15.4	6.2
Tax break	0.00	0.00	0.00	-104.30	-306.06	-327.68	-510.15	-680.23
Effective contributions by worker	900.00	900.00	1,324.00	1,855.71	1,701.94	2,116.32	2,573.85	2,403.77
Contributions as percent of income (%)	120	60	44	41	28	24	12.9	4.8
C: Remove tax break and replace with direct per capita subsidy equivalent to public sector expenditure per person								
Monthly contributions for family	900.00	900.00	1,324.00	1,960.00	2,008.00	2,444.00	3,084.00	3,084.00
Per capita subsidy	-483.38	-483.38	-483.38	-483.38	-483.38	-483.38	-483.38	-483.38
Effective contributions by worker	416.62	416.62	840.62	1,476.62	1,524.62	1,960.62	2,600.62	2,600.62
Contributions as percent of income (%)	56	28	28	33	25	22	*13.0*	*5.2*

D: Introduction of REF after per capita subsidy

Monthly contributions for family	900.00	900.00	1,324.00	1,960.00	2,008.00	2,444.00	3,084.00	3,084.00
Payment to REF at industry community rate	1,028.20	1,028.20	1,028.20	1,028.20	1,028.20	1,028.20	1,028.20	1,028.20
Payment to scheme from REF for PMBs	−572.99	−572.99	−795.27	−731.72	−820.70	−820.70	−1,294.66	−1,294.66
Net REF adjustment (+ve is net paid to REF)	455.21	455.21	232.93	296.48	207.50	207.50	−266.46	−266.46
Contributions after REF adjustment	1,355.21	1,355.21	1,556.93	2,256.48	2,215.50	2,651.50	2,817.54	2,817.54
Per capita subsidy	−483.38	−483.38	−483.38	−483.38	−483.38	−483.38	−483.38	−483.38
Effective contributions by worker	871.82	871.82	1,073.55	1,773.10	1,732.12	2,168.12	2,334.16	2,334.16
Contributions as percent of income (%)	116	58	36	39	29	24	11.7	4.7

E: Introduction of income cross-subsidy after per capita subsidy and REF

Original monthly contributions for family	900.00	900.00	1,324.00	1,960.00	2,008.00	2,444.00	3,084.00	3,084.00
Scheme cost of PMBs	325.37	325.37	489.59	632.90	776.22	944.76	1,256.72	1,256.72
Package in excess of PMBs	574.63	574.63	834.41	1,327.10	1,231.78	1,499.24	1,827.28	1,827.28
Payment to scheme from REF for PMBs	−572.99	−572.99	−795.27	−731.72	−820.70	−820.70	−1,294.66	−1,294.66
Cost of package after REF payment	327.01	327.01	528.73	1,228.28	1,187.30	1,623.30	1,789.34	1,789.34
Social security contribution: 4.1% of income	30.75	61.50	123.00	184.50	246.00	369.00	820.00	2,050.00
Effective contributions by worker	357.76	388.51	651.73	1,412.78	1,433.30	1,992.30	2,609.34	3,839.34
Contributions as percent of income (%)	48	26	22	31	24	22	13.0	7.7

Table 3. (*Continued*)

All Calculations in 2007 on a Monthly Basis for a Family of Four (Two Adults+Two Children) with One Income	Informal Workers	Formal Farm and Domestic Workers	Formal Workers below Tax Threshold	Worker Just above Tax Threshold	Low-Paid Civil Servants	Clerical and Service	Supervisory and Managerial	Professional
F: Introduction of common benefits (PMBs only) after per capita subsidy, REF and income-based contribution								
Revised PMB cost for family	883.89	883.89	883.89	883.89	883.89	883.89	883.89	883.89
Package in excess of PMBs	574.63	574.63	834.41	1,327.10	1,231.78	1,499.24	1,827.28	1,827.28
Total revised contribution for family	1,458.52	1,458.52	1,718.30	2,210.98	2,115.67	2,383.13	2,711.16	2,711.16
Payment to scheme from REF for PMBs	−838.71	−838.71	−838.71	−838.71	−838.71	−838.71	−838.71	−838.71
Cost of package after REF payment	619.81	619.81	879.59	1,372.27	1,276.96	1,544.42	1,872.46	1,872.46
Social security contribution: 4.1% of income	30.75	61.50	123.00	184.50	246.00	369.00	820.00	2,050.00
Effective contributions by worker	650.56	681.31	1,002.59	1,556.77	1,522.96	1,913.42	2,692.46	3,922.46
Contributions as percent of income 9%)	87	45	33	35	25	21	13.5	7.8

G: Expanded common benefits (PMBs including in-hospital benefits) after per capita subsidy, REF and income-based contribution

Revised PMB cost for family	1,276.65	1,276.65	1,276.65	1,276.65	1,276.65	1,276.65	1,276.65	1,276.65
Package in excess of revised PMBs	428.21	428.21	614.10	1,087.26	882.82	1,074.51	1,255.61	1,255.61
Total revised contribution for family	1,704.86	1,704.86	1,890.74	2,363.90	2,159.47	2,351.16	2,532.25	2,532.25
Payment to scheme from REF revised PMBs	−1,219.61	−1,219.61	−1,219.61	−1,219.61	−1,219.61	−1,219.61	−1,219.61	−1,219.61
Cost of package after REF payment	485.25	485.25	671.13	1,144.29	939.86	1,131.54	1,312.64	1,312.64
Social security contribution: 10.3% of income	77.17	154.34	308.67	463.01	617.34	926.01	2,057.81	5,144.52
Effective contributions by worker	562.41	639.58	979.80	1,607.30	1,557.20	2,057.56	3,370.45	6,457.17
Contributions as percent of income (%)	75	43	33	36	26	23	16.9	12.9

[a] data in 2005/2006

so that at the tax threshold, only 33% of beneficiaries in insurable family are covered. Below the tax threshold,[20] medical scheme membership rapidly falls below 10% of the eligible insurable family members.

Section A (Table 3) illustrates the affordability problem by placing all income groups on the highest comprehensive benefit option in the scheme. While the percentage of income is 6.2% for the professional family, the price of cover exceeds total income for those earning below the tax threshold. Even a substantial employer subsidy of 50% of the package makes the comprehensive package affordable only to the two highest income groups. In South Africa, affordable contributions have generally been taken to be below 16% of family income (Ministerial Task Team on Social Health Insurance, 2005).

One of the ways low-income workers have coped with the high cost of medical schemes is to choose a benefit option according to its affordability rather than according to need. Many of the younger and healthier members who belong to private medical schemes in South Africa belong to benefit options that currently cost less. This can be expected as healthier members consume less medical resources and therefore do not require a benefit option with such comprehensive benefits as an older or sicker person may need. Younger members are also typically in the earlier stages of their careers when incomes are lower, and thus, they are more price sensitive. Benefit design has been effective as a risk selection tool, and the benefit options used by these lower income members usually have a very young age profile.

Section B (Table 3) illustrates this phenomenon by placing only the highest income workers on a comprehensive benefit package and allocating the others to benefit packages that are more affordable.[21] This reduces the contributions as a percent of income to about 40% on either side of the tax threshold. This is clearly still unaffordable for these low-income workers, as demonstrated by the low take-up in the voluntary market earlier in the table. Section B, the current situation, becomes the base case for illustrating the impact of each step in the reforms. There are a range of ways an employer could choose to assist with a subsidy, but all subsidies eventually form part of the total remuneration package that can be afforded by employers. An increase in subsidy is typically offset by a reduction in cash salary. The remainder of the table is thus shown without employer subsidies to show the actual total cost of each benefit option.

Section C (Table 3) illustrates the very large impact on low-income workers of removing the existing tax subsidy and replacing it with a per capita subsidy.[22] The cells in which the family is worse off than the base case of Section B are shown in italic (see Tables 3 and 4). The highest income workers lose the effect of the tax break, but all other workers benefit substantially. For those earning below the tax threshold, the price of voluntary medical schemes falls about half from the current situation.

Section D (Table 3) indicates the impact of introducing REF after the per capita subsidy. This largely reverses the gains for the lowest income workers as they are on benefit options that have a younger profile than the industry, and those benefit options thus become net payors to REF. The only benefit option in this scheme, which is a net recipient from REF, is the one used for the two highest income groups. Compared to the base case in Section B, the middle-income groups are worse off than before with all others being close to the original position.

There are many other sequences of reform possible. The methodology of using sample families is very helpful in identifying the consequences for workers of these other trajectories and eliminating those that cause the most harm. Three possibilities are illustrated in Table 4.

Section X (Table 4) indicates the impact of attempting to introduce REF before the per capita subsidy. This scenario is highly detrimental to the lower income groups, and all groups are worse off except the two groups with the highest incomes (where the benefit option is a net recipient from REF). If REF is implemented before both mandatory membership and the income cross-subsidy are introduced, not only low-income workers but also many of these younger and healthier members will experience a significant increase in contributions to the sickness fund and may thus drop out of the private insured market. This could start a cost spiral as the industry community rate increases due to lower cross-subsidies from the younger and healthier members. This could in turn cause more people to opt out of the private insured market causing even further increases. The introduction of REF in a voluntary environment without other simultaneous reforms is clearly unworkable.

A mandatory health insurance system should improve affordability of healthcare for low-income workers through the introduction of income cross-subsidies. At present, a low-income worker with a family of four might need nearly 40% of income to be spent on medical cover and can only afford this if the employer subsidy is generous. Section E (Table 3) shows the impact of an income cross-subsidy for minimum benefits, using a social security contribution of a flat percent of income.[23] The outcome is improved for the low- and middle-income groups but is still higher than the target 16%, but this target is within reach for all except the very lowest income band if the cost of delivery can be reduced. The effects of a reduction in the scheme price of benefits due to changes in the demographic profile have not been modelled.[24]

Table 4. Impact on Workers of Some Alternative Trajectories of Reform.

All Calculations in 2007 on a Monthly Basis for a Family of Four (Two Adults+Two Children) with One Income	Informal Workers	Formal Farm and Domestic Workers	Formal Workers below Tax Threshold	Worker Just above Tax Threshold	Low-Paid Civil Servants	Clerical and Service	Supervisory and Managerial	Professional
Income range for phased National Health Insurance	Under R1,000 pm	R1,000 to R2,000 pm	R2,000 to tax threshold	Above tax threshold to R5,000 pm	R5,000 to R8,000 pm	R8,000 to R12,000 pm	R12,000 to R30,000 pm	Over R30,000 pm
Alternative trajectories (steps in trajectory abandoned if low-income workers in a worse-off position than section **B**)								
X: Introduction of REF before per capita subsidy								
Monthly contributions for family	900.00	900.00	1,324.00	1,960.00	2,008.00	2,444.00	3,084.00	3,084.00
Net REF adjustment (+ve is net not paid to REF)	455.21	455.21	232.93	296.48	207.50	207.50	−266.46	−266.46
Contributions after REF adjustment	1,355.21	1,355.21	1,556.93	2,256.48	2,215.50	2,651.50	2,817.54	2,817.54
Tax break	0.00	0.00	0.00	−104.30	−306.06	−327.68	−510.15	−680.23
Effective contributions by worker	1,355.21	1,355.21	1,556.93	2,152.19	1,909.44	2,323.82	2,307.39	2,137.31
Contributions as percent of income (%)	*181*	*90*	*52*	*48*	*32*	*26*	*11.5*	*4.3*
Y: Introduction of common benefits (PMBs only) before REF or per capita subsidy								
Revised PMB cost for family	883.89	883.89	883.89	883.89	883.89	883.89	883.89	883.89
Package in excess of PMBs	574.63	574.63	834.41	1,327.10	1,231.78	1,499.24	1,827.28	1,827.28
Total revised contribution for family	1,458.52	1,458.52	1,718.30	2,210.98	2,115.67	2,383.13	2,711.16	2,711.16
Tax break	0.00	0.00	0.00	−104.30	−306.06	−327.68	−510.15	−680.23

Effective contributions by worker	1,458.52	1,458.52	1,718.30	2,106.69	1,809.61	2,055.44	2,201.01	2,030.93
Contributions as percent of income (%)	*194*	*97*	*57*	*47*	*30*	*23*	11.0	4.1
Z: Introduction of common benefits (PMBs including in-hospital benefits) before REF or per capita subsidy								
Revised PMB cost for family	1,276.65	1,276.65	1,276.65	1,276.65	1,276.65	1,276.65	1,276.65	1,276.65
Package in excess of revised **PMBs**	428.21	428.21	614.10	1,087.26	882.82	1,074.51	1,255.61	1,255.61
Total revised contribution for family	1,704.86	1,704.86	1,890.74	2,363.90	2,159.47	2,351.16	2,532.25	2,532.25
Tax break	0.00	0.00	0.00	−104.30	−306.06	−327.68	−510.15	−680.23
Effective contributions by worker	1,704.86	1,704.86	1,890.74	2,259.61	1,853.41	2,023.47	2,022.10	1,852.02
Contributions as percent of income (%)	*227*	*114*	*63*	*50*	*31*	*22*	10.1	3.7

There are many other ways to organise the social security contribution, for example, an upper limit on family contributions; a percentage determined using only above threshold income or a progressive scale which is the same shape as general tax payments. However, the extent of the income cross-subsidy is an area that has not been debated in the health industry or discussed with the social partners (the community, organised labour and organised business). These alternatives can usefully be illustrated for stakeholders using the same approach but for brevity are not shown in this chapter.

A difficult issue remains on the reform agenda: the design of benefit options and the degree to which benefits should be pooled across each scheme. The draft legislation proposed in 2008 suggests a system of 'common benefits' across every scheme, and the effects are illustrated in Sections F and G, if these occur after mandatory membership. While conceptually this reform makes sense, the impact on middle- and low-income workers reverses the gains they had in Section E. The impact of introducing these reforms before the per capita subsidy and REF is indicated in Sections Y and Z (Table 4) to be clearly unaffordable for all except the highest income workers.

CONCLUSIONS ON THE SEQUENTIAL IMPLEMENTATION OF COMPLEX REFORMS

From an implementation point of view, there are considerable risks in implementing all the steps towards a system of mandatory membership at the same time. If all steps are not introduced at the same time, the order in which the steps are introduced will have a different impact on different stakeholders.

Fig. 7 has been used for some years in South Africa to indicate the policy flow from the mid-1990s to achieving a mandatory health system. Comprehensive PMBs were envisaged to include the existing definition of PMBs together with primary care in this figure but could equally be used for the extended common benefits that were illustrated earlier.

Fig. 7 is useful in that it shows the risk cross-subsidy axis separately from the reforms related to income cross-subsidies. While numbered sequentially, it was always envisaged that the actual trajectory would begin to incorporate elements of income cross-subsidy before all the risk cross-subsidy elements were completed.

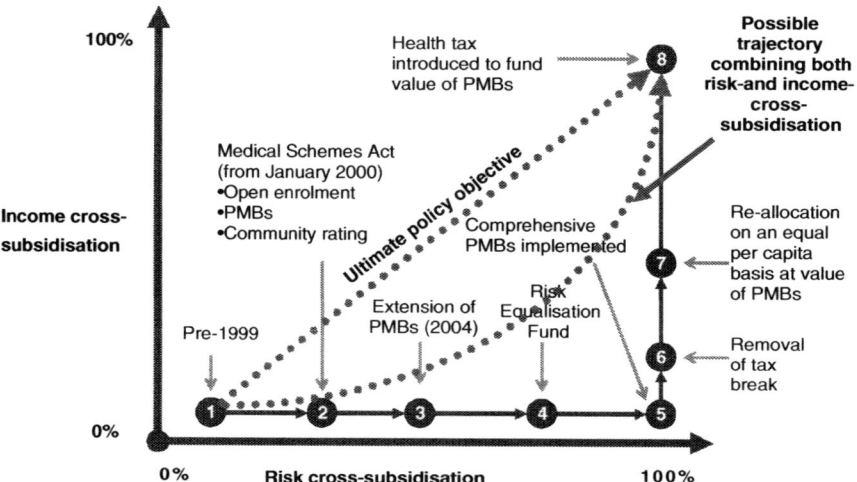

Fig. 7. Policy Flow in Medical Schemes to Achieve Social Health Insurance. *Source:* Ministerial Task Team on SHI, July 2005, with amended wording.

To retain stability within the current system as well as to attract new members into the system, it would be essential to introduce income cross-subsidies before the introduction of other reforms. As argued earlier, introducing the other reforms before income cross-subsidies are introduced will decrease the affordability of private health insurance for many members, thereby forcing them to opt out of the system.

If risk equalization is not introduced before a common benefit approach across a scheme is enforced, it could increase risk selection activity. This is because the common benefit package is likely to be similar for every scheme. Whereas benefits and thus prices are currently difficult to compare across benefit options due to the fact that benefits are not standardised, introducing a set of common benefits will make the comparison between different schemes much easier. In the absence of REF, a scheme with a better profile will be able to charge much less for the same set of common benefits.

It is demonstrated in Tables 3 and 4 that the sequence that will cause the least instability and seems most viable in terms of the impact on workers is as follows:

- Introduce open enrolment, community rating and minimum benefits (this has already been implemented, otherwise the sequence could have begun differently);

- Remove the tax subsidy for voluntary private health insurance membership and replace with a per capita subsidy;
- Introduce the REF to operate between benefit options;
- Introduce an income cross-subsidy;
- Introduce mandatory membership for all earning any income (however, the very lowest income would need some form of wage subsidy or subsidy of social security contributions if these are a flat percent of income);
- Deal with benefit option restructuring issues to improve community rating at scheme level and enlarging the package of minimum benefits (although a suitable trajectory for these reforms still requires further analysis).

The phased implementation of the mandatory system to achieve universal coverage, as summarised in Table 2, can also usefully be demonstrated using a similar approach.

IMPLICATIONS FOR POLICY IN OTHER COUNTRIES

The South African experience of risk equalization is of interest as it attempts to introduce more solidarity into a small but highly competitive private insurance market. The core principles of open enrolment, community rating, minimum benefits and risk equalization are typically found in competitive markets. The South African experience demonstrates the extent to which competing insurance funds can alter their risk profiles through risk selection and benefit design to compete on community rates in the absence of risk equalization.

The institution created for risk equalization also functions as a mechanism for pooling subsidies, value-added tax (VAT) funding, income tax funding, social health contributions or any other revenues earmarked for the mandatory system. As such, it is the core institutional component of a mandatory system. While it may be the first component to be built in legislative terms, it could be very de-stabilising on the voluntary system to switch on risk equalization before the income cross-subsidy components are in place. Affordability in a voluntary market is key to participation, and any reform that makes affordability worse for the lower income groups will probably result in them leaving the system. As lower income workers tend to be younger and chronic disease is related to age, this can exacerbate the effects on the voluntary system.

It is of critical importance when pricing in healthcare to work by at least age and gender. This is particularly so in moving from voluntary to mandatory systems as the age and gender profile of the voluntary system is likely to be very different from the country as a whole. If data is available, then pricing by age, gender and disease risk is advocated, but the evidence for variation in disease burden between the insured and the rest of the population may be poor.

Even when the end point of policy reform is agreed, such as universal coverage, the nature of reforms is that there are sequential elements. While the technical experts involved with pricing and design may understand the potential impacts of different reform trajectories, there is often enormous difficulty in conveying these concepts to policy-makers and politicians. Warnings about the impacts may be mistrusted as being merely to delay reform.

The methodology used here of demonstrating the impact on particular families makes the impacts more tangible and understandable. The table illustrated only a family of four with one income, but in practice, other family groups like single mothers, dual income households and large families would also be of interest. The form of analysis can readily be extended to cover the unemployed, by including elements such as unemployment benefits or other social security support. The analysis can also be shown in a simple graphical form by comparing the 'contributions as percent of income' lines at various stages of reform.

We advocate the creation of a common set of demographic data to be used for all analyses by any interested party. At the outset, a choice of illustrative families should be made that stakeholders agree will be used to demonstrate alternative reform trajectories. These measures reduce the discussion to the impact of core policy elements rather than focussing on the different assumptions being used by different advocacy groups.

The difficulties raised by the sequential implementation of complex reforms are significant in the transition from a voluntary to a mandatory health insurance system. The adverse impact of risk equalization on low-income workers in the absence of income cross-subsidies and mandatory membership was demonstrated in the South African situation, and a similar result could be expected in other countries.

Risk equalization is a critical institutional component in moving towards a system of social or national health insurance in competitive markets, but the sequence of its implementation needs to be carefully considered.

NOTES

1. International usage to describe a system of risk adjustment has become 'risk equalization'. However, the official name in South Africa is the 'Risk Equalisation Fund'.

2. This is a framework developed by Kutzin (2001) to describe a country's health system and to facilitate comparisons between countries. The vertical axis describes

the four components of healthcare financing, while the size of the element on the horizontal axis shows the sources and relative weight in monetary terms.

3. A statutory body with the Registrar and board appointed by the Minister of Health. An annual industry levy provides operating funds for the Council.

4. This is some 70% higher than the tax threshold; however, only 20.5% of income earners earn more than this amount.

5. The PMB package is a list of some 270 diagnosis-treatment pairs (DTPs) primarily offered in hospital (introduced January 2000); all emergency medical conditions (defined January 2003); diagnosis, treatment and medicine according to therapeutic algorithms for 25 defined chronic conditions on the Chronic Disease List (CDLs) (introduced January 2004).

6. Designated Service Providers or DSPs.

7. Lists of cost-effective medicines that the scheme will reimburse.

8. There have been changes in terminology over time, from 'National Health Insurance' in 1994 to 'Social Health Insurance' in subsequent papers with a return in 2008 to the description 'National Health Insurance'. McIntyre and van den Heever (2007) argue that there is substantial common ground amongst the proposals and advocate using the term 'mandatory insurance' instead.

9. Assuming the same efficiency in purchasing healthcare. Where efficiency levels differ, the difference is charged or repaid to members as discussed later.

10. A counter-proposal by organised labour in 2008 suggests that revenue collection should only be from tax-funding with pooling and purchasing entirely by the Department of Health. This proposal controversially envisages a single-payer system. This proposal features as a central platform for the ruling party in the elections in early 2009, but the details of the reforms required are not yet in the public domain.

11. Expected industry value uses the tables of prevalence developed for the REF.

12. An example of gaming the system would be for an administrator to make the diagnosis criteria for a disease less strict so that more members are identified with a particular disease and thus qualify for a higher REF payment. The problem is greatest with the highest cost diseases.

13. The tax threshold for those under age 65 was R3,583 per month in 2007 and R2,917 per month in 2005. The data used for illustrating the phases of mandatory insurance is from 2005.

14. Insurable spouse would include wife, husband or same-sex partner. There may be multiple spouses in traditional marriages. Insurable children for this illustration are all children under age 20 plus all children between age 20 and 30 who are living in the household and who are not earning in their own right.

15. There are many other factors that could have an impact on the actual price of minimum benefits. Estimates of the differences in disease burden between the currently covered population and those who would be added can be made, but there is seldom strong evidence to use in the calculations. Factors that require considerable judgement in the pricing include the issue of greater demand from moral hazard due to easier access and the impact of removing limits or co-payments on benefits included in the minimum package.

16. Actuarial Society of South Africa, ASSA2003 Model Results Provincial Output spreadsheet version 051129.

17. The higher the income threshold at which people become contributors, the lower the percentage of income needed. As more low-income workers are added, the

proportion of income paid by each needs to be higher. If the entire population were to be covered and not only the families of contributors, then the proportion of income needed would more than double from 4.1% to 9.5% of income. The cost of delivery of PMBs in a future, more efficient, public sector has not been taken into account in this estimate.

18. This could rise to 1.03% of income if the entire population is covered.

19. Patterns of incomes and coverage are derived from the General Household Survey of 2005, using the concept of an 'insurable family'. This allows for the working person to be the member of the scheme and to cover their spouse and children. The definition of child includes those under age 20 as well as children over age 20 living in the same household and either studying or not yet able to find work. The medical scheme data is the 2006 profile used for pricing the REF in 2007 (Risk Equalisation Technical Advisory Panel, 2007). The total population is from Statistics South Africa for the same time period in 2006.

20. Tax calculations are done using the 2007/2008 tax year tables and rules that would have applied in mid-2007. This includes the effects of the reform of the tax treatment of medical schemes during 2006. The tax threshold for those under age 65 was R3,583 per month in 2007.

21. The medical scheme contributions are from a large medical scheme for the benefit year 2007.

22. The per capita subsidy was estimated to be R1,300 per annum (Ministerial Task Team on Social Health Insurance, 2005) and this is inflated with CPIX (consumer inflation without the effect of mortgage rates) for a value of R1,450 per person per annum in 2007.

23. The effect on the price of mandatory membership for all earning any income is used to arrive at the social security contribution of 4.1% of income. If mandatory membership is restricted to (say) only those earning above the tax threshold, then the analysis needs to be split into the impact of the mandatory system on those above the tax threshold and the impact of continued voluntary membership on those below the tax threshold. The most favourable position for low-income workers is an immediate mandatory membership for all earning any income.

24. This is an area requiring many assumptions about the effect on an individual scheme. It would depend on the nature of the scheme (open or restricted), and if open, the target market in the future and the distribution of new members between existing and yet to be created schemes.

REFERENCES

African National Congress. (1994). *A national health plan for South Africa*. Johannesburg, SA: African National Congress. Available at http://www.anc.org.za

Armstrong, J., Deeble, J., Dror, D. M., Rice, N., Thiede, M., & Van de Ven, W. P. M. M. (2004). *The International Review Panel report to the South African Risk Equalization Fund Task Group*, 16 February. Available at http://www.medicalschemes.com/publications/ publications.aspx?catid = 23

Broomberg, J., & Shisana, O. (1995). *Restructuring the national health system for universal primary health care*. Report of the Committee of Inquiry into a National Health Insurance System. Executive Summary. June 1995

Council for Medical Schemes. (2008a). Guidelines for the identification of beneficiaries with REF risk factors in accordance with the REF entry and verification criteria, version 3.2. Applicable to all REF cases from 1 January 2008. Published 27 March 2008. Available at http://www.medicalschemes.com/publications/publications.aspx?catid = 23

Council for Medical Schemes. (2008b). Report of the Registrar of Medical Schemes, 2007/2008. Available at http://www.medicalschemes.com/publications/publications.aspx?catid = 7

Department of Social Development. (2002). *Transforming the present – protecting the future.* Report of the Committee of Inquiry into a Comprehensive System of Social Security for South Africa, March. Available at http://www.welfare.gov.za

Harrison, S., Bhana, R., & Ntuli, A. (Eds). (2007). The role of the private sector within the South African health system. In: *South African Health Review 2007.* Durban: Health Systems Trust. Available at http://www.hst.org.za/publications/711

Kirigia, J. M., Preker, A., Carrin, G., Mwikisa, C., & Diarra-Nama, A. J. (2006). An overview of health financing patterns and the way forward in the WHO African Region. *East African Medical Journal* (Supplement), Si–Siii, S1–S28. Available at http://www.who.int/health_financing/documents/eamj-health_financing_africa.pdf

Kutzin, J. (2001). A descriptive framework for country-level analysis of health care financing arrangements. *Health Policy, 56*(3), 171–204.

Low Income Medical Schemes Process. (2006). Low income medical schemes process. In: J. Broomberg (Ed.), *Consultative investigation into low income medical schemes* (Final Report, 7 April). Available at http://www.medicalschemes.com

McIntyre, D., & van den Heever, A. (2007). Social or national health insurance. In: S. Harrison, R. Bhana & A. Ntuli (Eds), *South African Health Review 2007.* Durban: Health Systems Trust Availale at http://www.hst.org.za/publications/711

McIntyre, D., & Thiede, M. (2007). Health care financing and expenditure. In: S. Harrison, R. Bhana & A. Ntuli (Eds), *South African Health Review 2007.* Durban: Health Systems TrustAvailable at http://www.hst.org.za/publications/711

McLeod, H., Matisonn, S., Fourie, I., Grobler, P., Mynhardt, S., & Marx, G. (2004). *The determination of the formula for the risk equalisation fund in South Africa.* Prepared for the Risk Equalisation Fund Task Group on behalf of the Formula Consultative Task Team, January. Available at http://www.medicalschemes.com/publications/publications.aspx?catid = 23

McLeod, H., & Ramjee, S. (2007). Medical schemes. In: S. Harrison, R. Bhana & A. Ntuli (Eds), *South African Health Review 2007.* Durban: Health Systems Trust Available at http://www.hst.org.za/publications/711

Ministerial Task Team on Social Health Insurance. (2005). *Social health insurance options: Financial and fiscal impact assessment,* June 2005. Unpublished technical report to the Department of Health, Pretoria.

Risk Equalisation Technical Advisory Panel. (2007). *Methodology for the Determination of the Risk Equalisation Fund Contribution Table 2007 [Base 2005, Use 2007].* Recommendations to the Council for Medical Schemes, 17 April. Report no. 9, Council for Medical Schemes, Pretoria. Available at http://www.medicalschemes.com/publications/publications.aspx?catid = 23

Söderlund, N., & Peprah, E. (1998). *An essential hospital package for South Africa: Selection criteria, costs and affordability.* Centre for Health Policy, Johannesburg, Monograph Number 52. Available at http://web.wits.ac.za/Academic/Centres/CHP/

World Health Organization. (2005). Sustainable health financing, universal coverage and social health insurance. *Resolutions and decisions.* Fifty-Eighth World Health Assembly WHA58.33, Agenda item 13.16, 25 May. Available at http://www.who.int/gb/ebwha/pdf_files/WHA58/WHA58_33-en.pdf

PURCHASING HEALTH CARE IN CHINA: EXPERIENCES, OPPORTUNITIES AND CHALLENGES

Winnie Yip and Kara Hanson

ABSTRACT

Objectives – *Purchasing has been promoted as a key policy instrument to improve health system performance. Despite its widespread adoption, there is little empirical evidence on how it works, the challenges surrounding its implementation, its impact, and the preconditions for it to function effectively, particularly in low- and middle-income settings. The objective of this chapter is to analyze critically the extent to which purchasing could be, and has been used strategically in China and to identify modifications that are needed for purchasing to be effective in assuring that the government's new funding for health care will result in efficient and effective health services.*

Methods – *We present a conceptual framework for purchasing, which identifies three critical principal–agent relationships in purchasing. We draw on evidence from secondary data, results of other research studies, interviews, and the impact evaluation of a social experiment in rural China that explicitly used purchasing to improve quality and efficiency. This information is used to examine purchasing relationships in urban*

Innovations in Health System Finance in Developing and Transitional Economies
Advances in Health Economics and Health Services Research, Volume 21, 197–218
Copyright © 2009 by Emerald Group Publishing Limited
ISSN: 0731-2199/doi:10.1108/S0731-2199(2009)0000021011

social health insurance (SHI), the rural medical insurance scheme, and purchasing of public health services.

Findings – *To date, use of strategic purchasing is limited in China. Both the urban and the rural health insurance schemes act as passive third-party payers, failing to take advantage of the opportunities to strengthen incentives to improve quality and efficiency. This may be because as government agencies, the extent to which the Ministries of Health and Labor and Social Security can act independently from provider interests, or act in the best interest of the population, is unclear. Other important challenges include ensuring adequate representation of the population's views and preferences and making better use of the leverage provided by purchasing to create appropriate provider incentives, through better integration of financing and improved coordination among purchasers.*

Implications for policy – *In designing purchasing arrangements, attention needs to be paid to all three principal–agent relationships. Successful purchasing appears to require mechanisms to mobilize and represent community preferences and more strategic contracting with providers. More research is needed to strengthen the evidence on which purchasing arrangements work, which do not work, and under what conditions different purchasing configurations can work most effectively.*

1. INTRODUCTION

Around the world, purchasing is promoted as a key policy instrument to improve health system performance, especially in terms of quality and efficiency. But establishing an effective system of purchasing is far from simple; its success depends on many variables such as who is the purchaser, the leverage this purchaser has over providers, and to what extent it represents the interests of the population on whose behalf it is purchasing. The provider market and regulatory environment are also important elements that can determine the success or failure of a purchasing scheme. Despite the widespread adoption of purchasing, there is, however, very little empirical evidence on how it works, the challenges surrounding its implementation, and much less on its impact and the preconditions for it to function effectively. The evidence is particularly scant in lower and middle income countries (LMICs), even though purchasing has gained currency in recent years in these countries. Using China as an illustration, this chapter aims to fill this gap.

In April, 2009, the Chinese government unveiled its health care reform plan, which promises an additional 850 billion RMB (123 billion US dollars) over the next three years to provide universal and affordable basic health care for its 1.3 billion population (Anonymous, 2009; Chen, 2009). This investment represents a doubling of government spending on health in 2009 and signals the government's increased role in financing health care.

In the years that led up to the announcement of the reform plan, a heated debate centered around one key question: How can China ensure that its new health care spending will result in effective and efficient health services? In other words, how can China improve efficiency and quality? Two major views prevailed, reflecting the international debate over the best model of health care provision. One school of thought advocated direct subsidies to government facilities, while the other supported reliance on a regulated market.

Proponents of direct provision argue that the root cause of China's rampant inefficiency is inadequate government funding for public facilities; therefore, increasing the government budget to providers will solve the problem. When China embarked on its economic reform in the late 1970s, the government experienced a significant reduction in revenue, reducing its capacity to fund health care. Government subsidies for public health facilities fell to a mere 10% of the facilities' total revenues by the early 1990s. To allow public facilities to survive financially, the government set a fee schedule such that prices for basic health care are set below cost and prices for drugs and high-tech services are set above cost. This has created perverse incentives for providers at all levels to overprescribe drugs and tests to increase profits (Liu & Mills, 1999; Blumenthal & Hsiao, 2005; Yip & Hsiao, 2008).[1] Moreover, hospitals receive kickbacks from drug companies for prescribing their products, and doctors' bonuses are often tied to these kickbacks, further exacerbating the problem of overprescribing. In rural areas, village doctors buy expired and counterfeit drugs at low cost and sell them as valid products at higher prices (Blumenthal & Hsiao, 2005). Advocates of a direct government provision approach argue that providing public providers with an *adequate* budget, combined with management, would eliminate their for-profit behavior.

Proponents of the regulated market approach argue that increasing government funding alone will not result in efficient and effective use of the government's new spending. They argue that because of serious market failures, a prudent purchaser is required to act on behalf of the population to select and contract with providers for the best quality of services. They advocate for the government's new funding to be channeled to the purchaser through a government demand-side subsidy. The purchaser would then strategically purchase services for the covered population based on price and provider performance. Providers, both public and private, would compete for the contracts.

The latest reform document, issued in April 2009 (Anonymous, 2009), indicates that China has identified five areas of reform: (1) increase demand subsidies for the rural population to enroll in the New Cooperative Medical Scheme (NCMS) (a form of rural health insurance) and for the urban uninsured to enroll in the Urban Resident Basic Medical Insurance (URBMI) Scheme; (2) increase government spending on public health services, especially in the lower income regions; (3) directly fund primary care facilities and basic staff salaries, focusing on community health centers in urban areas and township health centers in rural areas, and also make a substantial investment in infrastructure and the strengthening of these facilities, including village clinics; (4) reform the pharmaceutical market; and (5) finally, reform public hospitals.[2] The reform policy suggests that China will use both supply- and demand-side subsidy approaches. It also explicitly encourages the use of purchasing, especially through the expanded urban and rural health insurance schemes and government purchasing of public health, on which this chapter focuses.

We begin this chapter by reviewing the theoretical basis for purchasing in health and describe a conceptual framework on *strategic* purchasing adopted from Figueras, Robinson, and Jakubowski (2005), which we use to anchor our discussion. We then discuss China's rural health insurance, urban health insurance, and public health financing using this conceptual framework, and analyze the extent to which key components of strategic purchasing are used, in the Chinese context. Because many of China's reform initiatives are still in their early stages, they are not ready for rigorous impact evaluation. We draw our evidence from a number of information sources, including secondary data, results of other research studies, interviews, and the impact evaluation of a social experiment in rural China that explicitly used purchasing to improve quality and efficiency. The final section provides a critical examination of China's purchasing in the context of international experience, speculates on what China needs to do for strategic purchasing to be effective in improving the performance of its health care system, and finally identifies questions for future research.

2. PURCHASING: THEORETICAL ROOTS

Globally, purchasing has been identified as a key element of health system financing. Though differing across health systems, the aims of purchasing are typically to improve technical and allocative efficiency, to improve responsiveness to patients, and (in some cases) to improve equity. It is closely linked to, but broader than, notions of contracting (which we define here as representing the legal relationship that exists between a purchaser and a provider) and performance-based payments (which may be incorporated into a contracting relationship, but are not necessarily so). It involves decisions about *which* interventions should be purchased to meet the objectives of improving population health and satisfying user preferences; *how* interventions should be purchased, such as the specific contractual mechanisms and provider payment systems; and *from whom* interventions should be purchased, since public and private providers have relative advantages in terms of quality and efficiency (Figueras et al., 2005). The constituent elements of the purchasing relationship are described later.

Health service purchasing has its intellectual roots in two areas of economic thought. The first is related to the "make or buy" decision first explored by Williamson (1985) and used to explain how the boundaries of the firm are determined. In its application to for-profit firms, transaction cost economics hypothesizes that firms will choose the organizational form that is transaction cost minimizing. They will tend to "make" (i.e., produce internally, through "governance" arrangements) in circumstances where problems of opportunism and bounded rationality prevail, and together with high levels of asset specificity preclude the use of "classical" or "complete" contracts. In contrast, a firm will "buy" (contract with other firms) where bounded rationality and opportunism are less problematic and where problems of "hold up" due to asset specificity are less able to thwart efficient contracting.

This body of thought can be seen to have influenced the New Public Management (NPM) ideas that were developed in the 1980s and were influential in shaping public sector reforms in the UK and northern Europe (Walsh, 1995). NPM identified a role for market forces and competition to improve efficiency and responsiveness in public service delivery, to be achieved while maintaining public ownership through the development of a "purchaser–provider split" within internal (public) markets. Under these arrangements, the government is responsible for ensuring that services are provided (through financing and purchasing) but not necessarily for their direct provision. This entails a change in the role of government from "command-and-control" to one of "steer and negotiate" (WHO, 2008).

A second set of ideas linked to purchasing, and embedded in the NPM concept, is the economics of information and agency theory. While for most goods and services individuals make their own consumption decisions, the

complexity and uncertainty that surround decision-making in health care
and the difficulty that patients have in judging the quality of health care
providers mean that patients commonly depend on an informed agent to
make decisions on their behalf. In the traditional model in which patients
purchase care directly from providers, the providers act as the agent for the
patients. When providers seek to maximize their own income while at the
same time being tasked with making decisions that are best for the patients'
health, imperfect agency arises. The creation of a third-party purchaser, who
represents the collective interests of the users, can be effective at gathering
information and negotiating with the provider for the best price and quality
of services. Many forms of third-party purchasers exist around the world,
including insurance plans (e.g., the United States, Colombia), primary care
physicians (e.g., the UK), and independent government agencies (e.g.,
Thailand). A key question is who is in a position to act as the "best" agent
for the patient. Two important factors influencing this may be the
complexity of the services involved and the severity of the information gap.

A recent publication from the European Observatory on Health Systems
(Figueras et al., 2005) adopts a triple principal–agent framework in
analyzing the various components of *strategic* purchasing. The framework
consists of three relationships: between the purchasers and the users;
between the purchasers and the providers; and between the purchasers and
the government. We use this framework, organized along the following
questions, to describe and discuss China's purchasing arrangements.

1. *Organization of purchasing*: Who is the purchasing agency? Is purchasing
   centralized or decentralized? Is there competition among purchasers? If
   so, what is the degree of competition and on what basis do they compete?
2. *Purchaser–users relationship*: How are patients/users' needs and preferences reflected in purchasing decisions? What is being purchased? What
   role is played by the patients/users?
3. *Purchaser–provider relationship*: What types of contractual arrangements
   and provider payment methods govern their relationship? What other
   monitoring and regulatory mechanisms are used? What types of provider
   organizations are used (integrated public vs. autonomous public vs.
   private) and in what types of market structure do health care providers
   operate (competition vs. monopoly vs. oligopoly)? How much power
   does the purchaser have over the providers?
4. *Purchaser–government relationship*: To what extent does the purchaser, as
   an agent for the government, fulfil the government's objectives in terms
   of its purchasing activities? What role is played by the government in

regulating purchasing, including setting benefit packages, regulation of purchaser budgets, pricing, etc.?

3. PURCHASING IN RURAL CHINA

Since the beginning of the 2003, the Chinese government has allocated significant new resources to subsidize rural residents' enrollment in the NCMS. For the first waves of NCMS, the Chinese government subsidized each rural resident in poor Western and Central provinces by 20 RMB (US $2.50), shared equally between the central and local governments,[3] if he or she paid an annual premium of 10 RMB (US $1.25) to enroll in the NCMS. In 2006, the government subsidy was increased to 40 RMB (US $5), then again to 80 RMB in 2007, 100 RMB in 2008, and 120 RMB in 2009, with the individual's contribution increased to 20 RMB (Anonymous, 2009). Per capita total health expenditure in these provinces was about 160–200 RMB during this period. The local government's contribution is shared among the province, municipality and county, and the share paid by each level varies across provinces.

The government's stated goals for NCMS are to improve access to health care and reduce medical impoverishment. Conspicuously absent are improvements in health outcomes, efficiency, or quality. The national policy guidelines for NCMS have only two requirements: voluntary enrollment and coverage of major illness, which often is taken to mean hospitalization (Central Committee of CPC, 2002). Apart from these, each local NCMS can decide on the benefit package, provider payment method, and other administrative arrangements. As a result, many different models exist.[4] The majority of those in the Western and Central regions cover only hospitalization. All of them involve coinsurance rates, reimbursement caps, and many also require payment of a deductible (Mao, 2005).

This shift to the use of subsidized insurance plans represents a departure from China's traditional model of financing, shifting from a supply- to demand-side subsidy and thus creating a purchaser–provider split. The collected funds are managed by a NCMS management office, which sits within the county level Health Bureau. Risk is pooled at the county level, which has an average population size of 300,000.[5] This places the role of purchasing in the hands of the NCMS management office by default, with no other competing purchasers. As such, purchasing for health care is devolved to the county level.

The advantage of placing purchasing at the local level is that it is close to the people and therefore should, in theory, be better able to reflect the population's needs and preferences and more likely to be accountable to the local population. In practice, however, there is little evidence to suggest that people's preferences are solicited or that health needs are taken into account in deciding what services NCMS will cover. In fact, although interviews with households show that many rural residents would prefer coverage of primary health care at conveniently located health facilities, the majority of first-wave NCMS models primarily cover only hospitalization (Mao, 2005). Similarly, despite the fact that chronic conditions represent an increasing share of the disease burden among the rural population, until recently, most NCMS models did not cover chronic conditions unless they involved hospitalization (Ma, 2008; Wang, 2008; Wen, 2009; Yip & Hsiao, 2009). Finally, villagers have little, if any, representation in the NCMS management.

In terms of the purchasing relationship between the NCMS management office and health care providers, evidence suggests that most NCMS purchasers play a passive third-party payer role and continue to pay providers on a fee-for-service basis. There is no explicit contracting to delineate the scope of services or quality standards. Although there have been some efforts to introduce performance evaluation, in-depth interviews and reviews of performance indicators raise doubt about their effectiveness: indicators are largely tied to the number of visits and the volume of services provided and less so to quality of these services, and indicator measurements are frequently based on subjective assessment rather than objective evaluation. One possible reason for the failure of NCMS to adopt a more active purchasing role may be that the scope of services purchased by the NCMS management office is too limited. If only hospital services are covered, the NCMS management office cannot exercise any purchasing power over outpatient-based services, which are primarily delivered by township health centers and village doctors. Hospital services are provided by county hospitals, but since these facilities also serve patients covered by the Urban Employee Basic Medical Insurance (UEBMI) scheme (described below), NCMS may not have much leverage over them. Another possible reason for the limited purchasing role of the NCMS office is that prices in China are set by the Provincial Pricing Bureau. Although this can relieve the purchaser from the difficult job of negotiating prices, it also limits its effectiveness if the Pricing Bureau and the NCMS management office are not aligned in their objectives. Finally and perhaps most importantly, the fact that the NCMS management office is part of the Ministry of Health may have limited its purchasing function. Since the Ministry of Health represents the interests of both the providers and the patients, the separation of purchasing and provision is incomplete and the purchaser's management is unclear of their objectives.

In sum, up to now, strategic purchasing in rural China is limited even though the government's substantial increase in demand-side subsidies provides new opportunities and potential. Nonetheless, there are ongoing efforts to pilot feasible forms of purchasing, with the goal of improving efficiency and quality of health services for the rural population. We describe here one such pilot and its experience in detail.

3.1. A Pilot Experiment: Rural Mutual Health Care

Between 2002 and 2007, a group of researchers based at Harvard University designed and implemented a pilot experiment, Rural Mutual Health Care (RMHC), in two western provinces of China (Hsiao, 2004; Hsiao, Yip, & Wang, 2008). The study design matched intervention sites with control sites, and data were collected in the baseline and annually after the intervention started in 2003. RMHC followed the government's guidelines for voluntary enrollment and coverage of major illnesses. The project simulated the government subsidy for each villager who prepaid a premium to enroll in RMHC. However, the pilot had several major differences from the government's NCMS, especially in terms of its goals and the use of strategic purchasing.

Like the government's NCMS, RMHC aimed to improve access to health care and financial risk protection for the rural population. However, recognizing that rapid cost inflation is a root cause of unaffordable health care, RMHC also aimed to improve the efficiency of health care delivery and to improve the population's health status through better quality services.

In designing the role and functions of the RMHC fund office – the purchaser – a key concern was how to ensure that it would be accountable to the population, representing as well as possible their interests and preferences. RMHC used direct community participation to improve the agency function of the purchaser. Since villagers had an interest in ensuring that they would benefit from the scheme, it was felt that they were in a good position to monitor the use of funds and to influence the choice of benefit package to reflect the views of the community. A Fund Board was created, which included an elected representative from each village, government officials, township health center directors, and town financial auditors. The Board was responsible for selecting the benefit package that would best reflect villagers' preferences; for example, RMHC covered primary care and drugs at the village level because villagers desired basic health care and drugs to be geographically accessible. In addition, review of utilization data showed that a significant proportion of the population suffered from chronic conditions and experienced high levels of associated medical expenditure. As a result, the benefit package of RMHC covered outpatient and primary care services, in addition to the hospitalization coverage stipulated by the government guideline. The Board also managed and controlled the Fund Office that paid and contracted with service providers.

The Fund Office acted as a single purchaser and selected the best village doctors (when there are more than one village doctor in the village) on a competitive basis. Since no clinical performance records exist at the village level in China (as in most low- and middle-income countries), selection was based on a combination of qualifications and a village vote. The Fund Office contracted with selected village doctors, compensating them with a salary plus a bonus based on performance indicators, including conforming to established protocols for treatment of common diseases such as upper respiratory infections and diarrhea, proper maintenance of patient medical records, delivery of public health functions, and patient satisfaction ratings. Doctors who were not selected saw their patient loads drastically reduced because villagers enrolled in RMHC were reimbursed only for care provided by contracted village doctors. Because close to 80% of the villagers enrolled in the scheme, village doctors had very strong incentives to improve their performance to increase their chance of being selected. Provider contracts explicitly outlined provider responsibilities and payment. The delineation of responsibilities, combined with the salary plus bonus payment of village doctors, provided contracted doctors with incentives to focus on tasks within their level of competency (instead of competing with township and county providers) and to focus on primary care and prevention activities.

In addition, as a single purchaser with significant market power over village doctors, the Fund Office was able to establish bulk purchasing for drugs. Village doctors were no longer permitted to purchase drugs directly from drug manufacturers or distributors. Instead, they submitted to the Fund Office a list of the drugs needed for their practice. The Fund Office in turn worked with the local health bureau to conduct competitive bidding to select the lowest price and best quality suppliers. Drugs were then distributed to the village doctors directly. Bulk purchasing resulted not only in a reduction in drug prices but also much better monitoring of the use of fake and substandard drugs.

To monitor provider performance, each village organized a five-member volunteer committee. This committee monitored the availability of staff, drugs, and supplies in the village clinic; the day-to-day cleanliness of the health facilities; and other interpersonal aspects of care such as whether the doctors explained health conditions and drug side-effects to the patients. Because the villagers and their families and neighbors directly experienced the services of these providers, they were very effective monitors. Complaints of high expenditure for visits and other concerns were reviewed by the Fund Board, which then took action to investigate the complaints. For clinical service quality, the project relied on physicians in the upper level facilities to monitor the lower level facilities.

The changes in payment incentives and organization of service delivery brought about measurable improvements in efficiency and quality, especially at the primary care level. Total expenditure (scheme plus copayment) per visit to the village doctor in intervention sites dropped from 16 RMB in the baseline to only about 10 RMB the year after the intervention, whereas total expenditure per visit in the control sites actually grew to about 18 RMB over the same period. Using both household surveys and prescription studies, the study found that the reduction in expenditure per visit was attributed to several factors: a reduction in the number of drugs prescribed; reductions in the number of prescriptions for antibiotics and steroids; a reduction in the number of intravenous injections; and finally, a reduction in drug prices. After implementing the drug bulk purchasing policy and audits of the Fund Office, records from the RMHC's Fund Office showed that the use of fake and expired drugs had been eliminated, whereas the use of counterfeit drugs in the control sites remained at about 30%.

RMHC also improved villagers' access to basic health care, which household surveys had indicated as being a priority for the community. Specifically, villagers wanted access to primary health care, which is exactly what RMHC delivered. Measuring access to care as health care utilization rates adjusted for need, the pilot showed that RMHC increased the two-week probability of an outpatient visit by 70%. About 82% of the increase was in visits to village doctors. At the same time, RMHC reduced the probability of self-medication by about two-thirds, suggesting a shift from self-medication to seeking formal care (Yip, Wang, & Hsiao, 2008). Unsurprisingly, RMHC enjoyed high levels of villager satisfaction, with 85% of the enrolled satisfied with the scheme, and close to 90% wishing to continue their enrollment (Hsiao et al., 2008).

4. PURCHASING IN URBAN CHINA

At present, there are two health insurance programs in urban China – UEBMI for employees in the formal sector and government agencies, including retirees, and URBMI for those who are not covered by UEBMI, including children and the elderly. UEBMI was first piloted in Zhenjiang and Jiujiang cities in 1997 and was expanded to the entire country starting in 1999. It covers about 50% of the urban population. URBMI is a newer scheme that only began to be piloted in 2007 (Liu, 2008). This chapter therefore focuses its discussion on the UEBMI.

The UEBMI is a compulsory scheme in which employers and employees contribute 6% and 2% of the employees' wages, respectively, to enroll. Contributions are divided into two parts: two-thirds of the employer's contribution is allocated to a risk pooled fund, while the remaining one-third is combined with the 2% from employees and deposited in an individual savings account owned by the employee. There are coinsurance rates, deductibles, and ceilings applied to the risk pooled fund. The funds in the savings accounts can only be used to pay for health care.[6]

The UEBMI is managed by a Social Health Insurance (SHI) Bureau, housed within the Bureau of Labor and Social Security at the municipal level, where risks are pooled. The SHI is thus positioned to be the purchasing agency. In contrast to NCMS, the central government plays a stronger role in defining the benefit packages for UEBMI. There are three formularies: drugs, health services, and medical technology/equipment. The Ministry of Labor and Social Security determines the national essential drug list, while provincial local Bureau of Labor and Social Security define the formularies for health services and medical technology/equipment (Liu, 2008).

Once the formularies have been established, the SHIs selectively contract with providers, both public and private, to deliver the defined list of services and drugs to the UEBMI-insured population. There is a contractual agreement between the SHIs and the contracted providers that specifies not only the services to be delivered to the insured but also the right of the medical insurance agency to inspect and supervise the activities of these designated healthcare institutions. In practice, however, most public providers are contracted, and most contracts are renewed. This raises the question of whether selective contracting is effectively used by the SHI to provide incentives for providers to improve the quality of health care services.

Provider payment for designated providers is still largely on a fee-for-service basis, although some cities are experimenting with different forms of provider payment methods, including global budgets, case-based payment, and expenditure caps (Yip & Eggleston, 2001; Meng, 2008). The goal of these payment changes appears to be to control program expenditure, and there is little evidence to show that the provider payment changes introduced by the UEBMI aim to improve efficiency or quality. Given that UEBMI only covers 50% of most cities' population, SHI's leverage over hospitals is constrained.

It is important to note that under the UEBMI, the relationship between the purchaser and the users/patients within the triple principle–agent relationship is largely absent. The SHI is a government organization, with no beneficiary representation. As a result, beneficiaries are largely voiceless and the benefit package design does not necessarily reflect their preferences or health needs.

5. PURCHASING PUBLIC HEALTH

The Chinese government has committed significant resources to improving the provision of public health and preventive services such as vaccinations, maternal and child care, health promotion and health education, as well as the equitable distribution of public health services both between urban and rural areas and between rich and poor regions. Concerned that additional funding will not result in improved services under the traditional model of directly funding public providers, the Ministry of Finance and its counterparts in local government are particularly eager to experiment with feasible ways of purchasing public health services.

In the latest reform, government financing for public health services takes the form of a capitation payment (targeted to be 15 RMB and 20 RMB per person in 2010 and 2011, respectively) for a defined package of public health and preventive services, for a defined population (Anonymous, 2009; Chen, 2009). Local Health Bureaus hold the capitated budget and use it to purchase the defined package of services from community health centers in urban areas, and township health centers and village clinics in rural areas, paying them through some form of pay-for-performance payment method.

The government is currently conducting pilot studies on purchasing public health in two provinces – Shandong and Ningxia. In Shandong, the capitated budget for public health is 10 RMB per person. The defined package includes immunization and vaccinations, maternal and child health, health promotion (such as regular checkups), health education, infectious disease control and prevention, prevention and management of chronic diseases, creation and management of health records for the covered population, and treatment of common health problems in the community. Services included in the defined package are provided free of charge to the population.

In urban areas, health bureaus selectively contract with community health centres, both public and private. At this stage, selection is largely based on infrastructure and staffing, such as whether the facility satisfies the building size requirement and whether there are staff trained to provide services specified in the package, but as experience accumulates, there may be opportunities to select based on quality and delivery of defined services. Both parties sign a contract defining the services to be provided. Selected institutions are given 30%–40% of the capitated budget at the beginning of the contract period, with the rest disbursed based on assessment of performance. Examples of performance criteria include number of vaccinations and immunizations, number of pre- and post-natal care visits, number of health records created, number of health examinations conducted, number of seminars given on specific topics of health prevention, patient satisfaction based on a survey, and so on.

In rural areas, where there is only one township health center for each town, there is no selective contracting. Instead, pay-for-performance is the main tool purchasers use to ensure quality services. As in the urban areas, providers receive only a portion of the capitated budget upfront, with receipt of the rest dependent on performance assessment as described earlier.

Because this pilot project is still in progress, it is too early to conduct a rigorous impact evaluation study. Nevertheless, two issues have already emerged during field visits and interviews. First, contracted providers have not shown much motivation to improve services defined under the public health package beyond those indicators against which their performance will be measured. This may be because the public health budget only represents a small share of providers' total revenue; thus, the contracted providers' focus is still on the curative services for which they earn fee-for-service profits. This may also be due to the fact that performance criteria focus on quantity of services, for example, how many seminars are given and how many posters and pamphlets are printed for health education, rather than actually measuring how effective the education program has been in changing the health behavior of the population. Second, the public health package has services that overlap with the "basic" care services covered by the NCMS. This repetition is both ineffective and inefficient, as providers face different incentives from different purchasers. Both of these observations would suggest that integrating the public health spending with NCMS (Urban Insurance in the urban areas) would strengthen the purchasing function.

6. DISCUSSION

Strategic purchasing in China to date has been limited in scale and in scope. Despite a significant increase in government spending to subsidize the demand side, full advantage has not been taken of the potential opportunities of a regulated market approach to ensure that the government's new funding will result in efficient and effective health services. Both the urban and the rural health insurance programs have functioned as passive third-party reimbursement schemes.

Here, we revisit the three principal–agent relationships that govern the structure of purchasing arrangements and provide a critical examination of China's purchasing in the context of international experience. We speculate on what China needs to do to better realize the potential of strategic purchasing in assuring that the government's new spending will result in efficient and effective health services, and also identify areas for future research.

It is important to note that purchasing arrangements are complex: they involve at least three key principal–agent relationships, linking actors at different levels of the health system. The devil is in the detail: the specific features of each of these relationships will influence the ability of the arrangements as a whole to reach the desired outcomes. In addition, how well the purchasing arrangements work is likely to depend on a number of pre-conditions and contextual factors such as existing provider market structure, regulatory capacity and enforceability, and governance. Not only do the features of complexity and context-dependence pose a particular challenge for evaluation (especially impact evaluation), they also mean that it is difficult to apply generalizable lessons from one country's experience to other settings. Nonetheless, given the widespread adoption of purchasing and the yet limited empirical evidence around it, China's early experience adds value to the existing literature. One caveat is in order. China is a vast country, and the description in this chapter represents an overview of the situation. We acknowledge that there may be specific cases that we have not fully incorporated.

6.1. Who is the Purchasing Agency?

A critical determinant of the effectiveness of a regulated market approach in improving efficiency and quality is the nature of the purchaser. In particular, what type of organization is in the best position and motivated to be an effective purchaser, able both to meet the government's social objectives and to act in the best interest of the population? In China, purchasing organizations are primarily government agencies: the SHI Bureau located within the Ministry of Labor and Social Security and the NCMS management office located within the Ministry of Health. Most civil servants are, however, motivated by their individual interests, such as keeping their jobs, getting a promotion, and increasing their earnings, rather than achieving the social objectives of the insurance programs (Hsiao, 2007). As the experience of the SHI shows, during its 10 years of operation it has functioned as a passive purchaser, primarily reimbursing for care provided, and its main objective appears to have been to balance its books. For the rural sector, where the NCMS management office is placed under the Ministry of Health, it is even more questionable how well it can engage in effective purchasing to achieve the government's social objectives, since it also represents the interests of the providers, who form the constituency of the Ministry of Health. This incomplete separation between purchasers and providers is likely to further limit the effectiveness of purchasing.

Other LMICs have elected to adopt different types of purchasing organization and institutional arrangements. At the other end of the spectrum, Colombia operates a system of competing private purchasers (Escobar, Giedion, Acosta, Castano, & Pinto, 2009). Thailand chose to establish a quasi-public autonomous organization – the National Health Security Office. Even in many transitional countries of eastern Europe and the Former Soviet Union, the purchaser is a public but autonomous insurance fund. Given this diversity of experience, the questions of who will be the best "agent" for the government to achieve its social objectives, which types of organization are more effective purchasers in achieving the goals of health system, and under what conditions they are able to exercise this function effectively remain unanswered. The synthesis of European experience (Figueras et al., 2005) suggests that there is no single type of purchaser that will work best in all contexts; that there are some advantages to having purchasing power devolved (increased autonomy and innovation, improved responsiveness to local conditions, and more effective con-tracting); but that some functions need to be performed at higher levels (e.g., pursuit of equity goals and some public health functions). As well as considering the type of purchasing organization, research in this area should focus on identifying the factors that influence their ability to perform this function effectively.

6.2. Purchaser–User Relationship

At present, in both the urban and the rural insurance schemes, there is no mechanism by which consumer preferences and health needs are reflected in the design of the benefit package. However, the Harvard rural experiment has demonstrated that it is feasible to include citizen representatives on the board of the county level purchaser, even among very low-income populations. Clearly, such representation is not sufficient for effective participation and exercise of "voice" to influence purchaser behavior, but at least in this context, there are indications that this mechanism has provided an effective channel of accountability between the purchaser and the population.

A range of other potential "voice" mechanisms exist, such as public consultations, advocacy groups, and consumer organizations (den Exter, 2005). A review of experience from Europe, including the transition countries, suggests that empowering citizens is essential in the purchasing process (Figueras et al., 2005). However, the experience of these structures in low-income settings is highly varied, and their effects have not been widely studied.

In theory, "choice" or "exit" mechanisms, such as allowing competing plans, might help to strengthen accountability between the purchasers and the population. In the Colombian reforms, for example, multiple plans compete for enrollees, with the intention that competition will occur on quality, not price (Escobar et al., 2009). Competition among purchasers might create incentives to be more responsive and accountable to the population. However, with multiple competing purchasers, the reallocation of funds to address inequalities, for example, at the regional level, would require some form of additional higher level intervention. Furthermore, competition would inevitably raise the issue of risk selection. The evidence on the effectiveness of choice at the purchaser level is very limited. In Europe, there has generally been more emphasis on mechanisms of voice than exit (Figueras et al., 2005).

Future research efforts should focus on: What types of mechanism will help to ensure that the purchaser's actions are in the interests of the population? Under what circumstances are "voice" options likely to be effective (and what is needed to make these arrangements effective)? What are the advantages and disadvantages of exit options (multiple purchasers) in increasing accountability to the population, particularly in low-income settings?

6.3. Purchaser–Provider Relationship

The purchaser – provider relationship is perhaps one of the most important among the triple principal – agent relationships. In the Chinese experience to date, there has been little use of explicit contracting, and provider payment has predominantly taken the form of fee-for-service. While there has been widespread adoption of explicit links between budget and performance, these have mostly relied on indicators of quantity rather than quality; subjective, rather than objective, measurement of indicators; and indicators that are only loosely tied to the overall system objectives of improved efficiency and quality.

There is a rich literature reviewing the experience of contracting for health services in LMICs (for recent reviews, refer Loevinsohn & Harding, 2005; Liu, Hotchkiss, & Bose, 2008), and a variety of "toolkits" for effective contracting have been prepared (refer, e.g., England, 2000; Loevinsohn, 2008). The requirements for contracting to lead to efficient and high-quality services include payment methods that incentivize providers to produce efficient, high–quality, and responsive services and clear performance measures, with explicit and objectively measured indicators that are directly linked to the purchasing objectives. In practice, contracting for a comprehensive set of health care services will be complex, due to problems of incomplete information and uncertainty. While contracting for comprehensive services is quite common across a range of settings, most of the evidence about the impact of contracting in LMICs has examined programs focusing on a narrowly defined set of essential services (e.g. Loevinsohn & Harding, 2005).

A fundamental issue linked to the purchaser–provider relationship is whether the purchaser has sufficient leverage over the providers to allow it to effectively counteract incentives that underlie providers' inefficient behavior. In general, the larger the share of provider revenue that the purchaser controls, the more likely it is that the purchaser can leverage desired performance from providers. The Chinese experience shows that both the SHI Bureaus and the NCMS management offices have not been very effective in reducing inefficient provider behaviors that are a consequence of the distorted price schedule and drug mark up, which have created perverse incentives. This may be because in the urban areas UEBMI covers only about 50% of the population. As a result, revenue from the SHI only represents a fraction of providers' income. SHI Bureaus have mostly been passive reimbursement schemes and have not actively used provider payment methods or contracts to improve efficiency and quality. Despite some pilot efforts to try out new forms of provider payment methods, SHI largely pays providers on a fee-for-service basis. Similarly, although in theory, SHI could select providers to contract on an annual basis, in practice, all public providers in the city are contracted and their contracts have been renewed almost every year. Prescription and ordering of excessive and expensive drugs and high-tech diagnostic tests remain unabated. Likewise, in NCMS models that covered only the costs of hospitalization, the purchasers had no influence over the provision of outpatient care. Village doctors and township health centers continue to overprescribe drugs. Furthermore, county hospitals received revenue from both the NCMS and the scheme covering urban workers, limiting the leverage of the NCMS management office over the county hospitals. In contrast, in NCMS models that cover both inpatient and outpatient services, such as the RMHC experiment and NCMS models in the coastal areas, the purchaser is better placed to exercise selective contracting and change the provider payment mechanism, as it represents a significant share of provider income.

The early experience of public health purchasing in China also illustrates that fragmented purchasing can limit its effectiveness. Having multiple purchasers dealing with community level providers dilutes the purchaser's power, increases the transaction costs (with multiple purchasers purchasing different services from the same providers), and because of ambiguity in the definition of the public health service package may even lead to multiple payments for the same services. Integration of the public health service package into the basic NCMS service package would seem to be useful both to increase the purchasers' influence over how these services are delivered and to reduce transaction costs.

Such fragmentation of purchasing is likely to arise across a range of LMIC settings as many countries still rely on multiple sources of financing that are not necessarily consolidated into a single purchaser. Even in the case of Thailand, it has not yet been feasible to merge the public insurance schemes that existed before the implementation of Universal Coverage in 2001, and multiple purchasers remain. It will be valuable to study how separate purchasing by multiple purchasers has constrained their leverage over provider behavior.

6.4. Purchaser–Government Relationship

Assessing the extent to which the purchaser acts as the government's agent and fulfils the government's objectives in its purchasing activities is complicated in China by the integration of the purchaser (SHI Bureau or NCMS management office) with the Ministry of Labor and Social Security and the Ministry of Health. Because of this integration, the relationship between the government and the purchaser is not necessarily best analyzed as one between a principal and an agent. A more systematic analysis of the structure and factors that govern the relationship between these two parties is needed before meaningful recommendations can be made on how to strengthen the purchaser's role and function in achieving the government's social objectives. Another key role that the government plays in purchasing is that of a steward and a regulator (Figueras et al., 2005). In China, this transformation of government's role from direct provider to steward and regulator has not yet occurred, especially in rural areas. However, it is clear that the system is still in transition, and these relationships continue to evolve.

7. CONCLUSION

While strategic purchasing is a promising approach to strengthen health system performance, there is very little empirical evidence on how it works, the challenges surrounding its implementation, its impact, and the preconditions for it to function effectively. Using the triple principal–agent relationships that define strategic purchasing, this chapter critically examined the extent to which China is, or is not, using strategic purchasing to transform its new government spending into efficient and effective health services for the population. We found that strategic purchasing is still limited in China. A fundamental question is, being government agencies motivated to pursue bureaucratic interests, to what extent do, and can, the Ministry of Health and the Ministry of Labor and Social Security serve as the best agents for the population? In addition, we suggested a number of areas where further modification is needed if purchasing is to achieve meaningful outcomes. Our findings were consistent with those from other settings, which have demonstrated that health service purchasing is a broad systems intervention, and action must be taken in relation to all its various components for purchasing to achieve its desired results (Figueras et al., 2005). A major research effort is needed to examine the experience of existing purchasing arrangements to answer the questions of what works, what does not work, and under what conditions different purchasing configurations can work most effectively.

NOTES

1. For example, 75% of patients suffering from a common cold are prescribed antibiotics, as are 79% of hospital patients – over twice the international average of 30%. Consequently, China's health care expenditure has been growing at 16% per year – 7% faster than the growth of gross domestic product (GDP) – for the past two decades.

2. When this chapter was drafted, the government had not decided what specific reform measures it will introduce for reforming the public hospitals. It plans to use the next three years to pilot experiment.

3. Provinces in the eastern region do not receive subsidies from the Central Government.

4. A survey of 354 counties in China found that most NCMS models in the first few years covered only inpatient services, some covered inpatient plus several selected outpatient services for major acute illnesses, and a small proportion covered both inpatient and outpatient services. In the Western and Central regions, the most commonly found model combines a medical savings account and high-deductible catastrophic insurance for inpatient services (Mao, 2005).

5. Some counties have population size as large as 1 million, while smaller ones, especially those in mountainous areas, can be as small as 100,000.

6. In some cases, the savings account is used to pay for outpatient services while the risk pooled fund is used to pay for inpatient care. In other cases, funds in the savings account have to be exhausted before using risk pooled funds.

REFERENCES

Anonymous. (2009). *The standing conference of State Council of China adopted guidelines for furthering the reform of health-care system in principle. Ministry of Health of China.* Available at http://www.moh.gov.cn/publicfiles/business/htmlfiles/mohbgt/s3582/200901/38889.htm (in Chinese). Accessed on March 13, 2009.

Blumenthal, D., & Hsiao, W. C. (2005). Privatization and its discontents – The evolving Chinese health care system. *New England Journal of Medicine, 353*(11), 1165–1170.

Central Committee of CPC. (2002). *Decisions of the central committee of the communist party of China and the state council on further strengthening rural health work.* Beijing, China.

Chen, Z. (2009). Launch of the health-care reform plan in China. *The Lancet, 373*(9672), 1322–1324.

den Exter, A. P. (2005). Purchasers as the public's agent. In: J. Figueras, R. Robinson & E. Jakubowski (Eds), *Purchasing to improve health systems performance.* Maidenhead: Open University Press.

England, R. (2000). Contracting and performance management in the health sector: Some pointers on how to do it. DFID Health Systems Resource Centre, London. Available at http://www.dfidhealthrc.org/publications/health_service_delivery/Contracting.PDF. Retrieved on 17 March, 2009.

Escobar, M. L., Giedion, U., Acosta, O. L., Castano, R. A., & Pinto, D. M. L. (2009). Health care financing. In: A. Glassman, A. Giuffrida, M. L. Escobar & U. Giedion (Eds), *From few to many: Ten years of health insurance expansion in Colombia.* Washington, DC: Inter-American Development Bank and Brookings Institution.

Figueras, J., Robinson, R., & Jakubowski, E. (Eds). (2005). *Purchasing to improve health systems performance.* Maidenhead: Open University Press.

Hsiao, W. C. (2004). Disparity in health: the underbelly of China's economic development. *Harvard China Review, 5*(1), 64–70.

Hsiao, W. C. (2007). The political economy of Chinese health reform. *Health Economics, Policy and Law, 2*(3), 241–249.

Hsiao, W. C., Yip, W., & Wang, H. (2008). *A social experiment in rural China: Rural Mutual Health Care – A summary report.* Working Paper. Program in Health Care Financing, Harvard, Cambridge, MA.

Liu, G. G. (2008). *Urban medical insurance and financing in China: An update report.* Report for the World Bank, World Bank, Washington, DC.

Liu, X., Hotchkiss, D. R., & Bose, S. (2008). The effectiveness of contracting-out primary health care services in developing countries: A review of the evidence. *Health Policy and Planning, 23*(1), 1–13.

Liu, X., & Mills, A. (1999). Evaluating payment mechanisms: How can we measure unnecessary care? *Health Policy and Planning, 14*(4), 409–413.

Loevinsohn, B. (2008). *Performance-based contracting for health services in developing countries: A toolkit.* Washington, DC: The World Bank.

Loevinsohn, B., & Harding, A. (2005). Buying results? Contracting for health service delivery in developing countries. *The Lancet, 366*(9486), 676–681.

Ma, T. (2008). Guangxi's Liuzhou plans to add 20 chronic diseases to the NCMS. *Xinhua News, 17*(November), 2.

Mao, Z. (2005). *Pilot programme of NCMS in China: System design and progress.* Background paper for World Bank China Rural Health Study, Sichuan, China.

Meng, Q. (2008). *Provider payment reforms in China: an updated review.* Washington, DC: World Bank AAA Report, World Bank.

Walsh, K. (1995). *Public services and market mechanisms: Competition, contracting and the New Public Management.* London: Macmillan.

Wang, L. (2008). Fujian: 10 types of major chronic diseases to be added to the NCMS plan. *Xinhua News, 6*(April), 4.

Wen, J. (2009). Wen Jiabao: Will appropriately increase the scope of health insurance benefits, and increase the scale of benefits. *Renmin Wang, 6*(March), 1.

WHO. (2008). *World health report 2008: Primary health care – Now more than ever.* Geneva: World Health Organization.

Williamson, O. (1985). *The economic institutions of capitalism.* New York: Free Press.

Yip, W., & Eggleston, K. (2001). Provider payment reform in China: the case of hospital reimbursement in Hainan province. *Health Economics, 10*(4), 325–339.

Yip, W., & Hsiao, W. C. (2008). The Chinese health system at a crossroads. *Health Affairs, 27*(2), 460–468.

Yip, W., & Hsiao, W. C. (2009). Non-evidence-based policy: How effective is China's new cooperative medical scheme in reducing medical impoverishment? *Social Science & Medicine, 68*(2), 201–209.

Yip, W., Wang, H., & Hsiao, W. C. (2008). *The impact of rural mutual health care on access to health care: Evaluation of a social experiment in rural China.* Working Paper. Program in Health Care Financing, Harvard University, Cambridge, MA.

SECTION IV
MODIFYING DEMAND

THE IMPACT OF NEPAL'S NATIONAL INCENTIVE PROGRAMME TO PROMOTE SAFE DELIVERY IN THE DISTRICT OF MAKWANPUR

T. Powell-Jackson, B. D. Neupane, S. Tiwari, K. Tumbahangphe, D. Manandhar and A. M. Costello

ABSTRACT

Objective – *Nepal's Safe Delivery Incentive Programme (SDIP) was introduced nationwide in 2005 with the aim of encouraging greater use of professional care at childbirth. It provided cash to women giving birth in a public health facility and an incentive to the health provider for each delivery attended, either at home or in the facility. We aimed to assess the impact of the programme on neonatal mortality and health care seeking behaviour at childbirth in one district of Nepal.*

Methods – *Impacts were identified using an interrupted time series approach, applied to household data. We estimated a model linking the level of each outcome at a point in time to the start of the programme,*

Innovations in Health System Finance in Developing and Transitional Economies
Advances in Health Economics and Health Services Research, Volume 21, 221–249
ISSN: 0731-2199/doi:10.1108/S0731-2199(2009)0000021012

demographic controls, a vector of time variables and community-level fixed effects.

Findings – *The recipients of the cash transfer in the programme's first two years were disproportionately wealthier households, reflecting existing inequality in the use of government maternity services. In places with women's groups – where information about the policy was widely disseminated – the SDIP substantially increased skilled birth attendance, but failed to impact on either neonatal mortality or the caesarean section rate. In places with no women's groups, the SDIP had no impact on utilisation outcomes or neonatal mortality.*

Implications for policy – *The lack of any impact on neonatal mortality suggests that greater increases in utilisation or better quality of care are needed to improve health outcomes. The SDIP changed health care seeking behaviour only in those areas with women's groups highlighting the importance of effective communication of the policy to the wider public.*

INTRODUCTION

Under-utilisation of health care services is a familiar problem in developing countries. A combination of both supply- and demand-side barriers restrict access to services, particularly for poorer households who are in greatest need of health care (Ensor & Cooper, 2004; Travis et al., 2004). Overcoming these obstacles is especially challenging in maternal health, in part because the provision of and the reluctance to use maternity services are inextricably linked to deep-rooted issues such as the state of the health system and the place of women in society. This may explain, perhaps, why professional care at childbirth in sub-Saharan Africa and south Asia has stagnated over the past decade (Koblinsky et al., 2006).

A big part of the challenge, and one that is being increasingly recognised, is persuading the relevant agents to undertake changes in behaviour that promote the health of individuals and families. Many countries, particularly in Latin America, have sought to raise demand for health services by providing monetary incentives to households on the condition that they engage in certain health care seeking practices (Fiszbein & Schady, 2009). The most influential of these was the Mexican *Progresa* programme, introduced in 1997 to target poor households with cash transfers provided the children regularly attended school and made preventive health care visits

(Gertler, 2004). Other nationwide conditional cash transfer (CCT) programmes – *Red de Proteccion Socia* in Nicaragua, *Familias en Accion* in Colombia, *Bolsa Alimentacao* in Brazil, *Programa de Asignacion* in Honduras and *Bono de Desarrollo Humano* in Ecuador – were similar in design to the Mexican programme, also targeting poor household with a focus on human capital formation (Attanasio, Carlos Gomez, Heredia, & Vera-Hernandez, 2005; Maluccio & Flores, 2004; Morris, Flores, Olinto, & Medina, 2004a; Morris, Olinto, Flores, Nilson, & Figueiro, 2004b; Paxon & Schady, 2007). Many of these programmes were evaluated using randomised methods, providing a strong body of evidence that they can be an effective means to increase utilisation and, in some cases, improve health (Lagarde, Haines, & Palmer, 2007; Glassman, Todd, & Gaarder, 2007).

Also popular are schemes that incentivise health staff to work harder by linking payments to some measure of effort. Performance-based payment schemes have been implemented in Cambodia (Soeters & Griffiths, 2003), Rwanda (Meessen, Kashala, & Musango, 2007) and Haiti (Eichler, Auxila, & Pollock, 2001), modelled around the basic idea of paying or 'contracting' health providers to meet performance targets related to health outputs, punctuality or management capacity. The evidence regarding the success of provider-payment schemes is not only mixed but also, in the case of positive findings, questionable due to weaknesses in study design (Eldridge & Palmer, 2009).

In 2005, Nepal introduced the Safe Delivery Incentive Programme (SDIP) that combines the two types of incentive. It provides a CCT to households with an incentive to health staff for each delivery they attend. The SDIP grew out of concerns about the slow progress in raising coverage of skilled birth attendance and the prohibitively high cost faced by households trying to access professional care at childbirth (Borghi, Ensor, Neupane, & Tiwari, 2006). Latest figures show that over 80 percent of women in Nepal continue to deliver at home and only 19 percent deliver with a doctor or nurse in attendance (Government of Nepal, 2007). The SDIP marked a departure from past government policy that tended to focus on service provision only. Since the launch of the SDIP, India and Bangladesh have followed suit with similar programmes of their own reflecting growing interest in south Asia (Devadasan, Elias, John, Grahachary, & Ralte, 2008; Government of the People's Republic of Bangladesh, 2007). While these programmes fit the CCT label less well than the Latin American programmes – they are not intended as a social safety net – they still seek to change health seeking behaviour with cash transfers.

This chapter reports on a study that assessed the performance of the SDIP in Makwanpur, a district of Nepal where suitable data were available.

Specifically, it explored three related issues: the financial burden of health care at childbirth, the benefit incidence of the CCT and the impact of the SDIP. The study was by no means comprehensive; it was limited to a quantitative evaluation of the SDIP in one part of the country. The larger evaluation, of which this study was a part, was broader in its scope capturing, for example, the experiences of a wide range of stakeholders with a view to identifying the main factors that have impeded and facilitated implementation of the programme (Powell-Jackson, Neupane, Tiwari, Morrison, & Costello, 2008). Nevertheless, the study reported here seeks to assess programme impact, the key component of any evaluation. Moreover, the findings are likely to be applicable, in some measure, to the rest of the country. There is little hard empirical evidence on the health impact of CCT programmes in south Asia, where implementation is constrained by weak governance (Kaufmann, Kraay, & Mastruzzi, 2008). The existing body of evidence is limited largely to schemes in Latin American countries, where government systems to verify eligibility, pay beneficiaries and monitor activities are more developed.

The model used to estimate the impact of the SDIP looks for a discontinuity at the specific point in time the programme began in the district (Cook & Campbell, 1979). At this point in time, we would expect observations after the programme to be different from those before it if the programme is to have had any impact. Our dataset from a community surveillance system lends itself well to such an approach. It covers almost seven years of continuous data collection and contains household data, which is not able to be manipulated as easily as service data to make performance of a programme appear better. The absence of any non-programme areas to construct a comparison group, however, is a major limitation. With pre- and post-intervention data on both programme and non-programme sites, it would have been possible to use difference-in-difference (e.g. Wagstaff, 2009b) or even triple difference methods to estimate impacts (Moffitt, 1991; Wagstaff, 2009a). Instead, the approach is limited to identifying instantaneous impacts and must assume no change in the secular trend of the outcome in the no-treatment state. It is capable of providing *plausible* evidence of an impact (Habicht, Victora, & Vaughan, 1999; Victora, Habicht, & Bryce, 2004).

We were also interested in the disruptive effects of out-of-pocket (OOP) spending for institutional delivery care on household consumption. Our intention was not to look at changes over time, but instead provide estimates at one point in time, after the SDIP started. We might expect payments for delivery care to be more disruptive than other types of health care, since they are known to be particularly high in Nepal (Borghi et al., 2006). On the other hand, childbirth differs from your typical health shock in that the event is largely predictable, giving families time to prepare financially.[1]

In the next section, we describe the SDIP in Nepal and give a brief overview of implementation of the programme to-date. The subsequent sections outline the methods used to assess the performance of the programme and report the results of the study. Finally, implications of the findings are discussed.

SAFE DELIVERY INCENTIVE PROGRAMME

The Nepalese health care system is dominated by the public sector, although the number of private and charitable hospitals is growing. Maternity services in Makwanpur, as in the rest of the country, are delivered through a network of health facilities based around a district health system model, supported by regional and national hospitals providing specialised care.

Delivery care services are not free at the point of use; in fact, household OOP expenditures can be substantial, particularly in the case of emergency surgery. In Makwanpur, the mean cost to a household of a normal delivery was found to be 4,042 NRS ($63.2), compared with 22,780 NRS ($356.2) incurred by those with a caesarean section (Table 1). For both types of delivery, facility-based charges and the additional costs of goods and services purchased outside of the health facility together account for around two-thirds of the overall cost. Payments made to the health provider are retained at facility level and placed under the control of the health management

Table 1. Household Costs of Institutional Delivery Care by Cost Category in Makwanpur (Rupees).

Cost Category	Vaginal (n = 271)	95% CI	%	Caesarean Section (n = 29)	95% CI	%
Facility-based charges	1,492	(1,191–1,793)	36.9	7,913	(5,675–10,150)	34.7
Additional charges	1,185	(1,040–1,330)	29.3	7,071	(4777–9,405)	31.1
Transport costs	669	(565–773)	16.5	1,415	(845–1,985)	6.2
Debt to service provider	697	(474–920)	17.2	6,362	(2,995–9,730)	27.9
Total	4042	(3,522–4,562)	100	22,780	(17,045–28,516)	100

Source: Cost of delivery and living standards survey.

committee (if in place). Clearly, delivery care can be an important source of revenue for health facilities. Outstanding debts to service providers remain a sizable share of the total cost suggesting households, particularly those with women requiring a caesarean section, struggle to find any means to pay their bills at the time the service is received.[2] The transport cost associated with a caesarean section is almost double that of a normal delivery, presumably because families need to travel further and more urgently to hospitals sufficiently specialised to carry out surgery.

With a view to alleviating some of financial cost of delivery care, the Government of Nepal launched the SDIP nationwide in 2005.[3] The SDIP's package of financial benefits included (i) a CCT to women who delivered their baby in a health facility and (ii) an incentive to health workers for each delivery attended either at home or in a health facility (see Table 2); (Government of Nepal, 2005).[4] In this way, the programme sought to increase utilisation of professional care at delivery by influencing the behaviour of both households and health workers. The amount of cash offered to the woman varied across geographical regions to account for differences in the transport cost faced by households (Borghi et al., 2006).

The CCT, worth 1,000 NRS, is clearly not enough to cover the full cost of delivery care incurred by a household, representing one quarter of the cost of a normal delivery or one twentieth of the cost of a caesarean section. The intention of the SDIP was to share the cost, leaving the household still to pay for a substantial proportion of the costs of health care.

The provider incentive for attending a delivery at home was born out of a desire to improve care for those women wising to deliver at home. Despite being well-intentioned, this decision gave rise to a possible tension between the various incentives, with the CCT, on the one hand, incentivising women

Table 2. The Benefits Offered by the SDIP and the Eligibility Criteria Applied in Makwanpur.

Financial Benefit	Eligibility Criteria
1. Conditional cash transfer to women	
• 1000 NRS ($15.6)	• Woman delivered in a public health facility *and* had no more than two living children *or* an obstetric complication
2. Provider incentive	
• 300 NRS ($4.7) per delivery	• Doctor, nurse, midwife, health assistant, auxiliary health worker or maternal and child health worker attended a delivery at home or in a public health facility

to the health facility, and the provider incentive, on the other hand, encouraging health providers to attend deliveries at home[5]. The extent to which health workers can attend both deliveries at home and deliveries at the health facility depends on whether there is slack in the labour supply. If there is indeed a trade-off, how the incentive influences behaviour of the health worker will then depend in part on the income that would be forgone (both the provider incentive and the user fee from the patient) by not being present to attend a delivery in the health facility. Another interesting element to the design of the programme is the condition that the CCT is available only to those with two or fewer children (unless the woman has an obstetric complication). The restriction was put in place to reflect concerns that the programme might inadvertently increase fertility. In practice, however, health workers found it difficult to verify a woman's parity and the condition was later scrapped.

The programme was limited to public sector health facilities in the first two years (our study period) but has subsequently expanded to include both non-profit and private health facilities. Unlike many other demand-side programmes, the SDIP does not explicitly target the poor, despite the rhetoric of national policymakers sometimes suggesting otherwise.[6] Nor does the programme use vouchers, distributing the CCT as cash. Numerous types of health worker can claim the provider incentive, including those with no formal training in delivery care, reflecting the compromise that was required to make the programme workable in a country where human resources in health are scarce.

There has been substantial involvement of the central level in the implementation of the programme; the Ministry of Health is in charge of overall management of the programme and provides funds in instalments to each district and regional hospital. Implementation has been governed by a set of guidelines, developed at the central level then issued to districts, to explain the management of funds and the monitoring of activities, as well as the eligibility criteria for beneficiaries. Despite these guidelines, implementation was found to vary substantially between districts owing, in part, to widespread confusion amongst district officials and health workers. There were variations in the eligibility criteria applied to the CCT, the sharing of the provider payment among staff, the payment mechanisms used, the means of monitoring and so on.

The programme has faced a number of challenges related to lengthy delays in the disbursement of funds and hesitation on the part of the central government to promote the programme. As a result, the level of coverage achieved by the programme in its first three years was low. A household survey found that only 27 percent of households had ever heard of the programme and 29 percent of women who delivered in an eligible facility received the CCT at the time of delivery (Powell-Jackson et al., 2008). With this level of awareness, a substantial proportion of the population were not reached by the SDIP. In Makwanpur, there were no data on community awareness, but this is likely to have been substantially higher where women's groups were operating since efforts were made to publicise the programme widely through this existing channel.

METHODS

Estimation of Financial Burden

The purpose of this analysis is to show the financial burden of paying for delivery care at a health facility, once the SDIP had begun.[7] If the woman received the CCT, spending on delivery care is adjusted accordingly to include what is effectively a subsidy. The unit of analysis is the household, and financial burden is measured as the share of health spending for delivery care in household consumption.[8] A common extension of this approach uses measures of catastrophic spending to estimate the effect of health care payments on household material living standards (Wagstaff & van Doorslaer, 2003; Xu et al., 2003). Health spending is regarded as catastrophic if it exceeds a certain fraction of total household expenditure in any given time period. It is based on the premise that health spending is likely to displace consumption of other goods and services if it makes up a large proportion of total household resources.

Catastrophic payments have been defined in two ways. The first measures catastrophic payments as the share of health spending in total household consumption, while the other estimates health spending relative to household consumption net of spending on basic essentials (i.e. non-food consumption). The second measure reflects the view that non-discretionary expenditure may be a better indicator of a household's living standard or capacity to pay for health care (Wagstaff & van Doorslaer, 2003; Xu et al., 2003). The threshold above which health spending is classified as catastrophic is essentially arbitrary (O'Donnell, van Doorslaer, Wagstaff, & Lindelow, 2008). We use the most common thresholds of 10 percent in the case of the first measure of catastrophic payments and 40 percent in the second case. Results are stratified by type of delivery since spending on normal deliveries and caesarean sections is expected to diverge widely.

Identification of Impacts

Time is commonly used in the evaluation literature to establish a comparison group with which to assess a programme's impact. The most basic approach estimates impact by measuring the mean change in outcome before and after the programme commences. It is rarely able to permit reasonable causal inferences, as there is no a priori reason why the key assumption of no change in the absence of the programme should hold in practice. Unless the influence of non-programme factors can be ruled out with confidence, the conclusions from such a design can be weak. With more time periods, it is possible to test for an interruption at a specific point in time around the start of the programme, thereby providing more plausible causal inferences.

In the first instance, we plot outcomes against time to see if there is any evidence of a discontinuity in the time series around the month the SDIP began. From interviews with district programme managers, we know that Makwanpur district was able to start implementation of the SDIP in September 2005, two months after the official launch. The graphs also plot the three-month moving average to show with more clarity the underlying pattern by smoothing the data. While crude, the graphs provide a visual means of assessing the impact of the programme on the set of outcomes.

The second step involves estimation of a model that links the level of the outcome at a point in time to the start of the programme, contemporaneous values of a series of demographic controls, time and community-level fixed effects. The specification takes the form:

$$y_{it} = \gamma D_t + \beta X_{it} + \lambda T + \alpha_j + \varepsilon_{it},$$

where y_{it} is the outcome variable for individual i measured at time t, D_t is the treatment dummy at time t, X_{it} is a vector of individual and household characteristics measured at time t, T is time measured in months, α_j are community-level fixed effects and ε_{it} is a random error. The impact of the programme is given by the size of the coefficient γ. A value of γ equal to 0 indicates that the SDIP has had no impact on the outcome of interest. We include a full set of community dummies to control for influences at the village level such as the activities of non-governmental organisations (NGOs). We also include a vector of individual and household characteristics to capture other secular trends in the outcome: the woman's age, religion, ethnicity, educational attainment, the occupation of the household head, the size of the household, the materials used to make the house and the number of months the household had sufficient food in the previous year. The time variable(s) captures the secular trend in the outcome over time. How we specify this relationship between the outcome and time may affect the results. We, therefore, show results for two different specifications to assess the robustness of the results: a restricted model where time is a quadratic function and a more flexible model in which time is specified as a polynomial function of degree four.

The impact of the SDIP is assessed in relation to a set of outcomes that include a measure of health and various indicators of utilisation of delivery care services (Table 3). These outcome indicators are defined as probabilities. Our preference would have been to use maternal mortality as one of our main health outcomes, to be consistent with the main goal of the programme. However, given the rarity of a maternal death and the huge sample size required to detect even a large effect, we assess the impact of the SDIP on neonatal mortality only. About 25–45 percent of neonatal deaths occur around the first day of life and can, therefore, be prevented through direct medical intervention at the time of childbirth (Lawn, Cousens, & Zupan, 2005). Neonatal mortality is both of interest in itself and a reasonable proxy for maternal mortality. A prerequisite for there to be an effect of the SDIP on mortality is an increase in utilisation of maternity services and adequate quality of care. Put another way, a finding that showed an impact on neonatal mortality without any impact on utilisation of maternity services would, given our behavioural model, be difficult to rationalise.

Utilisation outcomes refer to the place of delivery (home, government facility or private facility) and the type of birth attendant (a skilled birth attendant or any health worker). We expect a positive impact of the programme on utilisation of government maternity services and skilled birth attendance. The CCT to the woman functions as a price subsidy reducing the cost of care and thereby raising demand, the extent to which depends on the household's price elasticity. The provider payment, however, should increase the availability of health workers to attend deliveries by providing additional motivation to work. We also include the probability of a caesarean section, although our expectation of an impact on this outcome is perhaps lower given that the SDIP does not address many of the supply-side constraints that explain the low rate of caesarean sections in Nepal. The final outcome is the number of antenatal care visits, whose inclusion is explained later. With the exception of this outcome, all outcomes are binary. Thus, an appropriate model is a probit. In presenting the results, we report

Table 3. Summary Statistics of the Community Surveillance System Dataset.

Variable	Pre-SDIP		Post-SDIP	
	Mean	Standard Error	Mean	Standard Error
Outcomes				
Neonatal mortality	0.029	0.002	0.023	0.002
Delivery at home	0.946	0.003	0.870	0.004
Delivery at government facility	0.042	0.002	0.108	0.004
Delivery at private facility	0.002	0.001	0.010	0.001
Delivery with skilled birth attendant	0.044	0.002	0.109	0.004
Delivery with any health worker	0.061	0.003	0.170	0.004
Delivery by caesarean section	0.003	0.001	0.010	0.001
Number of ANC visits	1.235	0.020	2.116	0.024
Characteristics of woman and household				
Age of woman during birth of child	27.918	0.075	25.619	0.075
Education grade	1.028	0.027	1.998	0.037
HH size	6.899	0.035	7.192	0.038
Months of sufficient food in previous year	9.222	0.031	9.637	0.033
Hindu	0.336	0.005	0.321	0.006
Buddhist	0.653	0.005	0.656	0.006
Muslim	0.000	0.000	0.001	0.000
Christian	0.010	0.001	0.014	0.001
Other religion	0.001	0.000	0.008	0.001
Brahmin/Chhetri	0.156	0.004	0.156	0.004
Newar	0.023	0.002	0.018	0.002
Janajati	0.777	0.005	0.778	0.005
Other caste	0.003	0.001	0.007	0.001
Cement house	0.022	0.002	0.044	0.002
Brick/mud house	0.020	0.002	0.031	0.002
Stone/mud house	0.630	0.006	0.589	0.006
Planks house	0.312	0.005	0.254	0.005
Brushwood house	0.009	0.001	0.009	0.001
Thatch house	0.004	0.001	0.006	0.001
Other type of house	0.003	0.001	0.046	0.002
Agricultural work	0.910	0.003	0.927	0.003
Salaried/government work	0.019	0.002	0.015	0.001
Small business	0.014	0.001	0.017	0.002
Wage labourer	0.058	0.003	0.040	0.002
Other work	0.000	0.000	0.002	0.001
HH in women's group intervention area	0.499	0.006	0.461	0.006
N	7,613		7,186	

the change in probability associated with a given change in the treatment variable rather than the estimated coefficient.

The identification strategy relies on there being no other change at the time of the programme's introduction that could account for a discontinuity or shift in the relationship between the outcome and time. Changes in non-programme factors such as health infrastructure, staffing levels, government policy and the activities of NGOs working in maternal health are a particular concern. One way of testing the plausibility of this assumption is to estimate the impact of the SDIP on the use of antenatal care, an outcome unrelated to the SDIP but closely linked to maternal health more broadly. If the explanation for a discontinuity in the use of delivery care is a factor other than the SDIP, it is likely this same factor would also affect antenatal care seeking.

A further limitation is that the regression model is only able to identify impacts that surface instantaneously. Thus, the question is whether the SDIP would be expected to have an immediate effect on the set outcomes. The CCT and the provider payment in principle *should* have an instantaneous impact on utilisation and neonatal mortality, but if implementation has been slow, the effects may be incremental or simply delayed. On the demand side, the critical factor is awareness of the CCT in households. In those villages where women's groups were running (i.e. approximately half of the sample), we are confident that awareness was high from the outset due to the widespread promotion of the SDIP through this channel, as stated earlier. For this reason, when presenting the results, we stratify according to those villages that did and those that did not have women's groups at the time the SDIP was implemented.

Data

This chapter draws on data from a community surveillance system that has been running in rural areas of Makwanpur district, as part of a randomised control trial to assess the effectiveness of a participatory intervention with women's groups (Manandhar et al., 2004). In the surveillance area, every woman was interviewed one month postpartum about her health seeking behaviour at childbirth, the survival status of the newborn, her household's socioeconomic status and receipt of the CCT. The questionnaire recorded ownership of assets, with which an asset wealth index was constructed using principal components analysis (Filmer & Pritchett, 1998). Over the period 2001–2007, complete data were collected on 14,799 deliveries in the 24 local administrative areas or Village Development Committees (VDC) covered by the surveillance system.[9] This period includes five years before the SDIP started and almost two years of programme implementation.

After the SDIP had begun, women who delivered in a health facility were asked additional questions on general household consumption and the cost of delivery care. The recall period remained one month, except for expenditures on durable items. Over a six-month period, every household (300 in total) in the surveillance area with a woman who delivered in a health facility was interviewed. The additional module captured general household expenditure, following closely the Nepal Living Standards Measurement Survey (Government of Nepal, 2004), as well as household expenditures on delivery care and outstanding debt. The approach to measuring household living standards was comprehensive, capturing information on not just household expenditures but also the value of home production and those goods or services received in kind. This allows computation of household consumption, a proxy for permanent income (Deaton & Grosh, 2000). The cost of delivery covered facility-based charges (registration; delivery fee; operating theatre; bed charge; drugs; medical supplies; diagnostic tests; food, gifts to health staff and spending on traditional practitioner if sought during labour), additional charges (lodging and food of accompanying family and drugs, medical supplies and food bought outside) and transport charges (Borghi et al., 2006).[10] Outstanding payments to health providers were also included. A summary of these data was presented in the previous section.

Table 3 reports descriptive statistics of the outcome and socioeconomic variables for the five-year period before and the two-year period after the start of the SDIP. Neonatal mortality fell from 29 deaths per 1,000 live births in the first period to 23 deaths per 1,000 in the second period. Utilisation of maternity services and skilled birth attendance were both low in the first period but have risen markedly over time. The proportion of women delivering at a government health facility, for example, increased from 4.2 percent to 10.8 percent between the two periods, and skilled birth attendance rose from 4.4 percent to 10.9 percent. Also, women in the second period were far more likely to deliver in the presence of a health worker. There was an increase in the caesarean section rate from 0.3 percent to 1 percent and an increase in the mean number of antenatal care visits from 1.2 to 2.1.

In the X_{it}, we include a number of characteristics of the woman and her household. There have been notable changes in some of these characteristics over time. While women are more likely to give birth at a younger age and household size has increased, there has been little change in the religion or caste of families. The education level of women is low, although it has increased over time. Similarly, food sufficiency and the type of house have both improved. Almost 50 percent of the sample was resident in areas that received the women's group intervention.

RESULTS

Financial Burden of Delivery Care

We estimate the OOP health care budget share as an indicator of the financial burden associated with giving birth in a health facility. Table 4 indicates that OOP payments for normal delivery care accounted for 3.6 percent of total annual household consumption, while those for a caesarean section accounted for a much higher 19.3 percent, even with the SDIP in place. Clearly, spending on a caesarean section places an enormous strain on the household budget. The concentration indices of OOP budget shares for both types of delivery are negative indicating that better-off families spend a smaller fraction of total household resources on delivery care. The quintile

Table 4.   Out-of-Pocket Spending on Institutional Delivery Care as a Percentage of Household Consumption.

	Vaginal Delivery	Caesarean Section
OOP delivery care spending as % of total household consumption		
Mean (%)	3.6	19.3
Quintile mean		
Poorest (20%)	5.1	22.9
Poorer (20%)	5.6	18.9
Middle (20%)	2.7	22.1
Richer (20%)	2.5	16.3
Richest (20%)	1.9	16.2
Concentration index	−0.23	−0.058
Incidence of catastrophic spending (>10%)	7.4	72.4
OOP delivery care spending as % of household non-food consumption		
Mean (%)	9.9	35.9
Concentration index	−0.21	−0.075
Incidence of catastrophic spending (>40%)	2.6	41.4

Source: Cost of delivery and living standards survey.
Notes: Vaginal deliveries ($N = 271$); caesarean section ($N = 29$).

means also show a similar pattern, although the gradient is less steep in the case of caesarean sections. Given that our sample covered only households seeking delivery care, it is perhaps to be expected that the OOP budget share decreased with household resources. If we had included those who did not seek any care – that is, women who delivered at home – it is likely we would have found that wealthier households spend proportionately more on health care, consistent with other studies (van Doorslaer et al., 2007). The proportion of households that incur catastrophic spending is considerable. Using a 10 percent threshold, the incidence of catastrophic spending was 7.4 percent for normal delivery care and 72.4 percent for caesarean sections.

The mean OOP budget share of non-food expenditure offers an alternative measure of the disruptive effect of OOP payments on living standards. The mean share rises considerably to 9.9 percent for normal deliveries and 35.9 percent for caesarean sections reflecting the large fraction of household resources devoted to food (basic necessities) in our sample. Again, the concentration indices are negative suggesting that richer households spent a smaller fraction of their discretionary resources on delivery care. The incidence of catastrophic spending, as defined by a 40 percent threshold, was 2.6 percent in the case of normal delivery care and 41.4 percent for caesarean sections.

While we are unable to comment on how the SDIP has affected the financial burden of delivery care, health spending, and particularly that on surgery, appears to be highly disruptive to the living standards of households, despite the financial assistance offered by the SDIP.

Uptake and Benefit Incidence of the Conditional Cash Transfer

Women who meet the conditions of the SDIP should receive the CCT on the day of discharge from the health facility. During our study period, only two-fifths of eligible women received the CCT after childbirth. There are likely to be factors other than the official conditions laid down in the policy that influence the chances of a woman receiving the CCT. We explored this possibility using a probit model, the results of which are reported in Table 5.

In accordance with the official eligibility criteria, if a woman had two or fewer children or delivered in a public health facility, she was more likely to receive the CCT. In addition, a number of other factors were statistically significant. The chances of receiving the CCT varied by type of public health facility, suggesting differences in uptake were related to where the woman delivered. Women who delivered in a primary health care centre were most

Table 5.   Results of Probit of Determinants of Receiving the
Conditional Cash Transfer.

Variable	Coefficient	Z score
Two or fewer living children	0.833	6.75
Home delivery	*Reference category*	
District hospital delivery	2.362	19.88
Other public hospital delivery	2.035	16.00
Primary health centre delivery	2.575	20.42
Health post delivery	1.679	4.00
Private health facility delivery	0.885	3.12
Asset wealth	0.013	0.67
Ethnically marginalised	0.132	1.56
No education	*Reference category*	
Primary education	0.397	3.54
Some secondary	0.471	3.98
Secondary or higher education	0.561	4.06
Woman attended women's group	0.124	1.07
Agricultural work	*Reference category*	
Salaried work	−0.248	−1.49
Small business	−0.004	−0.03
Waged labour	0.288	1.69
Other occupation	0.381	0.72
constant	−3.982	−23.35
N observations	9,801	
Pseudo R^2	0.524	

Source: Community surveillance system 2005–2007.
Notes: Data include additional villages that were included in the surveillance system from 2005 onwards. Table 3 does not report summary statistics for these villages.

likely to receive the cash, while those using a health post were least likely. Those who delivered in a private health facility rather than at home were more likely to receive the CCT. This could be explained by women receiving the cash after childbirth during a visit to a public health facility to manage postpartum complications. Women with at least some education had a higher chance of receiving the CCT. Given the administrative procedures, women with no education (i.e. illiterate women) may have found it difficult – and health staff unwilling to assist – to complete the required form to apply for the CCT. The explanatory variables in the model do not fully capture administrative problems in the management of funds and undoubtedly, as reported elsewhere, delays in the disbursement of funds higher up the system prevented women getting access to the CCT (Powell-Jackson et al., 2008).

With no explicit targeting built into the SDIP, we would expect the same factors that influence use of public health facilities at delivery also to affect the chances of a woman receiving the CCT. Indeed, if we omit the variables relating to place of delivery in the probit model mentioned earlier (results not shown), wealth becomes significant – that is, richer households are much more likely to receive the CCT because they have a higher chance of delivering in a public health facility.[11] Another way of showing this is with concentration curves. In Fig. 1, we see that receipt of the CCT is heavily concentrated among richer households, reflecting the fact that users of government maternity services are also disproportionately wealthier.[12] Inequality in the benefit incidence of the CCT is simply illustrative of an existing inequality in the use of delivery care services. The main purpose of the CCT is to raise demand for health services, but it is also a transfer of resources to households. In this

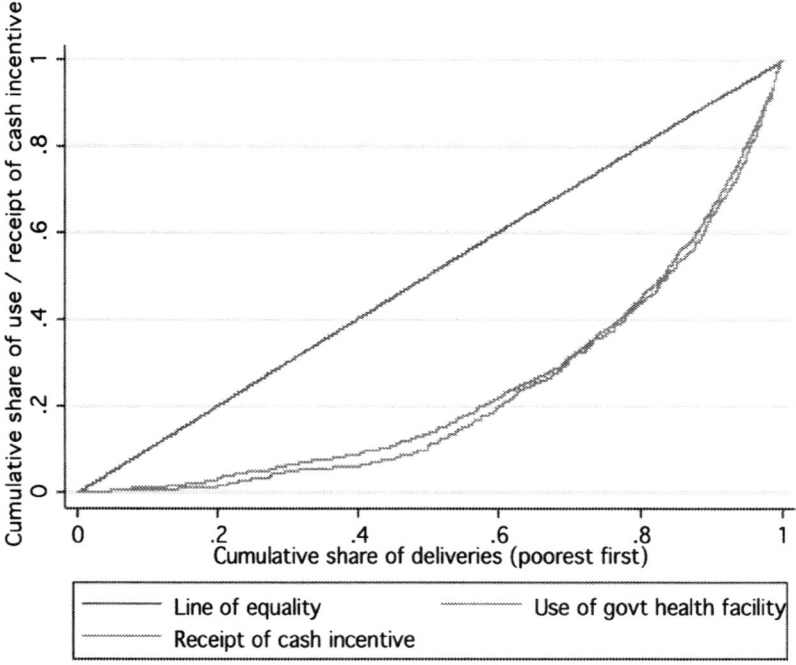

Fig. 1. Concentration Curves for Use of Institutional Delivery and Receipt of Conditional Cash Transfer in the Entire Population of Delivering Women. *Source:* Community Surveillance System 2005–2007.

second regard, it may be considered inequitable, benefiting relatively wealthier groups within our sample of rural women.

Impacts

Figs. 2–5 plot selected outcomes over time, showing the three-month moving average and a vertical line to indicate the point at which implementation of the SDIP began. Visual inspection of the time series data provides a useful starting point to identify impacts.

An interruption in the time series at the month of the programme's introduction can be seen in the case of a delivery at home and a delivery with a skilled birth attendant. The shifts are in the expected direction: a reduction in the probability of a home delivery and an increase in the chances of a delivery with a skilled birth attendant. In contrast, there is no obvious shift in the probability of a neonatal death or the number of antenatal care visits at around the time of the programme's introduction, but rather a consistent trend over the entire period.

Next, we turn to the regression analysis, starting with the most flexible specification of the relationship between the outcomes and time. The

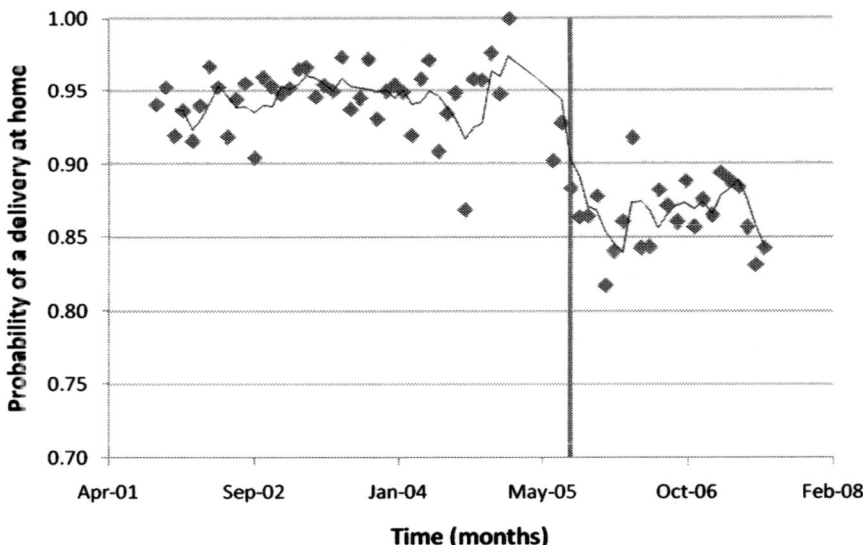

Fig. 2.   Probability of a Delivery at Home Over Time: The Three-Month Moving Average and Start of the SDIP.

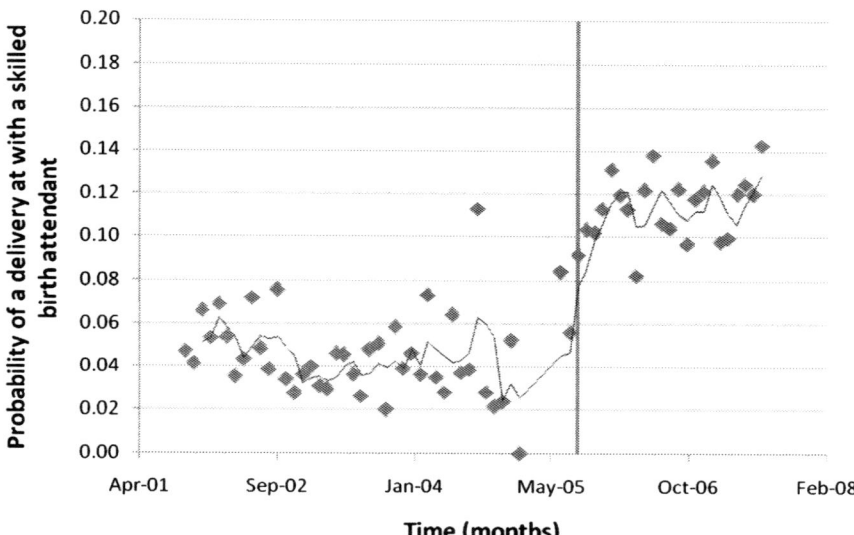

Fig. 3. Probability of a Delivery with a Skilled Birth Attendant Over Time: The Three-Month Moving Average and Start of the SDIP.

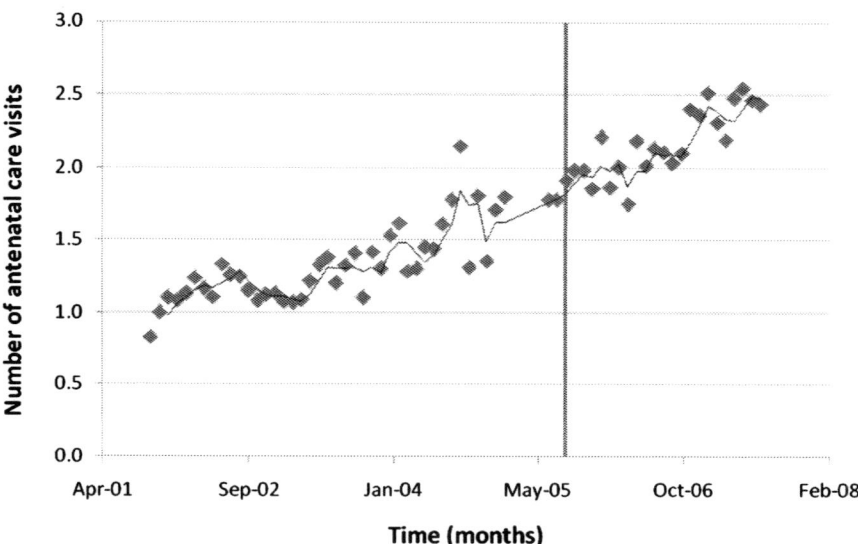

Fig. 4. Number of Antenatal Care Visits Over Time: The Three-Month Moving Average and Start of the SDIP.

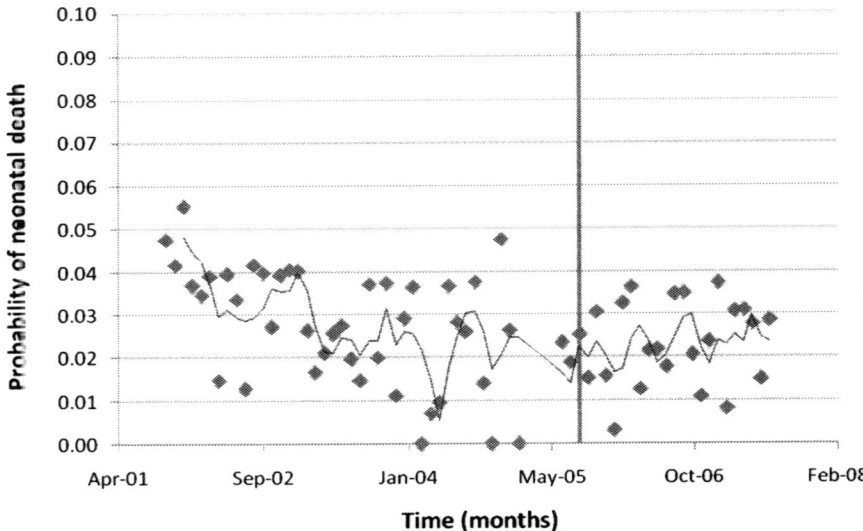

Fig. 5. Probability of a Neonatal Death Over Time: The Three-Month Moving
Average and Start of the SDIP.

regressions based on the full sample (i.e. including all villages) confirm the
results of the visual inspection. Table 6 illustrates that the SDIP had a
significant impact on a number of outcomes. The SDIP reduced the probability of a home delivery by 4.2 percentage points and increased the chances
of a delivery in a government health facility by 2.6 percentage points.
Estimates also suggest a positive impact on skilled birth attendance (2.3
percentage points) and attendance by any health worker (4.4 percentage
points). There is no evidence that the SDIP had any impact on neonatal
mortality, utilisation of private health facilities and the caesarean section rate.

When we stratify the results between the villages that were receiving the
women's group intervention at the time the SDIP began and those that were
not, substantial differences in the impacts are revealed (Table 6). In the
villages without women's groups, the SDIP had no impact on any of the
outcomes. In the villages with women's groups, however, the SDIP
increased skilled birth attendance by 5.3 percentage points and raised the
chances of a delivery in a government health facility by 6.3 percentage
points. The results from the full sample are driven by the villages with
women's groups. The possibility remains that some factor other than the
SDIP was responsible for these impacts. In Table 7, estimates show that

Table 6. Effect of the SDIP on the Probability of a Neonatal Death and the Use of Health Care Services at Childbirth (Quartic Time Function).

Outcome	All Villages			Villages with Women's Groups			Villages without Women's Groups		
	Effect		Pseudo R^2	Effect		Pseudo R^2	Effect		Pseudo R^2
	dy/dx	z		dy/dx	z		dy/dx	z	
Neonatal mortality	−0.0004	−0.05	0.019	−0.002	−0.20	0.020	0.001	0.11	0.025
Delivery at home	−0.042	−3.49	0.212	−0.091	−3.82	0.201	−0.009	−0.82	0.189
Delivery at government facility	0.026	2.78	0.244	0.063	3.25	0.225	0.004	0.45	0.235
Delivery at private facility	0.002	1.17	0.337	0.000	0.41	0.409	0.000	0.57	0.197
Delivery with skilled birth attendance	0.023	2.34	0.245	0.053	2.72	0.223	0.005	0.52	0.253
Delivery with a health worker	0.044	3.46	0.247	0.088	3.51	0.219	0.016	1.29	0.240
Delivery by caesarean section	−0.001	−0.69	0.186	−0.003	−1.00	0.182	0.000	0.43	0.225

Notes: Regressions include 24 community-level fixed effects, dummies capturing ethnicity, religion, occupation of household head, and materials used to make house, as well variables for age of the woman at childbirth, educational attainment and number of months in the previous year for which household had enough food. The time function is a polynomial of degree four.

Table 7. Effect of the SDIP on the Number of Antenatal Care Visits (Quartic Time Function).

Outcome	All Villages			Villages with Women's Groups			Villages without Women's Groups		
	Effect		R^2	Effect		R^2	Effect		R^2
	Coeff.	t-Stat.		Coeff.	t-Stat.		Coeff.	t-Stat.	
Number of antenatal care visits	0.031	0.38	0.380	0.128	1.01	0.357	−0.054	−0.53	0.332

Notes: Regressions include 24 community-level fixed effects, dummies capturing ethnicity, religion, occupation of household head, and materials used to make house, as well variables for age of the woman at childbirth, educational attainment and number of months in the previous year for which household had enough food. The time function is a polynomial of degree four.

there was no discontinuity in the number of antenatal care visits at the time of the SDIP's introduction, strengthening the plausibility of the overall findings. It seems unlikely that non-programme factors would have affected utilisation of maternity services without having an impact on antenatal care.

Tables 8 and 9 provide impact estimates using the more restricted specification where time is modelled as a quadratic function. Some important differences in impact estimates between the two sets of regressions emerge. The regressions based on the full sample indicate that the SDIP had a positive impact on the probability of a delivery at a private health facility. In practice, such a finding is difficult to explain, unless there was a misunderstanding in the community that the SDIP was also covering the private sector. The other major difference is the finding of a positive impact of the SDIP on utilisation of government maternity services in villages that did not receive the women's group intervention. The two specifications remain consistent in their finding of no impact on either neonatal mortality or the caesarean section rate.

Table 8.   Effect of the SDIP on the Probability of a Neonatal Death and the Use of Health Care Services at Childbirth (Quadratic Time Function).

Outcome	All Villages			Villages with Women's Groups			Villages without Women's Groups		
	Effect		Pseudo R^2	Effect		Pseudo R^2	Effect		Pseudo R^2
	dy/dx	z		dy/dx	z		dy/dx	z	
Neonatal mortality	0.0001	0.01	0.019	0.002	0.27	0.020	0.000	0.00	0.025
Delivery at home	−0.049	−5.25	0.212	−0.073	−4.33	0.201	−0.033	−3.17	0.186
Delivery at government facility	0.029	4.18	0.244	0.045	3.33	0.225	0.020	2.68	0.232
Delivery at private facility	0.004	2.25	0.330	0.002	1.86	0.402	0.000	0.77	0.188
Delivery with skilled birth attendance	0.031	4.16	0.245	0.046	3.32	0.222	0.021	2.74	0.251
Delivery with a health worker	0.069	6.60	0.245	0.110	5.58	0.218	0.042	3.74	0.236
Delivery by caesarean section	−0.0004	−0.30	0.185	−0.002	−0.79	0.181	0.001	0.93	0.224

Notes: Regressions include 24 community-level fixed effects, dummies capturing ethnicity, religion, occupation of household head, and materials used to make house, as well variables for age of the woman at childbirth, educational attainment and number of months in the previous year for which household had enough food. The time function is a polynomial of degree two.

Table 9. Effect of the SDIP on the Number of Antenatal Care Visits (Quadratic Time Function).

Outcome	All Villages		Villages with Women's Groups		Villages without Women's Groups	
	Effect	R^2	Effect	R^2	Effect	R^2
	Coeff. *t*-Stat.		Coeff. *t*-Stat.		Coeff. *t*-Stat.	
Number of antenatal care visits	−0.046 −0.75	0.379	−0.013 −0.14	0.356	−0.072 −0.91	0.332

Notes: Regressions include 24 community-level fixed effects, dummies capturing ethnicity, religion, occupation of household head, and materials used to make house, as well variables for age of the woman at childbirth, educational attainment and number of months in the previous year for which household had enough food. The time function is a polynomial of degree two.

DISCUSSION

While CCT programmes in Latin America have been well-documented, there is little empirical evidence on whether large-scale cash incentive programmes in south Asia can improve health care seeking behaviour and health outcomes. This chapter provides evidence of the SDIP's impact in one district of Nepal.

The results suggest that the SDIP had a significant impact on utilisation of maternity services, despite known problems in the administration and uptake of the CCT. The programme raised skilled birth attendance and reduced the chance of a woman delivering at home. Even though the CCT represented a small proportion of the cost of delivery care to a household, it acted as a powerful enough signal for behavioural change. The programme, however, failed to have any impact on the caesarean rate, suggesting supply-side barriers constrain utilisation of emergency obstetric services rather than a lack of demand. The results also showed no impact on neonatal mortality. The SDIP changed health care seeking behaviour at childbirth but not the health outcomes of the newborn. It may be the case that the impact on utilisation was too modest to produce a detectable effect on mortality, or inadequate quality of care was the constraining factor in translating increases in utilisation into improved health.

A closer examination of the results from the most flexible model shows that the impact estimates from the entire sample are driven by the villages with women's groups. In these villages, the impact of the SDIP on utilisation of maternity services and skilled birth attendance was substantial. There remained, however, no impact of the programme on the caesarean section rate or neonatal mortality. These findings point towards the women's groups in Makwanpur as a useful means to communicate the SDIP to the public and highlight the importance of having a communication strategy as an integral part of implementation. There are implications for the impact of the programme in the rest of country, where indications are that awareness has been low. If the public are unaware of the programme's benefits, they cannot be expected to change behaviour as a consequence. It is conceivable that public awareness of the programme in the villages without women's groups spread slowly, causing a change in health care seeking behaviour over time that could not be identified using our approach.

There are reasons to believe that the impact estimates in our study area were greater than the country as a whole. Geographical access to health facilities in the district is relatively good, whereas in many other districts in Nepal, poor access represents more than simply a high transport cost – it is a physical barrier to getting to the health facility. Moreover, our sample included only rural households who are typically poorer than urban households. Economic theory would predict that poorer households are likely to be more incentivised by the CCT.

Of concern is the high incidence of catastrophic expenditure associated with OOP spending on institutional delivery care, despite the inclusion of the CCT in the estimates.[13] It implies that the SDIP, by incentivising greater use of institutional delivery, risks exposing more households to catastrophic payments. Moreover, there is no reason to assume that the health benefits of professional care necessarily outweigh the economic costs. CCT programmes in other countries have rarely encountered this tension because they have focused on low-cost preventive interventions (typically given free of charge) such as immunisation or growth monitoring. But evidence from China suggests that health insurance can increase the risk of catastrophic expenditure by raising utilisation of care (Wagstaff & Lindelow, 2008).

Further to this issue of cost, there was anecdotal evidence showing that providers may have price discriminated between patients, charging more to women who were given the CCT.[14] With such behaviour, the CCT provides no subsidy to the cost of care or protection against catastrophic payments. Greater transparency in the charging of user fees in Nepal would limit the extent to which health providers can price discriminate. More importantly, though, the SDIP should be linked to policies that offer better financial protection to households, focusing in particular on obstetric complications and poorer households – which are both associated with a higher incidence of catastrophic payments. The Government of Nepal recently abolished user fees for delivery care in the public sector. If implemented well, the change in policy should offer considerable financial protection to households. Any further evaluation of the SDIP will need to be wary of this policy change as a possible confounder in any analysis of utilisation.

The analysis of the determinants of uptake of the CCT suggest more households would be able to access the cash if the administration process were simplified so that it did not work against those with no education. Problems in the disbursement of funds at the central level are widely acknowledged, but the results suggest administration at the facility level also matters. It may be the case that certain types of health facility, such as health posts, need additional administrative support from the district health office to improve management of the SDIP.

The study raises the issue of targeting. One of the major differences between the SDIP and Latin American CCT programmes is its universal nature. In Mexico, de Janvry and Sadoulet (2006) has highlighted the inefficiencies associated with paying people to do what they would have done anyway. Since the CCT is given to those who meet the condition, irrespective of whether they would have met the condition in the absence of the programme, the cost per marginal visit can be very high. These inefficiencies are likely to be greater in the SDIP, as utilisation of delivery care services is higher amongst the better-off who remain eligible for the CCT. Also, we demonstrated another, if unsurprising, consequence of choosing not to target. The distribution of the CCT was skewed heavily in favour of relatively better-off families since they are most likely to attend health facilities. An obvious implication for the fine-tuning of the programme would be to target poor households. However, the evidence regarding the feasibility of targeting in low-income countries is not encouraging, and the cost of administration can be substantial. Given existing difficulties in the administration of the CCT, it is reasonable then that the SDIP does not target specific households; policymakers must accept the drawbacks and costs that this entails. Whether the SDIP represents value for money is a pressing question for further research, particularly given the additional inefficiencies that come hand in hand with not being able to target.

NOTES

1. An obstetric complication represents more of a health shock since it is, to some extent, unforeseen.

2. While we include debt to the service provider in the total cost, it is not known whether households paid the amount still owed after the time of survey.

3. A small number of large tertiary hospitals in Kathmandu were not part of the programme in its first two years.

4. In the least developed districts, women were also offered free care in addition to the CCT. Our study district was not one of the districts in which women from that district could benefit from the free delivery care component of the SDIP.

5. A related concern is that health workers attending a home delivery, worried that they could forgo the provider incentive, might be reluctant to refer women to a health facility in the case of an emergency.

6. An information pamphlet, for example, explains that 'more benefits reach to [the] poor, disadvantaged and marginalised women' and 'the [SDIP] contributes to mitigate the barrier in seeking care, provides relief to the poor families ...' (Government of Nepal, 2006).

7. In the absence of pre-implementation data, this chapter is not able to shed light on the question of whether the SDIP has affected delivery care spending and the financial burden it places on households.

8. Otherwise referred to as the OOP health care budget share.

9. Mean number of deliveries per month captured by the surveillance system was 221.

10. Unlike (Borghi et al., 2006), we did not include the opportunity cost of time.

11. Note that there was no independent effect of wealth in Table 5, once we controlled for the place of delivery.

12. As measured by a wealth index derived using principal components analysis from information about the ownership of assets.

13. We acknowledge that the estimates of catastrophic expenditure may exaggerate the short-term disruptive effects of paying for delivery care since childbirth typically is not a health shock and households can plan financially for the event. However, there are likely to be important longer term effects that are not captured in measures of catastrophic expenditure.

14. Among women who received the CCT, the mean OOP payment to the health provider for a normal delivery was 1,774 NRS (95% CI: 1304–2245), compared with 968 NRS 95% CI: 791–1145) among those who did not receive any cash.

ACKNOWLEDGMENTS

Part of the study received funding from the Support to Safe Motherhood Programme in Nepal, managed by Options UK and funded by the Department for International Development.

REFERENCES

Attanasio, O., Carlos Gomez, L., Heredia, P., & Vera-Hernandez, M. (2005). *The short term impact of a conditional cash subsidy on child health and nutrition in Columbia*. London: The Institute for Fiscal Studies.

Borghi, J., Ensor, T., Neupane, B. D., & Tiwari, S. (2006). Financial implications of skilled attendance at delivery in Nepal. *Tropical Medicine & International Health, 11*, 228–237.

Cook, T., & Campbell, D. (1979). *Quasi-experimentation. Design and analysis issues for field settings*. Boston: Houghton Mifflin Co.

de Janvry, A., & Sadoulet, E. (2006). Making conditional cash transfer programs more efficient: Designing for maximum effect of the conditionality. *The World Bank Economic Review, 20*(1), 1–29.

Deaton, A., & Grosh, M. (2000). *Consumption*. Washington DC: World Bank.

Devadasan, N., Elias, M., John, D., Grahachary, S., & Ralte, L. (2008). A conditional cash assistance programme for promoting institutional deliveries among the poor in India: Process evaluation results. In: F. Richard, S. Witter & V. Brouwere (Eds), *Reducing financial barriers to obstetric care in low-income countries*. Antwerp: ITG Press.

Eichler, R., Auxila, P., & Pollock, J. (2001). Promoting preventive health care: Paying for performance in Haiti. In: P. Brook & S. Smith (Eds), *Contracting for public services: Output-based aid and its applications* (pp. 65–72). Washington DC: World Bank.

Eldridge, C., & Palmer, N. (2009). Performance-based payment: Some reflections on the discourse, evidence and unanswered questions. *Health Policy Plan, 24*(3), 160–166.

Ensor, T., & Cooper, S. (2004). Overcoming barriers to health service access: Influencing the demand side. *Health Policy Plan, 19*, 69–79.

Filmer, D., & Pritchett, L. (1998). *Estimating wealth effects with no expenditure data-or tears: An application to educational enrollment in states of India*. Washington DC: World Bank.

Fiszbein, A., & Schady, N. (2009). *Conditional cash transfers: Reducing present and future poverty*. Washington DC: World Bank.

Gertler, P. (2004). Do conditional cash transfers improve child health? Evidence from PROGRESA's control randomised experiment. *American Economic Review, 94*, 336–341.

Glassman, A., Todd, J., & Gaarder, M. (2007). *Performance-based incentives for health: conditional cash transfer programs in Latin America and the Caribbean*. Washington DC: Center for Global Development.

Government of Nepal. (2004). *Nepal living standards survey 2003/04*. Central Bureau of Statistics, Government of Nepal, Kathmandu.

Government of Nepal. (2005). *Operational guidelines on incentives for safe delivery services*. Kathmandu: Government of Nepal, Ministry of Health and Population.

Government of Nepal. (2006). Information kit on cost sharing scheme for the promotion of safe delivery service. Government of Nepal and Support to Safe Motherhood Programme, Ministry of Health and Population, Kathmandu.

Government of Nepal. (2007). *Nepal Demographic and Health Survey*. Kathmandu, Nepal: Government of Nepal and ORC Macro.

Government of the People's Republic of Bangladesh. (2007). *Demand side financing pilot maternal health voucher scheme proposal*. Dhaka: Ministry of Health and Family Welfare, Government of the People's Republic of Bangladesh.

Habicht, J. P., Victora, C. G., & Vaughan, J. P. (1999). Evaluation designs for adequacy, plausibility and probability of public health programme performance and impact. *International Journal of Epidemiology, 28*, 10–18.

Kaufmann, D., Kraay, A., & Mastruzzi, M. (2008). *Governance matters VII: Aggregate and individual governance indicators, 1996–2007*. World Bank Policy Research Working Paper no. 4654. World Bank, Washington DC.

Koblinsky, M., Matthews, Z., Hussein, J., Mavalankar, D., Mridha, M. K., Anwar, I., Achadi, E., et al. (2006). Going to scale with professional skilled care. *Lancet, 368,* 1377–1386.

Lagarde, M., Haines, A., & Palmer, N. (2007). Conditional cash transfers for improving uptake of health interventions in low- and middle-income countries: A systematic review. *JAMA, 298,* 1900–1910.

Lawn, J. E., Cousens, S., & Zupan, J. (2005). 4 Million neonatal deaths: When? Where? Why? *Lancet, 365,* 891–900.

Maluccio, J., & Flores, R. (2004). *Impact evaluation of a conditional cash transfer program: The Nicaraguan red de proteccion social.* Discussion Paper, 184. International Food Policy Research Institute, Washington DC.

Manandhar, D. S., Osrin, D., Shrestha, B. P., Mesko, N., Morrison, J., Tumbahangphe, K. M., Tamang, S., et al. (2004). Effect of a participatory intervention with women's groups on birth outcomes in Nepal: Cluster-randomised controlled trial. *Lancet, 364,* 970–979.

Meessen, B., Kashala, J. P., & Musango, L. (2007). Output-based payment to boost staff productivity in public health centres: Contracting in Kabutare district, Rwanda. *Bulletin of the World Health Organization, 85,* 108–115.

Moffitt, R. (1991). Program evaluation with nonexperimental data. *Evaluation Review, 15,* 291–314.

Morris, S., Flores, R., Olinto, P., & Medina, J. M. (2004a). Monetary incentives in primary health care and effects on use and coverage of preventive health care interventions in rural Honduras: Cluster randomised trial. *Lancet, 364,* 2030–2037.

Morris, S. S., Olinto, P., Flores, R., Nilson, E. A., & Figueiro, A. C. (2004b). Conditional cash transfers are associated with a small reduction in the rate of weight gain of preschool children in northeast Brazil. *Journal of Nutrition, 134,* 2336–2341.

O'Donnell, O., Doorslaer, E., Wagstaff, A., & Lindelow, M. (2008). *Analysing health equity using household survey data: A guide to techniques and their implementation.* Washington DC: World Bank.

Paxon, C., & Schady, N. (2007). *Does money matter? The effects of cash transfers on child health and development in rural Ecuador.* Washington, DC: World Bank.

Powell-Jackson, T., Neupane, B. D., Tiwari, S., Morrison, J., & Costello, A. (2008). *Evaluation of the safe delivery incentive programme: Final report of the evaluation.* Kathmandu, Nepal: Support to Safe Motherhood Programme.

Soeters, R., & Griffiths, F. (2003). Improving government health services through contract management: A case from Cambodia. *Health Policy Plan, 18,* 74–83.

Travis, P., Bennett, S., Haines, A., Pang, T., Bhutta, Z., Hyder, A. A., Pielemeier, N. R., Mills, A., & Evans, T. (2004). Overcoming health-systems constraints to achieve the Millennium Development Goals. *Lancet, 364,* 900–906.

van Doorslaer, E., O'Donnell, O., Rannan-Eliya, R. P., Somanathan, A., Adhikari, S. R., Garg, C. C., Harbianto, D., et al. (2007). Catastrophic payments for health care in Asia. *Health Economics, 16,* 1159–1184.

Victora, C. G., Habicht, J. P., & Bryce, J. (2004). Evidence-based public health: Moving beyond randomized trials. *Ameircan Journal of Public Health, 94,* 400–405.

Wagstaff, A. (2009a). Estimating health insurance impacts under unobserved heterogeneity: The case of Vietnam's Health Care Fund for the Poor Health Economics. *Health Economics,* in press.

Wagstaff, A. (2009b). Extending health insurance to the rural population: An impact evaluation of China's new cooperative medical scheme. *Journal of Health Economics, 28*, 1–19.

Wagstaff, A., & Doorslaer, E. (2003). Catastrophe and impoverishment in paying for health care: With applications to Vietnam 1993–1998. *Health Economics, 12*, 921–934.

Wagstaff, A., & Lindelow, M. (2008). Can insurance increase financial risk? The curious case of health insurance in China. *Journal of Health Economics, 27*, 990–1005.

Xu, K., Evans, D. B., Kawabata, K., Zeramdini, R., Klavus, J., & Murray, C. J. (2003). Household catastrophic health expenditure: A multicountry analysis. *Lancet, 362*, 111–117.

SERVICE- AND POPULATION-BASED EXEMPTIONS: ARE THESE THE WAY FORWARD FOR EQUITY AND EFFICIENCY IN HEALTH FINANCING IN LOW-INCOME COUNTRIES? ✩

Sophie Witter

ABSTRACT

Objective – *The first wave of experiences of exemptions policies suggested that poverty-based exemptions, using individual targeting, were not effective, for practical and political economic reasons. In response, many countries have changed their approach in recent years – while maintaining user fees as a necessary source of revenue for facilities, they have been switching to categorical targeting, offering exemptions based on high-priority services or population groups. This chapter aims to examine the impact and conditions for effectiveness of this recent health finance modality.*

✩The funders have no responsibility for the information provided or views expressed in this paper. The views expressed herein are solely those of the author.

Innovations in Health System Finance in Developing and Transitional Economies
Advances in Health Economics and Health Services Research, Volume 21, 251–288
ISSN: 0731-2199/doi:10.1108/S0731-2199(2009)0000021013

Methodology/approach – *The chapter is based on a literature review and on data from two complex evaluations of national fee exemption policies for delivery care in West Africa (Ghana and Senegal). A conceptual framework for analysing the impact of exemption policies is developed and used. Although the analysis focuses on exemption for deliveries, the framework and findings are likely to be generalisable to other service- or population-based exemptions.*

Findings – *The chapter presents background information on the nature of delivery exemptions, the drivers for their use, their scale and common modalities in low-income countries. It then looks at evidence of their impact, on utilisation, quality of care and equity and investigates their cost-effectiveness. The final section presents lessons on implementation and implications for policy-makers, including the acceptability and sustainability of exemptions and how they compare to other possible mechanisms.*

Implications for policy – *The chapter concludes that funded service- or group-based exemptions offer a simple, potentially effective route to mitigating inequity and inefficiency in the health systems of low-income countries. However, there are a number of key constraints. One is the fungibility of resources at health facility level. The second is the difficulty of sustaining a separate funding stream over the medium to long term. The third is the arbitrary basis for selecting high-priority services for exemption. The chapter therefore concludes that this financing mode is unstable and is likely to be transitional.*

INTRODUCTION

User fees – direct payment by patients at the point of treatment – have always been a feature of health care finance but became more common in public health systems in developing countries from the late 1980s onwards, as a response to under-funding. At the time, a number of arguments were made in favour of them – in particular, that they would reduce frivolous use, that they would improve quality and that they would make services more responsive to users (Akin, Birdsall, & de Ferranti, 1987; Griffin, 1988). However, as user fee experiments progressed and were documented, it was noted that utilisation was being seriously reduced and that the utilisation of the poor was particularly badly affected (Gilson, 1997).

The need for exemptions was therefore recognised early on, and most health care systems with user fees claimed to offer exemptions for a variety of categories of services or patients. Most, particularly in low-income countries, were not funded and were poorly targeted and therefore not effective (Bitran & Giedion, 2003; Gilson, Russell, & Buse, 1995). The evidence that exemption systems were failing has generated support for a campaign for the abolition of user fees in general. Indeed, when user fees were removed recently, in South Africa (for primary care) and in Uganda (for all public health care), substantial increases in utilisation across all socio-economic groups were noted (Deininger & Mpuga, 2004). At the same time, there are pre-conditions for the success of this policy in terms of the supply-side changes, which are needed to ensure that quality does not drop even further (and, preferably, increases) when the small but important revenues from user fees are lost (Save the Children (UK), 2008; Yates, 2004b).

An alternative approach is to try to make exemptions work more effectively – addressing the main weaknesses identified with previous exemption schemes, which were lack of funding, poor targeting and the incentives that health workers faced to withhold exemptions. One innovation has been the use of Health Equity Funds, which make community groups, rather than health workers, responsible for identifying beneficiaries, and are funded from external sources (Noirhomme et al., 2007). A second response has been to experiment with funded national exemptions schemes that do not rely on individual (usually poverty-based) targeting, but use broader characteristics of services or populations. This chapter examines how effective this second approach has been, using secondary literature and recent evaluation data from two national delivery exemption policies in West Africa.

METHODS

A literature review was undertaken using the search terms: (deliver* OR caesarean*) AND (fee OR fees OR charge*) AND (remove* OR abolition OR reform OR waiver OR exemption*) AND (Africa OR Asia OR Latin America OR Central America OR developing). The period of analysis was 1990–2007 and was limited to publications in English. We searched Ovid Medline, AMED, British Nursing Index, EMBASE, HMIC, International Bibliography of the Social Sciences, Pub Med, Eldis and id21. In addition, the search tools were used on websites of organisations known to be active in this field, including bi- and multilateral donors (such as the World Bank and the Department for International Development (DFID)); United

Nations (UN) organisations (World Health Organisation (WHO), United Nations Childrens Fund (UNICEF), United Nations Fund for Population Activities (UNFPA), International Labour Office (ILO)) and research, implementation or consultancy projects (such as Partnerships for Health Reform, Harvard International Health Systems Programme, London School of Hygiene and Tropical Medicine, Family Care International, Initiative for Maternal Mortality Programme Assessment (Immpact) and Averting Maternal Death and Disability (AMDD)). Relevant papers' references were reviewed for additional studies. Searches were also undertaken of a selection of journals, including Reproductive Health Matters, WHO Bulletin, Social Science and Medicine, Health Policy and Planning and the International Journal of Health Planning and Management.

The data for the case studies are drawn from two evaluations conducted by Immpact in the two countries (Table 1). The evaluation in Ghana included a number of components, including key informant interviews for managers; a health worker incentive survey; financial flows tracking; two household surveys looking at utilisation and costs changes; focus group discussions and in-depth interviews amongst providers and communities; clinical case notes extraction in health centres and hospitals and confidential enquiry techniques to look at the quality of care changes (Immpact, 2005). These tools were applied in 12 focal districts of two regions (Central and Volta) between 2005 and 2006.

In Senegal, a much more limited set of research tools was applied. This included key informant interviews; community focus group discussions; financial flows tracking; and analysis of changes in clinical indicators (MSPM, Immpact, UNFPA, & CEFOREP, 2006). In Senegal, data were gathered from all of the five regions that had implemented the policy.

CONTEXT

Characteristics of Delivery Exemptions

An exemption is defined here as an official reduction in direct payments for health care, which is targeted by group, area or service. The current literature distinguishes between waivers (which are granted to individuals, entitling them to free or reduced cost access to all services) and exemptions (which make certain services free or free for broad categories of users) (Bitran & Giedion, 2003). Most studies have focussed on the difficulties of targeting waivers at needy individuals and households. The practical

Table 1. Summary of Research Methods (Ghana and Senegal Delivery Exemption Evaluations).

Research Component	Description of Tool	Variables Examined	Sample Size
Ghana evaluation			
Key informant interviews	Semi-structured interviews with stakeholders ranging from national level decision-makers and donors down to facility managers	Perceptions of policy, its implementation, successes, failures and recommendations for improvements	65 key informants, at national level, in 2 regions and 12 districts
Health worker incentive survey	Structured questionnaire (with some open questions at the end on motivation and views on policy)	Self-reported income, working hours, number of clients and changes to these variables over the period of policy implementation, along with views on impact of policy	374 respondents in 12 districts (21 doctors; 11 medical assistants; 117 public midwifes; 16 private midwifes; 50 nurses; 108 trained TBAs; 51 untrained TBAs)
Financial flows tracking	Set of forms used to extract financial information from national down to facility level	Total expenditure; unit costs; adequacy of financing; allocation by area and facility type; timeliness of transfers; impact on facilities	National; 2 regions; 12 districts; 11 facilities (covering different types and sectors)
Utilisation survey	Structured questionnaire administered to women of reproductive age (15–49 years)	Personal characteristics, place of delivery, person attending delivery	2,922 respondents from 100 enumeration areas in 12 districts in 2 regions
Household cost survey	Structured questionnaire administered to women who had had (1) vaginal delivery at a health facility; (2) vaginal delivery at home with a traditional birth attendant (TBA); (3) caesarean section	Out-of-pocket payment for delivery care: (a) payment to delivery service provider (drugs, supplies, inpatient stay; (b) items purchased outside health facility; (c) transportation costs; (d) amount spent on gifts; (e) other costs incurred in the course of the delivery	1,500 respondents from Volta (750 before and 750 after the introduction of the exemption); 750 respondents from Central (all from the period of implementation)

Table 1. (*Continued*)

Research Component	Description of Tool	Variables Examined	Sample Size
Focus group discussions/ Provider and community in-depth interviews	Unstructured discussions at community level	Views of policy and its impact on barriers to utilisation and on costs and quality of care	100 interviews and group discussions in 8 communities in 2 regions
Clinical case note extraction	Structured data extraction from clinical records	(1) Quality of clinical care in hospitals: best practice, timing and vigilance for management of haemorrhage, pregnancy-induced hypertension and emergency caesarean sections (2) Quality of care in health centres: scoring for selected activities of labour and delivery care	(1) 2 regions; 2 regional hospitals; 12 district hospitals (2) 49 health centres; 12 districts
Confidential enquiry	Review of records/ case notes and completion of maternal death assessment form by eight-member panel	Panel opinion of adverse and favourable events for the following: woman/ patient and community factors; administrative/ health system factors; clinical care provided; degree of availability of information	(3) 2 regional hospitals; 12 district hospitals; 20 cases of maternal deaths
Senegal evaluation			
Key informant interviews	Semi-structured interviews with stakeholders ranging from national level decision-makers and donors down to facility managers	Perceptions of policy, its implementation, successes, failures and recommendations for improvements	54 key informants from 5 regions (10 national; 12 regional; 17 district; 15 facilities)
Financial flows tracking	Set of forms used to extract financial and activity information from national down to facility level	Total expenditure; unit costs; adequacy of financing; allocation by area and facility type; timeliness of transfers; impact on	National; 5 regions; 6 districts; 10 health posts (all public)

Table 1. (*Continued*)

Research Component	Description of Tool	Variables Examined	Sample Size
		facilities; costing of services; changes to activities and staffing at facility level	
Focus group discussions/in-depth interviews	Unstructured discussions at community level	Views of policy and its impact on barriers to utilisation and on costs and quality of care	Qualitative research conducted in 4 districts. Included 4 in-depth interviews on policy with young women; 4 in-depth interviews on gender; 10 focus group discussions with young women, elderly women and men
Clinical record extraction	Structured questionnaire applied to clinical records	Changes in indicators of absolute need for emergency obstetric interventions	761 major obstetric interventions

difficulty of assessing income and deterring cheats brings high transaction costs and problems of both undercoverage (or false negatives – needy people wrongly excluded) and also leakage (or false positives – better off people wrongly included). The focus of the general literature on waivers and exemptions has been on how the targeting can be improved (Tien & Chee, 2002; Willis & Leighton, 1995). In practice, some schemes combine characteristics of both waivers and exemptions – for example, by making some services free but only to certain types of household.

The most common argument made for the use of exemptions has been for services with positive externalities such as immunisation (England, Kaddar, Nigam, & Pinto, 2001; Ensor & Cooper, 2004). These have features that make them particularly suited to the use of exemptions:

• They aim for universal coverage
• Demand for them is limited
• Supply-induced demand is not generally a problem as the interventions are low cost and not profitable for suppliers

The attraction of exemptions for obstetric services (and other service-based exemptions), in principle, is that they subsidise a high-priority service for an easily identified group. The targeting is therefore not the main challenge, and transaction costs should be lower. Unlike waivers, there are few opportunities for staff to discriminate between patients in return for funds or favours (Owino & Were, 1999). Moreover, pregnancy is a time-bound state, and therefore, there is no need for periodic reassessment of eligibility.

On the contrary, deliveries and delivery-related complications are relatively expensive and pregnancy is a common event, particularly in countries with high fertility rates, and therefore, financing exemptions for delivery care is likely to be challenging. In addition, there is a potential for supply-induced demand, especially for more expensive and profitable interventions, such as caesareans (Harris et al., 2007)

The exemptions approach assumes that financial, rather than geographical, barriers are the main constraint to skilled delivery. Services need to be available and of acceptable quality. Remoteness from facilities reduces the chance that a household will benefit from exemptions policies, which typically do not cover informal care. In remote areas, the decision to visit a facility may add to delays in reaching staff, compared to opting for a home delivery. In Nepal, for example, all attendants, both trained and untrained, reached households within an hour of being called to attend the delivery, which compared to an average of 2.8 hours travel time to facilities in the lowland districts, and over 8 hours in mountain districts (Borghi, Ensor, Neupane, & Tiwari, 2004). In this situation, financial support for skilled deliveries at home might be a better approach, with development of facilities as a medium-term plan.

The Drivers Behind Recent Delivery Exemption Policies

A number of countries have recently started experimenting with various ways of reducing financial barriers for delivery services, although these are as yet poorly documented. The objectives are generally a combination of reducing maternal mortality and morbidity, raising supervised delivery rates and reducing poverty (Alam, 2007; ICH & SSMP, 2006; Ministry of Health, 2004a; Ministry of Health, 2004b; Ministry of Health and Family Welfare, 2001). Reducing inequalities is mentioned more rarely.

One of the main drivers has been the Millennium Development Goals (MDGs) and the slow progress made towards MDG 5 in particular, which calls for a three-quarters reduction in maternal mortality ratios between 1990 and 2015. These led to the development of regional and national roadmaps, which cover a range of strategies, including, in some cases, commitments to reduce access costs (WHO-AFRO, 2004) (Ministry of Health, 2004b; WAHO, 2004).

Donor politics is also likely to be a significant driver. An institutional analysis of safe motherhood policy-making processes in Burkina Faso, for example, found that international agencies played a key role in influencing domestic policies (Marchal, Arcens, Coates, & De Brouwere, 2007). It concludes that the policy of removing fees for emergency caesareans in Burkina Faso was directly linked to World Bank grant conditionality and technical advice. In one case (Nepal), there is anecdotal evidence that research on the high costs to households of delivery care contributed to the formulation of a new policy on 'cost-sharing' (Ensor, Clapham, & Prasai, 2008).

Scale of Delivery Exemptions

A number of countries have recently introduced delivery- and other service- or population-based exemption policies (e.g. providing free care for the under-fives). Few have yet been formally evaluated and their impact published. A summary of some recent examples of delivery exemption policies are given in Table 2.

What are the Different Modalities for Exemptions?

There are many possible modalities for delivery exemptions, affecting the range of services covered, the types and level of facilities, the cost components covered and the system for reimbursing providers. Exempted packages can include the full range of pregnancy services or focus on the intra-partum period. Exemptions may apply to all delivery types or just complicated deliveries (or just 'normal' deliveries). Free care may be provided through certain facility types or certain sectors (such as public sector facilities only). The choice of facility type will affect the benefit incidence – whether they are predominantly rural or urban, higher level or primary and public or private. Different types of costs (such as registration, services, drugs, food and supplies) can be explicitly included or excluded from the exemption. Payment systems can include budgeting for funds to

Table 2. Summary of Features of Some Recent Delivery Exemption
Policies.

Date Started	Country	Eligible Group	Exemption Package	Eligible Facilities	Payment Mechanism	Financing Source
2003	Ghana	All women (in five poor regions at first; now whole country)	All facility costs are exempted for all delivery types (including immediate post-partum care)	All public, private and mission facilities. Private midwives included but not TBAs. Non-referred cases at regional hospitals have to pay	Retrospective reimbursement of facility claims at end of each month by district. Tariff set according to average costs of different facility types, with allowance for increased subsidy received by public facilities	Highly indebted poor countries (HIPC) (recycled debt repayment funds)
2005	Senegal	All women (in five poor regions at first; now whole country apart from the capital city)	All facility costs are exempted for normal deliveries and caesarean sections	Public sector only (regional and district hospitals for caesarean sections and health centres/ health posts for normal deliveries)	Prospective payment according to fixed tariff for regional hospitals. For lower level facilities, delivery kits are sent according to expected number of deliveries	General government budget
2005	Nepal	Women in low human development index (HDI)-districts eligible for free deliveries (no facility fees). All women eligible for subsidy towards general costs (e.g. transport) if deliver with skilled attendant (if < 2 children, or complicated delivery)		Public facilities down to Health Post level. Home deliveries also covered by subsidy, if attended by skilled attendant	Cash transfers to eligible women attending facilities, varied according to ecological zone (three tiers). Incentive payments to health workers for each delivery at facility or at home. Retrospective payment to facilities for free deliveries in low-HDI districts, according to fixed tariff	Donor funds (DFID) initially, though with growing contribution from government
2006	Mali	National	Caesareans	Public hospitals	Not known	Not known

Table 2. (*Continued*)

Date Started	Country	Eligible Group	Exemption Package	Eligible Facilities	Payment Mechanism	Financing Source
2006	Niger	National	Caesareans, uterine rupture, family planning (FP), antenatal care (ANC), care for under-fives	Not known	Not known	Half government funding; half French cooperation assistance
2006	Burundi	National	All care for pregnant women and under-fives	Public sector	Not known	Not known
2007	Malawi	All within areas where service agreements signed with Christian Health Association of Malawi (CHAM)	ANC and facility deliveries	Church mission facilities only	Not known, but specified in service agreement between government and CHAM	Donor funds (DFID)
2008	Sudan	National	Caesareans and care for under-fives	Not known	Not known	Public funds from oil revenues

Sources: Witter, Arhinful, Kusi, & Zakariah-Akoto (2007a), Witter, Dieng, Mbengue, Moreira, & De Brouwere (2008b), ICH & SSMP (2006), FCI (2006), DFID (2007), and Ridde, Moha, Tourigny, & Rauland (2008).

support free care (input subsidies, such as used for TB services and immunisation); prospective payment with a fixed tariff per act or retrospective reimbursement according to services provided.

By definition, exemptions cannot be targeted by individual characteristics (such as income levels) but can be combined with some forms of group targeting (e.g. by geographic area) or with some form of self-selection (e.g. if free care is offered only at facility types that are designed not to appeal to the rich). They can also be combined with other demand-side approaches (e.g. cash payments to compensate families for travel costs to reach facilities). Exemptions may also be combined with incentive payments to health workers, possibly to reach certain targets, or per delivery carried out. The Skilled Delivery Incentive Programme in Nepal combined exemptions for women in the poorest districts with health worker incentives and demand-side finance for transport (Barker, Bird, Pradhan, & Shakya, 2007; Powell-Jackson,

Neupane, Tiwari, Morrison, & Costello, 2008). It is now being refined to provide a national exemption approach, combined with ongoing transport assistance for households (Ensor & Witter, 2008).

The policies in Ghana and Senegal shared many characteristics and therefore do not illustrate all of the possible different modalities for an exemption scheme. A general typology is discussed in Table 3. Looking at the table, it is clear that countries can adopt a 'pick and mix' approach, selecting one or several options per dimension, and also that there are no limits to how the different dimensions can be combined. Clearly, the choice will depend on policy objectives, context and financial means.

In relation to targeting, both Ghana and Senegal used a service-based approach, with geographic targeting as a way of introducing the policy, followed by full or partial scale-up to national level. Other countries, such as

Table 3.   Main Modalities for Exemption Policies.

Dimension	Main Options			
Targeting Approach	Geographic	Based on Specified Facilities	Service-Based	Combined with Waivers
Package of services	Preventive care (e.g. antenatal)	Primary care (e.g. normal deliveries; postnatal care)	Secondary care (e.g. complicated deliveries)	Tertiary care (e.g. restorative surgery)
Cost components included	In facility costs: • Fees • Registration • Tests • Accommodation • Drugs • Supplies • Food	Option of combining with one or more of: Supplementary costs: • Drugs from outside pharmacy • External supplies • Informal payments	Other direct costs: • Travel • Accommodation • Expenses of companions	Incentives to health workers: • Facility-based • Outreach-based
Levels of service delivery	Outreach	Primary	Secondary	Tertiary
Choice of sector	Public	Private	Mission/Private not-for-profit	Informal
Funding mechanism	Central government budget	Aid/health partners	Local government	Insurance scheme
Channel of funding	Payments via facilities	Payments via patients (cash, vouchers)	Payments via third-party (NGO, local government, etc.)	
Payment systems	In advance, as input into budgets	In advance; per act (with fixed tariff)	Retrospectively, with fixed tariff	Retrospectively, fee for service

India, have combined service-based targeting with individual characteristics (such as poverty or caste status) (Devadasan, Elias, John, Grahacharya, & Ralte, 2008).

In relation to the package of care, both Ghana and Senegal excluded preventive care (i.e. family planning) but offered primary and secondary cover (with restrictions on which kinds of facilities could be visited for each type, in the case of Senegal). Ghana also included tertiary services, if a woman was referred.

Both countries aimed to cover all in-facility costs, though neither was very explicit about this, and in reality, many gaps were observed. Neither offered support for non-facility demand-side costs such as transport. Neither officially offered incentives to health workers, although one region in Ghana did improvise, giving a small portion of reimbursements to delivery staff.

Levels of service overlap to some extent with the package of care on offer, though they can be distinct. In Ghana, for example, primary and secondary delivery care (normal deliveries and complicated or emergency obstetric care) were exempted at all facilities, while in Senegal, primary care could only be accessed free at primary facilities and secondary care at secondary facilities.

In Ghana, the exemptions package covered public, private and non-governmental organization (NGO) services, while in Senegal, only the public sector was eligible to participate. In one district of Ghana, the informal sector had been included as a local innovation, despite this not being provided for in national guidelines. This reflected the local situation (a remote district, with strong links between the grassroots facilities and the traditional birth attendants (TBAs)).

In relation to funding sources, both schemes were funded through central government budgets, although the system in Ghana changed in 2008 to route delivery exemptions through the national health insurance system. Funding sources and channels can of course be multiple and multi-layered.

In Ghana and Senegal, the main payment channel was through facilities. The theory in Senegal was that funds and kits would be provided in advance, according to estimated caseload. The reality appears to have been a combination of advance payments and retrospective claims, according to an agreed fixed tariff. In Ghana, by contrast, all payments were made retrospectively, and the claims were calculated based on delivery numbers, using a tariff that set upper limits for payments per delivery, according to fixed categories of delivery type and sector (recognising the varying subsidies already received by public, mission and private facilities).

CONCEPTUAL FRAMEWORK FOR ANALYSIS OF EXEMPTIONS

A conceptual framework was developed to inform the evaluations of the exemption schemes (Fig. 1), though it can easily be adapted to examine any health financing change. It presents the policy objectives (on the right), the intermediate outputs that would be needed to feed into the objectives (in the centre) and the preconditions for effective implementation (on the left). The top half is focussed on demand-side features, while the bottom half is focussed on the health system. All of the nodes are connected, and each presents an important aspect to consider during evaluation. There is, however, no hierarchy, and it is possible that policy changes might have a positive impact on some aspects and negative on others.

The evaluation findings are presented, starting from the right of the conceptual framework with the evidence on their impact in relation to the policy objectives, followed by lessons relating to implementation, on the left. The impact on maternal mortality is not discussed as this evaluation was not able to measure this aspect. It is generally accepted that raising supervised delivery rates is a prerequisite for reducing maternal mortality and morbidity (Graham, Bell, & Bullough, 2001).

IMPACT

Impact on Utilisation of Services

The evaluations showed a significant response in both Ghana and Senegal – coincidentally, a 12% increase in facility deliveries in both Central Region (Penfold, Harrison, Bell, & Fitzmaurice, 2007) and in the selected facilities from which data was obtained in Senegal. (Volta Region showed a lower increase of 5%, but the short time frame and very partial implementation of the policy in that region makes this arguably a less reliable result.)

While significant, this change is of a lower magnitude than reported in other contexts of user fee removal. In Uganda, for example, which is one of the best-documented examples, administrative data showed that the abolition of fees resulted in a doubling of utilisation (mainly in the form of outpatient visits) at public hospitals and a 77% increase at lower level units between 2000 and 2001 (Yates, 2004a). The difference in magnitude may be linked to a number of issues, including the nature of the data, the

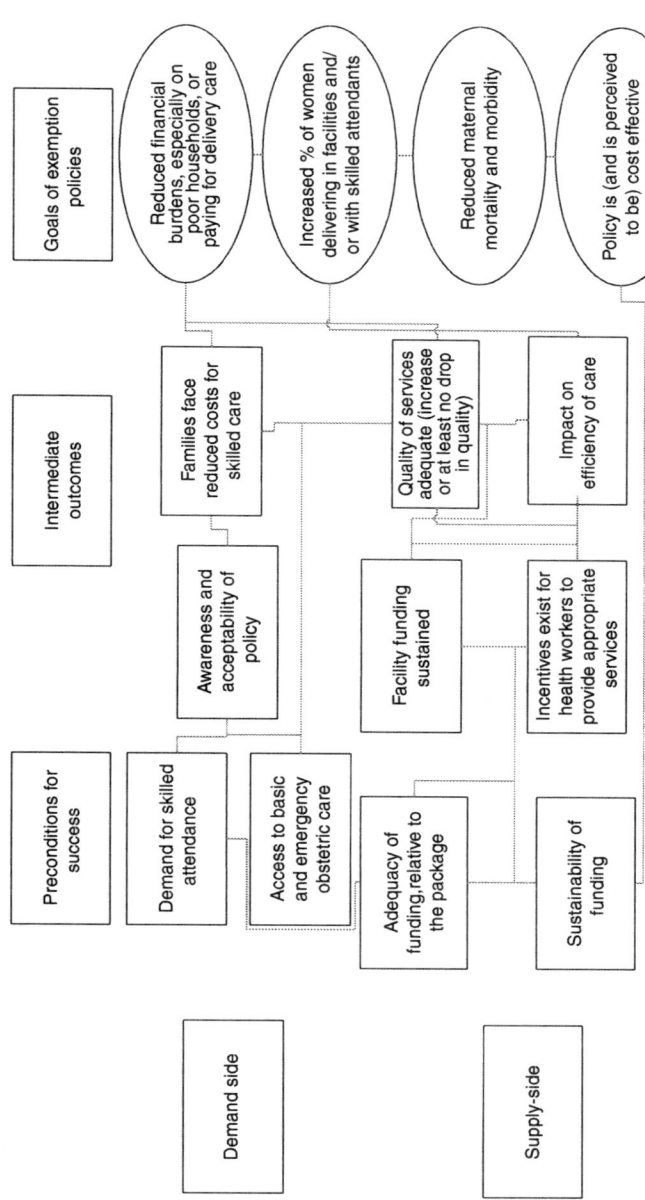

Fig. 1. Conceptual Framework for Assessing Impact of Delivery Exemptions.

context, the degree of effectiveness of the exemption in reducing costs and the nature of the service. Estimates for increases in facility deliveries, based on household data for Uganda, for example, suggested an increase of 28%, accompanied by a 16% decrease in TBA deliveries nationally (Deininger & Mpuga, 2004). The context of total fee abolition is also clearly different. In particular, it is easier to communicate the message of full removal of fees than of exemptions for one particular service. Moreover, the combination of fee removal with increases in funding for salaries and drugs was one which is judged to have rendered this particular policy change effective in reaching its goal of reducing household access costs (Nabyongo et al., 2008). Analysis of survey data from 1999 and 2002 found that the proportion of households reporting that they were charged for health consultations decreased from 29% before user fee abolition to 3% after (Deininger & Mpuga, 2004). This suggests a high degree of implementation effectiveness.

Whether there is something particular about delivery care, compared to other health care consumed, is harder to establish. There are few studies that report price or cost decreases and utilisation increases for delivery care specifically. In Uganda, there were no data for changes in out-of-pocket payments for deliveries specifically, although overall household health care expenditure decreased by 42% over 1999–2002 (with the highest proportion in the second quintile – 48%) (Deininger & Mpuga, 2004).

A study using Living Standards Measurement Survey data from urban areas of Bolivia found that price elasticities for obstetric care were low, ranging from −0.002 for the bottom quintile to –0.068 for the top one for public health centres (Li, 1996). In general, elasticities fall with rise in income, but the reverse was found in this data set for obstetric care (but not antenatal care). The Ghana data present a different picture, with price elasticity of demand higher for both normal deliveries (−0.26 in one region and −0.63 in another) and caesarean sections (−0.22). Moreover, analysis of the Volta data suggests that poorer households have much greater sensitivity to changes in the price of deliveries, comparing the utilisation responses by quintile with the changes of out-of-pocket payments as a proportion of household income (Table 4). The estimated price elasticity was 23 times higher for the poorest quintile, compared to the least poor. This suggests that equal price reductions across the quintiles will have a two-fold pro-poor effect: first, by constituting a larger proportion of household income for lower quintiles and, second, because the response to a given proportionate reduction will be greater amongst the poor.

As in Bolivia, income and education are both important determinants of demand for facility deliveries in Ghana. Women with secondary education

Table 4. Utilisation Response to Changes in Costs, by Quintile, Volta Region, Ghana.

Volta Region Quintile	% Delivering in Facility			Change in % of Household Income Before/After Delivery Exemption Policy (%)	Price Elasticity
	Before	After	% Change (%)		
1	12.4	23.8	92	−25	−3.72148
2	28.4	33.8	19	−21	−0.89596
3	51.4	55.9	9	−13	−0.69143
4	62.3	62.5	0	−29	−0.01108
5	80.8	85	5	−33	−0.15943

Source: Author's calculations, based on utilisation data from Penfold, Harrison, & Bell (2006) and expenditure data from Asante, Chikwama, Daniels, & Armar-Klemesu (2007). The change in expenditure was calculated for all delivery types and would be higher for facility deliveries alone.

were found to be five times more likely to deliver in a facility than those with none in Central Region, and nearly 12 times more likely in Volta (Penfold et al., 2007). For income, the odds ratio for a facility delivery was three times higher for top compared with bottom quintile in Volta and six times in Central.

In Bolivia, elasticities for private sector services were found to be higher than for public services. Data were not disaggregated by sector in Ghana, and therefore, no comparison with this finding can be made. In a study based on one area of the Philippines, price was found to be significant for poorer households in choosing obstetric services, and elasticity was low but increasing as income fell (Hotchkiss, 1993). Demand was, however, inelastic for all services except private hospitals.

In general, it is debateable whether a study of price elasticity of demand based on a horizontal analysis of prices charged by different providers can be directly compared with analysis of responses to a simultaneous price change for a whole category of providers. In the first, price may to some extent be seen as a marker of quality, whereas in the second scenario, the cost reduction may be seen as a 'windfall'. Whether this 'windfall' is sufficient to trigger longer term behaviour change (reflecting a shift in individual and social preferences over place of delivery) is more debateable, and clearly the interaction with perceptions of quality will be key. Evaluation data based on 18 months of patchy implementation is not sufficient to make an assessment of this longer term response.

In relation to place of delivery and type of attendant, in Central Region, the largest increase was in health centre deliveries, and in deliveries conducted by midwives, while in Volta, the largest increase was in hospital deliveries and deliveries by midwives (Penfold et al., 2007). Before and after, midwives were the most common attendant, and hospitals were the most common location for deliveries.

For Senegal, the data suggest a strong response overall, particularly in light of the variable implementation of the Free Delivery and Caesarean Policy (FDCP), but with considerable variation between areas and facilities. The response at the Health Post level appeared to be weaker than at higher facilities: overall facility delivery numbers increased by 20% at regional level over 2004–2005, by 31% at district level, but only by 8% at sub-district level. However, referrals increased by 49% from the Health Posts, which is consistent with the larger increase at district level. This pattern is promising in relation to skilled attendance, as the health posts generally lack midwives, and has no implication for costs, as both Health Posts and Health Centres receive the same support (delivery kits) at present.

The increase in caesarean sections (49%) was greater in Senegal than the increase in normal deliveries (12%), over 2004–2005, which is encouraging given the extremely low levels of caesarean sections being carried out in Senegal before the FDCP (3.3% nationally, but as low as 0.5% in some of the FDCP regions (Ndiaye & Ayad, 2006)). Quantative data on household cost changes was not available to indicate the price elasticity of demand for caesareans (and to allow comparison with Ghana), but the results of the analysis of financial flows and qualitative data at community level indicated that the absolute and proportionate out-of-pocket payment reductions may have been greater for caesareans than for normal deliveries, due to better financing mechanisms for caesareans. This would affect incentives for both demand and supply: reducing financial barriers for users while also rewarding providers for increasing their activity. If so, there is a risk in the longer term of inappropriate medicalisation of deliveries.

Impact on the Quality of Care

Quality of care is a diverse concept, encompassing features relating to health care inputs, processes, outputs and outcomes, judged from both a 'hard' angle of evidence-based medical protocols and also a 'soft' angle of perceptions and relationships. The evaluation data in Ghana was able to shed light on most of these features, while in Senegal, it relied mainly on perceptual information.

The short-term impact in both cases appeared negligible, but this does not indicate what the long-term effects might be, depending on long-run demand and supply responses. Moreover, the stability of quality during financing changes may rely on the safety valve of patient contributions. If funding for a policy is inadequate, for example, facilities may revert to a variety of strategies for charging, which, while subverting the original goals of reducing financial barriers, will nevertheless maintain the functioning of services. This scenario appears to have been illustrated by responses at lower level facilities in Senegal, where prices for other services were raised in direct response to the loss of revenue in some facilities (Witter, Armar-Klemesu, & Dieng, 2008a; Witter et al., 2008b; Witter, Richard, & De Brouwere, 2008c).

A summary of the findings on different aspects of quality of care are summarised in Table 5. While inputs are not generally used as a measure of quality of care, they tend to correlate quite closely with hard and soft quality measures and perceptions – they are therefore included.

Contribution of Delivery Exemptions to Poverty Reduction and Other Equity goals

In Ghana, the incidence of catastrophic out-of-pocket payments associated with delivery care was found to fall (Asante et al., 2007). For the poorest quintile, the proportion paying more than 2.5% of their income dropped from 55% before the policy to 46% after. Using the poverty head count, the proportion of households falling into extreme poverty as a result of their delivery payments reduced from 2.5% before the policy to 1.3% after. However, the proportionate decrease in out-of-pocket payments was greater for the richest households (22%), compared to the poorest (13%). This supports the conclusion that across-the-board price cuts are likely to benefit rich households as well as poor (and may benefit richer households more, in relation to their previously higher expenditure and better access to services); however, the significance of the reduction can still be greater for poorer households, given their greater resource constraints.

There is a further argument that emphasises the importance of increasing overall access and coverage of health care. Borrowing from infectious disease control terminology, some argue that there can be a protective 'herd effect': 'Although we might want to look at the poor in isolation, the reality is that improving health behaviours amongst the poorest requires improving health behaviours across all income levels. Poor-rich differentials are least in those countries with the best overall health outcomes, such as Sri Lanka,

Table 5. Summary of Impact of Delivery Exemptions on Quality of Care.

Dimensions		Ghana		Senegal	
		Positive	Negative	Positive	Negative
Hard	Inputs	– Facility revenue increased, during period when funding available – Health worker income increases with increased hours (though not in direct connection with the policy) – Inputs for comprehensive emergency obstetric care (CEmOC) found to be generally good	– Debts built up when funding ran out – Uncertainty for managers about timing and amount of funding – No increase in staffing to match increased workload – Staff working long hours before and after	– Regional hospitals benefited from increased reimbursement of caesareans	– Lower level facilities lost funding of the act of performing normal deliveries – Community staff paid from delivery user fees, so alternative funding had to be found – Value of funding and supplies reduced by delays and mismatch of supply and demand – No increase in staffing to match increased workload
	Processes	– No change in duration of admission in hospitals – No significant change in quality of care scores in health centres in Central Region. – Women arriving earlier in hospitals.	– Significant decrease in average quality of care scores in Volta – Processes for handling complications found to be poor, before and after Delivery Exemptions Policy	No tools to examine this aspect	No tools to examine this aspect

Table 5. (*Continued*)

Dimensions		Ghana		Senegal	
		Positive	Negative	Positive	Negative
	Outcomes	– No significant change in institutional Maternal Mortality Ratio (MMR) or cause of maternal deaths in hospitals – No significant change in stillbirth rates in health centres	None recorded	– Fresh still birth rate decreased (but not significantly) – Significant reduction in still births for women with caesareans in districts for which data available	None recorded
Soft	Inputs	– Health workers relieved that problem of inability to pay is solved – Staff report improved supplies	– Health workers feel policy has exacerbated staff shortages – Variable charges cause concern to clients	None recorded	Concern about impact on facility funding and ability to pay community staff
Processes		Health workers report no change in overall quality of care	Varied reports of relationship between health workers and clients, before and after	Consensus by communities and managers that quality of care overall unaffected by the policy (though not always viewed as acceptable before)	None recorded
Outcomes		All stakeholder groups report that women are able to access care quicker and so there are fewer deaths	None recorded	Perceived improvement due to increased and quicker access	None recorded

Sources: Author's summary, including findings from Armar-Klemesu et al. (2006) and MSPM & U. I. C (2007).

Viet Nam and Philippines' (Rannan-Eliya & Somanathan, 2005). These authors argue that universalism is the most effective route to reduced inequality. This suggests that increased uptake across the quintiles, as was documented in response to the Delivery Exemption Policy (DEP) in Ghana, is not a finding that policy-makers should worry about.

In addition, the distribution of health risks is likely to mean that even universal exemption measures will have a pro-poor effect. Although it is hard to measure need for obstetric care (most measures, like caesarean section rates, will reflect access as much as need), indirect determinants such as malnutrition weigh more heavily on poorer households, with women in the bottom quintile almost twice as likely on average to be malnourished, compared to the top quintile (Gwatkin et al., 2007). In addition, the tendency for poorer households to have larger families – an average of six children for the bottom quintile, compared to three for the top, in developing countries (Gwatkin et al., 2007) – should make maternal exemptions progressive. (This feature is however negated by policies that restrict eligibility to those of low parity, as has been the case in Nepal and India.) The household survey in Ghana, which examined changed costs per delivery, does not capture this fertility effect.

Set against these pro-poor features is the current huge differential in utilisation – a woman in the top quintile in a developing country is three times more likely on average to deliver with a medically trained attendant or in a public facility, compared to a woman in the bottom quintile (Gwatkin et al., 2007). This indicates that public subsidies to deliveries are likely to be disproportionately beneficial to wealthier households, at least initially.

Balancing the pro-poor risk and fertility factors against the pro-rich utilisation patterns suggests that on average a universal DEP should have a mild pro-poor impact, even in the short term, which may accelerate as utilisation patterns change and overall coverage of skilled birth attendance increases. Moreover, universal policies can be rolled out in a pro-poor manner by targeting deprived areas first (as was the case in both case study countries).

Analysis of context is also clearly critical to the decision to use a universal approach. Where there is 'marginal deprivation', with only the poorest lacking access to services, then a targeted approach is more justified, contrasted with 'massive deprivation', in which the bulk of the population lacks access (as is the case in many sub-Saharan African countries for skilled attendance at delivery[1]). In this context, a universal exemption is likely to be more equitable as well as more efficient.

Cost and Cost-Effectiveness of Delivery Exemptions

Summary figures for total expenditure, unit costs and cost per additional delivery are given in Table 6.

Costs can be compared with other similar schemes, although the basis for calculating costs and the cost structures varies, making this a relatively meaningless exercise. One review found that a normal delivery with a skilled attendant can cost as little as $2 in poor countries, but tends to range from $7 to $15 at health centres in Africa and Latin America (Leighton, 2000). It found that costs of a normal delivery at a hospital ranged from $10–35, and caesarean sections and complicated deliveries can cost from $50 to $100. The Uganda voucher scheme has budgeted $33 per 'safe delivery', to include all care during pregnancy and during and after the delivery (Nonay, 2007), while in Kenya, the delivery vouchers are costed at $70 per normal delivery and $292 per caesarean (Awiti, 2007). Bangladesh's vouchers are estimated to cost an average of $24 per delivery, including funds for transport.

The Ghana and Senegal estimates are consistent with these different costings. In some respects, they appear to offer good value for money. An expenditure of $2.2 per normal delivery in Senegal, for example, is very low. However, this masks the degree to which the exemption has become a subsidy (possibly very low) in practice, with limited support to facilities passed on in ongoing costs for households. Moreover, the expenditure data for the DEP in Ghana was limited (based on returns for one region and one year).

Table 6. Summary Figures on Expenditure and Cost-Effectiveness of Delivery Exemption Policies in Ghana and Senegal (USD, 2005).

Indicator	Ghana	Senegal
Total annual expenditure on policy (nationwide implementation for Ghana; five regions for Senegal)	$2,999,944	$308,389
Expenditure on policy as proportion of total annual health expenditure	0.64% 2004 (four regions) 0.7% 2005 (national) 2% in 2005 if fully funded	0.6% 2005 0.5% 2006
Expenditure per capita per annum	$0.16	$0.10
Expenditure per normal delivery	$22	$2.2
Expenditure per caesarean section		$154
Cost per additional normal delivery	$62	$21
Costs per additional caesarean section		$467

Source: Witter, Armar-Klemesu, Dieng (2008a).

Assessing cost-effectiveness is also not straightforward, as this depends on the opportunity costs of the resources, which are rarely clear. However, given the large 'sunk costs' of wider subsidies to health systems, any measure that stimulates demand for services at relatively low cost is likely to improve technical efficiency. One costing study in Tanzania, for example, found that the cost of a normal delivery at a dispensary was twice that of a normal delivery at a hospital. This finding – the reverse of the expected relationship – was directly related to low utilisation at dispensary level (Von Both, Jahn, & Flessa, 2007).

Increased technical efficiency is not necessarily linked to improved outcomes. However, in the context of a high burden of maternal mortality and morbidity (such as are found in both Ghana and Senegal), the returns to subsidising safe delivery are likely to be high, if a minimum quality threshold is reached. Returns are likely to range from reduced numbers of deaths to reduced ill-health (including mental), improved productivity, reduced impoverishment and benefits for children and families that span the health, education, economic and social spheres (Storeng et al., 2007).

IMPLEMENTATION AND POLICY LESSONS

Feasibility of Implementation

The settings for the evaluations in Ghana and Senegal were very realistic, in the sense that the policies were national initiatives, funded from national funds (poverty reduction funds in Ghana, the general health budget in Senegal) and implemented without any external support. These same features probably explain some of the implementation difficulties. In Senegal, these focussed around lack of consensus on the policy at high levels, lack of specific guidance on implementation and failure to develop full reimbursement systems. In Ghana, the central difficulty was failure to secure reliable and adequate funds, particularly for going to scale, and competition with other financing initiatives (including the National Health Insurance system) (Witter & Adjei, 2007).

Are the implementation problems documented in Ghana and Senegal peculiar to delivery exemptions? In many respects, they are illustrations of the difficulties faced by all policies, especially in a resource-constrained context where not only funds but also information and skilled time to plan and manage are very limited.

On the contrary, there are some features of the exemptions approach adopted by the two countries, which increase the complexity and risk. Clearly, exemptions require on-going funding, which is hard to sustain (this is true of most approaches to reduce financial barriers, but not all – some, such as insurance, can have internal risk-pooling). With retrospective reimbursement, there is uncertainty about the final cost, which adds to uncertainty and risk for the implementer, which in both cases was the Ministry of Health. With this retrospective reimbursement, the total cost to government of the subsidy can be increased by providers, which adds to the need for careful auditing.

Lessons for Effective Implementation

The Ghana experience emphasises the importance of adequate funding and the need for an agency with clear responsibility and interest in effective management of the scheme. In that case, there is potential for a positive impact on utilisation. But this will not bring down maternal mortality ratios unless quality of care is also assured, which includes an understanding of how policy will affect health workers' work patterns and incentives.

The importance of reimbursing actual costs is well supported by the case study of Senegal, where regional hospitals were overpaid and lower level facilities underpaid for the services that they were asked to provide for free. Fees for maternity care can form an important part of facility revenues and pay for essential service inputs. A problem with funding mechanisms lay at the root of the difficulty in channelling resources to the lower level facilities. Planning, budgeting, cash flow systems and accounting were once again poor. The case study also raises the importance of proper specification of the package of benefits: in this case, caesareans and normal deliveries were covered at specified facility types, but assisted deliveries of other types fell through a gap in the policy. This and the patchy implementation of the policy added to price uncertainty for users.

In Nepal, the process evaluation of the Safe Delivery Incentive Programme suggested similar themes: funding delays (mainly from the centre), difficulties communicating a complex scheme to staff and communities and poor monitoring (Powell-Jackson, Tiwari, Neupane, Morrison, & Costello, 2007).

It appears from many of these case studies that coverage is expanded too quickly, without first road-testing implementation and establishing the systems that need to be in place for effective functioning. Based on the experiences in Ghana and Senegal, a checklist has been developed, to help policy-makers to think through the necessary steps for implementing any policy addressing financial barriers (Witter et al., 2008c). This includes policy design, the policy development process, dissemination of the policy, resource allocation, payment systems, management, monitoring and evaluation.

For these policies to be sustained, an overall increase in public expenditure on health is also desirable, as the funding for the delivery care exemption should be additional, rather than being moved from some other priority area in already under-funded health systems.

Acceptability for Key Stakeholder Groups

Although the research was not able to probe in depth the original drivers of the delivery exemption policies, it appears in both case studies that the policies were perceived by technical staff within Ministries as being politically motivated. This was also the case with earlier fee abolition in Uganda (Yates, 2004b) and appears to be repeating itself now in Ghana with the Presidential announcement of free pregnancy care through the National Health Insurance Scheme (NHIS) in May 2008. This raises a number of interesting wider questions about how incentives may differ at different levels of the health and political system. Does risk aversion increase as you descend the pyramid? Are politicians and senior government figures rewarded for exciting new initiatives, while lower level public servants have to suffer if implementation does not follow rhetoric? Removal of fees, being an inherently attractive idea to the public, arguably constitutes the archetypal 'free lunch', for politicians and, apparently, the public – with health facilities and staff left at risk of paying the bill.

There has been a growing literature recently on the importance of trust as a facilitator of relationships within a health system, which can significantly reduce transactions costs (Ozawa, 2008). Trust is based largely on previous experiences. In the case of exemptions in Ghana, the previous experiences of exemptions for other services were largely negative, with facilities not receiving adequate funding from central government, and government perceiving facilities as circumventing the exemptions policies in the search for profit (Garshong, Ansah, Dakpallah, Huijts, & Adjei, 2001). In that respect, managers and health workers were sceptical from the start of the process of introducing delivery exemptions, and their expectations were fulfilled. Community responses, while positive towards the exemptions approach in principle, showed concerns with sustainability too.

In Ghana and Senegal, health workers (at least, those on the public payroll) do not derive their income directly from user fees, which should increase the acceptability of the exemptions policy for them. This may also explain the lack of provision for any payments linked to the DEP and FDCP to health workers. In the short term, and in the context of other developments (which included rising public pay levels in Ghana), this did not affect overall motivation (Witter, Kusi, & Aikins, 2007b). However, a higher dependence on fees and stagnant pay levels and increased utilisation over the medium term would pose challenges to motivation. While health workers presented themselves as altruistic in answer to motivation questions in the health worker incentives survey, their actions (a series of strikes for extra wages shortly after data collection) and other studies suggest that they are not and that minimum pay and pay for extra duties is important to motivation (Chandler, Chonya, Mtei, Reyburn, & Whitty, 2008).

Comparing Exemptions with Alternative Approaches to Reducing Financial Barriers

There is a wide range of potential strategies to address financial barriers for the poor, which should be developed in a context-specific way. It is well recognised that complex interventions, such as health financing or policy changes, do not operate in a simple cause-and-effect way, but interact with contextual factors to produce sometimes unexpected results (Penn-Kekana, McPake, & Parkhurst, 2007). Simplistic messages on which strategies are 'best' should not therefore be drawn, but we can nevertheless learn from experience on issues that frequently arise in relation to any particular mechanism (Table 7).

In addition to strategies that target financial barriers directly, there are many indirect strategies that can have highly significant effects on financial barriers. On the supply side, for example, investment that produces a reduction in distance to facilities or to trained staff can be effective in reducing access costs and increasing supervised delivery rates (Hatt et al., 2007). In China, one study found that the rural health insurance had not reduced catastrophic payments, while another concluded that supply-side measures (including the introduction of essential drug lists and treatment protocols) had been effective in reducing them (Wagstaff, 2008).

Resource reallocation to poorer areas is another supply-side measure that could reduce real prices faced by households. The distribution of public resources for health was inequitable in both case study countries, and

Table 7. Summary of Strengths and Weaknesses of Different
Mechanisms for Addressing Financial Barriers to Accessing Health Care.

Direct Strategies	Strengths	Weaknesses
Fee exemption	Universal, non-discriminatory	Official costs at facility may not be main barrier
	Low transaction costs	Tendency to under-fund exemptions programmes (relying on facilities to pick up the costs)
	Shown to increase utilisation, including for poor, though rich also benefit	
Waivers	Lower 'leakage' of benefits	Targeting problems (identifying poor)
	Can separate identification of poor and fund management from health services (e.g. Health Equity Funds)	Impact on near-poor
		Lack of protection for general population against catastrophic costs
		Stigma deters the eligible
		Tendency to under-fund
		Conflict of interest for staff (if they are identifying poor)
Formalising informal payments	Can reduce uncertainty and increase official resources	Not inherently pro-poor, unless combined with waiver or exemption scheme
Conditional cash transfers	Can empower poor clients	Tend to be targeted, so raise issues of identification and stigma (as under waivers)
	Can address non-facility costs	Complex to manage and requires high transparency
		High transaction costs (identification; administration)
Vouchers	Gives client choice (if choice is available)	Tend to be targeted, so raise issues of identification and stigma (as under waivers)
		High transaction costs
Loans	Can assist with immediate needs, including for non-facility costs such as transport	Poor not generally regarded as creditworthy
		Schemes smooth rather than reducing costs – address immediate constraints at risk of long-term indebtedness, especially for complex procedures
		Financial sustainability and scale-up are challenging

Table 7. (*Continued*)

Direct Strategies	Strengths	Weaknesses
Community health insurance	Can be subsidised to provide cover for poor and for delivery care	Financial sustainability and scale-up are challenging – often dependent on government or donor support
	Potential for greater community involvement in management	Tendency to exclude poorest (socially marginalised, etc.)
	Eligibility is assessed less frequently	Often exclude predictable costs of pregnancy, which 'self-induced' (adverse selection/ moral hazard)
	Most potential for obstetric emergencies	
Social health insurance	Can be designed to cross-subsidise the poor and delivery care	Getting cards to the poor can be problematic (depends on local networks, attitudes, etc.)
	Can have graduated premia (though this raises the question of assessing informal incomes)	Does not cover non-facility costs
	Can give stronger entitlement to poor (also longer term and potentially wider package)	Financial viability poor in context of low formal employment
		Complex to establish and manage
		Tend to increase service use by members (generally better off groups) – perverse effects

especially in Senegal, where public resources were not only biased to certain regions (e.g. Dakar) but also to the hospital sector. (Hospitals received 61% of state funding, while district services received 39%, while providing 91% of consultations.) However, in Senegal, for 1998–2002, the state provided only 34% of total resources for the health sector, with 55% coming from user fees (CEFOREP, 2003), and therefore, reallocation of official resources would only achieve a limited pro-poor effect.

In addition, there are supply-side measures that can raise utilisation of services with or without addressing financial barriers to users. In Rwanda, for example, incentive payments to health staff have been linked to a significant increase in supervised deliveries (although the payments were combined with other strategies, including extension of Community Health Insurance (CHI) and investments in the health system generally) (Logie, Rowson, & Ndagije, 2008).

In general, direct approaches that use individual targeting tend to be more complex and to incur higher running costs. Non-individually targeted ones are more suitable for areas with high poverty and access problems, though by definition these are the areas that can least afford to sustain such a scheme – hence the need for potentially long-term external support. While it might seem intuitively obvious that individual targeting focuses resources on the poor more effectively, there are important political economy arguments for universal access to services. A degree of benefit capture by better-off groups may in some circumstances be justified in terms of the social solidarity and pressure to maintain the quality of services that is generated by universal participation (Hanson, Worrall, & Wiseman, 2007).

All initiatives to reduce financial barriers to delivery, as to other, care share certain broad pre-conditions for success. On the health service side, these include the following:

- Understanding of the schemes by managers and staff
- Adequate budgeting and planning for the scheme
- Good monitoring and evaluation
- Reimbursement schemes that cover the real costs of services
- Measures in place to control supply-induced demand and inappropriate treatments (e.g. unnecessary caesareans)
- Services that are available and of acceptable quality (including Comprehensive and Basic Emergency Obstetric Care)
- Adequate staffing with appropriate skills and attitudes
- Incentives for health workers to serve in poor areas and serve the poor
- Availability of appropriate drugs, supplies and equipment
- Resource allocation systems to poor areas functioning
- Functional referral systems

On the community side, they include the following:

- Geographical access by the poor
- Cultural acceptability of services
- Gender barriers addressed
- Good dissemination of schemes to communities

The different approaches have more in common than not. All have shown the potential to increase utilisation of services, including by the poor *if well implemented*. All, if effective, have the potential to reduce delays in seeking care and reduce household indebtedness. Some however are easier to operate at scale (social insurance, exemption schemes and social transfers) than others (community health insurance and loans). Some (formalising informal payments) are complementary to all others (all schemes are undermined if informal charges continue). All should face similar costs for services, though their administrative costs will vary. More important are the funding sources (household, community, employer, donor and government), which are constrained in terms of volume and sustainability in differing ways.

Generalisability of Lessons from Delivery to Other Service-Based Exemptions

There are few comparable studies that have evaluated funded, service-based exemptions. It is therefore hard to assess how far the experience of delivery exemptions is likely to be exceptional. Deliveries certainly present some unusual features. Eighty-five percent of those who visit facilities could have delivered safely at home or with community-based support, but because of the unpredictable risk of being in the 15% who will face complications, which require skilled care, all women are encouraged to deliver in an environment where swift access to emergency care is possible. Emergency obstetric care, if it is required, is potentially life-saving, requires urgent provision and has the potential to cause catastrophic costs for a large proportion of households. Given these features, the case for public finance of emergency care is strong. One of the main arguments for subsidising access to routine delivery care is that it enables women to access emergency care as and when it is needed (Graham et al., 2001). However, these features are not unique: much health care involves facility-based triage of routine care, which can be largely managed by patients, from urgent cases, requiring intensive medical attention.

Many of the lessons learned on the implementation and effects of delivery exemptions in Ghana and Senegal are therefore likely to be shared with exemptions targeted by other services, groups, facilities or areas. However, deliveries, as a core reproductive activity, do have particular cultural significance, which increases the strength of traditional beliefs, which in turn affect uptake of services. In Ghana, for example, the qualitative research picked up local beliefs that delivering at home shows a woman's fidelity to her husband (Arhinful, Zakariah-Akoto, Madi, Mallet-Ashietey, & Armar-Klemesu, 2006). These indicate why price elasticity of demand may be lower than for other health care services. However, over time, reduced economic barriers are likely to affect beliefs and to mitigate cultural ones.

In addition, deliveries are, to some extent, self-induced. This makes exemptions more problematic: key stakeholders in both countries perceived women to be likely to take advantage of them by increasing their fertility.

This assumption can be questioned, on the grounds that the delivery cost is by no means likely to be the main factor in the decision to get pregnant. Moreover, in context of high unmet need for family planning and low gender status, the notion of women 'deciding' to get pregnant is in itself highly debatable. However, the perception does affect how the policy is viewed.

The burden of coping with payments may also be subtly different for deliveries, compared to many other health services. Evidence from Senegal suggests that women have to set aside funds to prepare for their own delivery (but that they rarely anticipate the possibility of complications). It is possible (but not investigated in depth by these studies) that the burden of paying for maternal and child health care falls more heavily on women.

Sustainability of Exemptions

As indicated in Table 5, the delivery exemptions policies absorbed a very small proportion of total health expenditure (between 0.5% and 0.7%, though this proportion would have been higher if the policy had been adequately funded in Ghana). They are therefore financially sustainable, if seen as effective tools towards a goal that has national significance. Cost-effectiveness can obviously be assessed in different ways, economic and political, and judged differently by different actors, according to their perspective. For a policy reform to last, and be embedded, requires that key stakeholders – those who influence policy decisions and resource allocation – see a positive return on the investment (technical, political and personal), and also concur with the goal. In the two case studies documented here, there were doubts about commitment to the policy from the start, which contributed to poor implementation, which in turn undermined commitment to the policy – a classic vicious circle. One factor may be that in both cases, the 'free care' approach clashed with other health financing trends – in Ghana, the development of the NHIS, and in Senegal, the encouragement of *mutuelles* at community level.

CONCLUSION

User fees offered the promise of raising income for health care, while offering exemptions for those who could not afford to pay. The first wave of experiences of exemptions policies suggested that poverty-based exemptions, using individual targeting, was not effective, for practical and political economic reasons – the poor were hard to identify and those carrying out the identification did not have incentives to do so effectively. This resulted in well-documented inequities and reduced utilisation. In response, many countries have changed their approach in recent years – while maintaining user fees as a necessary source of revenue for facilities, they are offering exemptions based on high-priority services or population groups. Common categories include young children, pregnant women and TB patients and are accompanied by recognition of the need to reimburse facilities for their lost revenues.

The Ghana and Senegal delivery exemption policies are part of a wave of similar schemes, across West Africa and other regions, in which the issue of user fees is addressed in a partial way through prioritising certain services for universal free access. Their lessons are therefore of wider international interest.

Delivery exemptions will be most appropriate in contexts where:

- Maternal mortality is high
- Fertility is high, especially in poorer households
- Poverty rates are high
- Official user fees for health care are high
- Skilled attendance rates are low, and inequalities are high
- Caesarean rates are low, and inequalities are high
- Financial barriers are a major constraint for skilled attendance (rather than poor geographical access, cultural barriers or poor quality of care within facilities)
- Gender imbalances are significant, and women lack financial autonomy or decision-making powers over health care

Unfortunately, these are also the contexts where the policy will be most costly to implement, most difficult to sustain and where substantial investments in the provision of quality care are likely to be needed. In particular, the high dependence of facilities in countries like Ghana and Senegal on revenue generated from user fees make exemptions policies hard to enforce.

Where staff benefit directly from user fees, as is the case for some staff in Senegal but not in Ghana, there is a direct personal incentive to maintain revenue flows through one means or the other. In Senegal, there was evidence that fees for other services were increased to compensate for lost delivery-related revenue. Had the funding mechanisms existed to fully reimburse facilities for lost revenue, this might not have occurred. However, the situation of partial abolition of fees (for some services), with continued charging for others, is arguably unstable, in that there will always be an incentive and opportunities for providers to capture some or all of the benefits. Evidence from Ghana suggests that partial capture did occur, although again there were mitigating circumstances (reimbursement was adequate, when funds were available, but overall funds were not adequate, particularly when the policy was scaled-up). Where fee abolition is total and clearly publicised, it is arguably harder for facilities to levy formal or informal charges (though clearly the revenue substitution burden for the public purse is much higher in this context).

The exemptions approach is consistent with the current trend towards 'output-based aid' and 'results-oriented financing'. In line with the shift towards giving greater managerial freedom to achieve defined targets, it might be preferable to adapt the payment method, so that facilities have additional subsidies built into their budgets in advance, and are then monitored for desirable outputs and outcomes. This approach does not however remove the need to audit reports, monitor quality of care and make periodic assessments of the impact on household payments.

While there has been a lot of debate over the relative merits of different targeting approaches and design of policies to reduce financial barriers to health care (maternal and general), the Ghana and Senegal evaluations suggest that the details of implementation and their interaction with contextual factors are more significant than design of the policy per se.

The evaluation evidence suggests that funded service- or group-based exemptions offer a simple, potentially effective route to mitigating inequity and inefficiency in the health systems of low-income countries. However, there are a number of key constraints. One is at health facility level, where the presence of continued charging for other services creates an opportunity for providers to absorb some or much of the exemption subsidy by increasing charges for other services or shifting costs to users. The second is the difficulty of sustaining a separate funding stream over the medium to long term, if it is not integrated with mainstream subsidies to facility running costs. The third is the arbitrary basis for selecting high-priority services for exemption, which can be based on a number of criteria, including public good characteristics, group vulnerability, the high incidence of catastrophic costs or worsening outcome indicators. (In the case of the delivery exemptions, the last three criteria were met, but many health care services could argue for similar prioritisation.) This financing mode is therefore inherently unstable and is likely to be transitional, leading to the extension of financial protection through more general risk-pooling, including wider user fee removal.

NOTE

1. A recent estimate of average skilled attendance at delivery for sub-Saharan Africa, based on analysis of the latest Demographic and Health Survey (DHS) estimates for a sample of 29 countries, was 39% (Gwatkin et al., 2007).

ACKNOWLEDGMENTS

This work was undertaken as part of an international research programme, Immpact (Initiative for Maternal Mortality Programme Assessment), funded by the Bill & Melinda Gates Foundation, Department for International Development, European Commission and USAID.

REFERENCES

Akin, J., Birdsall, N., & de Ferranti, D. (1987). *Financing health care in developing countries: An agenda for reform.* Washington, DC: World Bank.

Alam, D. A. (2007). *Maternal health voucher scheme* (Presentation to seminar on Targeting resources for health care of the poor: experiences with different financing options). Dhaka: WHO.

Arhinful, D., Zakariah-Akoto, S., Madi, B., Mallet-Ashietey, B., & Armar-Klemesu, M. (2006). *Effects of free delivery policy on provision and utilisation of skilled care at delivery: Views from providers and communities in Central and Volta regions of Ghana.* Aberdeen & Accra: Immpact.

Armar-Klemesu, M., Graham, W., Arhinful, D., Hussein, J., Asante, F., Witter, S., Deganus, S., et al. (2006). *An evaluation of Ghana's policy of universal fee exemption for delivery care.* Aberdeen & Accra: Immpact.

Asante, F., Chikwama, C., Daniels, A., & Armar-Klemesu, M. (2007). Evaluating the economic outcomes of the policy of fee exemption for maternal delivery care in Ghana. *Ghana Medical Journal, 41*(3), 110–117.

Awiti, C. (2007). *Output-based aid in Kenya: The implementer's perspective.* Presentation to Women Deliver conference, London.

Barker, C., Bird, C., Pradhan, A., & Shakya, G. (2007). Support to the safe motherhood programme in Nepal: An integrated approach. *Reproductive Health Matters, 15*(30), 81–90.

Bitran, R., & Giedion, U. (2003). *Waivers and exemptions for health services in developing countries.* Washington, DC: World Bank.

Borghi, J., Ensor, T., Neupane, B., & Tiwari, S. (2004). *Coping with the burden of the costs of maternal health.* London: DFID; Options; Nepal Safer Motherhood Project.

CEFOREP. (2003). *Evaluation finale du PDIS, 1998–2002: Rapport finale.* Dakar: MSPM.

Chandler, C., Chonya, S., Mtei, F., Reyburn, H., & Whitty, C. (2008). *What motivates public hospital clinicians in Tanzania?* London: LSHTM/Joint Malaria Programme.

Deininger, K., & Mpuga, P. (2004). *Economic and welfare effects of the abolition of health user fees: Evidence from Uganda.* Washington, DC: World Bank.

Devadasan, N., Elias, M., John, D., Grahacharya, S., & Ralte, L. (2008). A process evaluation of the Janani Suraksha Yojana in India. In: F. Richard, S. Witter & V. De Brouwere (Eds), *Financing obstetric care*. Antwerp: ITM.

DFID. (2007). *DFID's maternal health strategy. Reducing maternal deaths: Evidence and action. Second progress report*. London: DFID.

England, S., Kaddar, M., Nigam, A., & Pinto, M. (2001). *Practice and policies on user fees for immunisation in developing countries*. Geneva: World Health Organisation.

Ensor, T., Clapham, S., & Prasai, D. (2008). What drives health policy formulation? Insights from the Nepal maternity incentive scheme. *Health Policy, 90*, 247–253.

Ensor, T., & Cooper, S. (2004). Overcoming barriers to health service access: Influencing the demand side. *Health Policy and Planning, 19*(2), 69–79.

Ensor, T., & Witter, S. (2008). *Proposed revisions to the SDIP-strengthening a major national initiative for safe motherhood in Nepal*. London: Options for DFID and MoHP.

FCI. (2006). *Safe motherhood: A review. The save motherhood initiative 1987–2005*. New York: Family Care International.

Garshong, B., Ansah, E., Dakpallah, G., Huijts, I., & Adjei, S. (2001). *'We are still paying': A study on factors affecting the implementation of the exemptions policy in Ghana*. Accra: Health Research Unit, Ministry of Health.

Gilson, L. (1997). The lessons of user fee experience in Africa. *Health Policy and Planning, 12*(4), 273–285.

Gilson, L., Russell, S., & Buse, K. (1995). The political economy of user fees with targeting: Developing equitable health financing policies. *Journal of International Development, 7*(3), 369–401.

Graham, W., Bell, J., & Bullough, C. (2001). Can skilled attendance at delivery reduce maternal mortality in developing countries? In: V. De Brouwere & W. Van Lerberghe (Eds), *Sate motherhood strategies: A review of the evidence* (No. 17). Antwerp: Studies in Health Services Organisation and Policy.

Griffin, C. (1988). *User charges for health care in principle and practice*. Washington, DC: World Bank.

Gwatkin, D., Rutstein, S., Johnson, K., Suliman, E., Wagstaff, A., & Amouzou, A. (2007). *Socioeconomic differences in health, nutrition and population in developing countries: An overview*. Washington, DC: World Bank.

Hanson, K., Worrall, E., & Wiseman, V. (2007). Targeting services towards the poor: A review of targeting mechanisms and their effectiveness: from understanding to action. In: S. Bennett, L. Gilson & A. Mills (Eds), *Health, economic development and household poverty*. London: Routledge.

Harris, A., Gao, Y., Barclay, L., Belton, S., Yue, Z., Min, H., Aiqun, X., Hua, L., & Yun, Z. (2007). Consequences of birth policies and practices in post-reform China. *Reproductive Health Matters, 15*(30), 114–124.

Hatt, L., Stanton, C., Makowiecka, K., Adisasmita, A., Achadi, E., & Ronsmans, C. (2007). Did the strategy of skilled attendance at birth reach the poor in Indonesia? *WHO Bulletin, 85*(10), 733–820.

Hotchkiss, D. (1993). *The role of quality in the demand for health care on Cebu Island province, The Philippines* (Health Financing and Sustainability Project (HFS)). Bethesda, MD: Abt Associates.

ICH & SSMP. (2006). *Maternal health cost-sharing scheme in Nepal: Evaluation protocol*. London: ICH.

Immpact. (2005). *An evaluation of the policy of universal fee exemption for delivery care: Ghana operational protocol.* Aberdeen & Accra: Immpact.

Leighton, C. (2000). *How to pay for skilled attendance at delivery: Costs of intervention and financing schemes.* New York: Safe Motherhood Inter-Agency Group/Family Care International.

Li, M. (1996). *The demand for medical care: Evidence from urban areas in Bolivia.* Washington, DC: World Bank.

Logie, D., Rowson, M., & Ndagije, F. (2008). Innovations in Rwanda's health system: Looking to the future. *The Lancet,* July 10, 2008. DOI: 10.1016/S0140-6736(08)60962-9.

Marchal, B., Arcens, M., Coates, A., & De Brouwere, V. (2007). An institutional analysis of the safe motherhood policymaking process in Burkina Faso. Submitted for publication.

Ministry of Health. (2004a). *Guidelines for implementing the exemption policy on maternal deliveries* (MoH/Policy, Planning, Monitoring and Evaluation-59). Accra: Ministry of Health.

Ministry of Health. (2004b). *Road map for accelerating the attainment of the MDGs related to maternal and newborn health in Nigeria.* Abuja: Ministry of Health.

Ministry of Health and Family Welfare. (2001). *Bangladesh national strategy for maternal health.* Dhaka: MoHFW.

MSPM, Immpact, UNFPA, & CEFOREP. (2006). *An evaluation of the policy of fee exemption for deliveries and caesareans in Senegal: Operational protocol.* Aberdeen: Immpact.

MSPM & U. I. C. (2007). *Evaluation des strategies de reduction des barrieres economiques, socioculturelles, sanitaires et institutionnelles a l'acces aux soins obstetricaux et neonataux au Senegal.* Dakar: MSPM, FUNUAP, Immpact, CEFOREP.

Nabyongo, J., Karamagi, H., Atuyambe, L., Bagenda, F., Okuonzi, S., & Walker, O. (2008). Maintaining quality of health services after abolition of user fees: A Uganda case study. *BMC Health Services Research,* 8(102). Available at http://www.biomedcentral.com/1472-6963/8/102.

Ndiaye, S., & Ayad, M. (2006). *Enquête Démographique et de Santé au Sénégal 2005.* Maryland, MD: Centre de Recherche pour le Développement Humain & ORC Macro.

Noirhomme, M., Meessen, B., Griffiths, F., Ir, P., Jacobs, B., Thor, R., Criel, B., & Van Damme, W. (2007). Improving access to hospital care for the poor: Comparative analysis of four health equity funds in Cambodia. *Health Policy and Planning,* 22, 246–262.

Nonay, C. (2007). Designing output-based aid projects in the health sector. Women Delivery conference presentation.

Owino, W., & Were, M. (1999). *Enhancing access to health care among vulnerable groups: The questions of waivers and exemptions* (Discussion Paper no. 14/99). Nairobi: Institute of Policy Analysis and Research.

Ozawa, S. (2008). *The role of trust in health care settings: Does trust matter?* Oxford: OPI.

Penfold, S., Harrison, E., & Bell, J. (2006). *Evaluation of the free delivery policy in Ghana: Population estimates of changes in delivery service utilisation.* Aberdeen & Accra: Immpact.

Penfold, S., Harrison, E., Bell, J., & Fitzmaurice, A. (2007). Evaluation of the delivery-fee-exemption policy in Ghana: Population estimates of changes in delivery service utilisation in two regions. *Ghana Medical Journal,* 41(3), 100–109.

Penn-Kekana, L., McPake, B., & Parkhurst, J. (2007). Improving maternal health: Getting what works to happen. *Reproductive Health Matters,* 15(30), 28–37.

Powell-Jackson, T., Neupane, B., Tiwari, S., Morrison, J., & Costello, A. (2008). *Final report of the evaluation of the safe delivery incentive programme.* London: DFID.

Powell-Jackson, T., Tiwari, S., Neupane, B., Morrison, J., & Costello, A. (2007). *Evaluation of the maternity incentive scheme: Report of the process evaluation.* Kathmandu, Nepal: SSMP.

Rannan-Eliya, R., & Somanathan, A. (2005). *Access of the very poor to health services in Asia: Evidence on the role of health systems from Equitap.* London: DFID.

Ridde, V., Moha, M., Tourigny, C., & Rauland, C. (2008). *The abolition of user fees increases women's health care utilisation in Niger.* Unpublished manuscript.

Save the Children (UK). (2008). *Freeing up healthcare: A guide to removing fees.* London: Save the Children (UK).

Storeng, K., Baggaley, R., Ganaba, R., Ouattara, F., Akoum, M., & Filippi, V. (2007). Paying the price: The cost and consequences of emergency obstetric care in Burkina Faso. *Social Science & Medicine, 66*(3), 545–557.

Tien, M., & Chee, G. (2002). *Literature review and findings: Implementation of waiver policy.* Bethesda, MD: Abt for PHRplus.

Von Both, C., Jahn, A., & Flessa, S. (2007). Costing maternal health services in South Tanzania: A case study from Mtwara Urban District. *The European Journal of Health Economics, 9*(2), 103–115.

Wagstaff, A. (2008). *Measuring financial protection in health.* Washington, DC: World Bank.

WAHO. (2004). *WAHO strategy for the reduction of maternal and perinatal mortality in West Africa 2004–8.* Bobo, Burkina Faso: WAHO.

WHO-AFRO (2004). WHO says that maternal mortality is a 'silent emergency'. http:// www.afro.who.int/press/2004/pr2004100502.html

Willis, C., & Leighton, C. (1995). Protecting the poor under cost-recovery: The role of means testing. *Health Policy and Planning, 10*(3), 241–256.

Witter, S., & Adjei, S. (2007). Start-stop funding, its causes and consequences: A case study of the delivery exemptions policy in Ghana. *International Journal of Health Planning and Management, 22*(2), 133–143.

Witter, S., Arhinful, D., Kusi, A., & Zakariah-Akoto, S. (2007a). The experience of Ghana in implementing a user fee exemption policy to provide free delivery care. *Reproductive Health Matters, 15*(30), 1–11.

Witter, S., Armar-Klemesu, M., & Dieng, T. (2008a). National fee exemption schemes for deliveries: Comparing the recent experiences of Ghana and Senegal. In: F. Richard, S. Witter & V. De Brouwere (Eds), *Financing obstetric care.* Antwerp: ITM.

Witter, S., Dieng, T., Mbengue, D., Moreira, I., & De Brouwere, V. (2008b). The free delivery and caesarean policy in Senegal – how effective and cost-effective has it been? Submitted for publication.

Witter, S., Kusi, A., & Aikins, M. (2007b). Working practices and incomes of health workers: Evidence from an evaluation of a delivery fee exemption scheme in Ghana. *Human Resources for Health, 5*(2).

Witter, S., Richard, F., & De Brouwere, V. (2008c). Learning lessons and moving forward: How to reduce financial barriers to obstetric care in low-income contexts. *Studies in Health Services Organisation and Policy, 24*, 277–304.

Yates, R. (2004a). *Should African governments scrap user fees for health services?* Pretoria: DFID.

Yates, R. (2004b). The Ugandan health SWAP: Improving efficiency and equity. Presentation to World Bank, Washington, DC.

SECTION V
THE UNIVERSAL INTEGRATED
HEALTHCARE SYSTEM

FROM SCHEME TO SYSTEM: SOCIAL HEALTH INSURANCE FUNDS AND THE TRANSFORMATION OF HEALTH FINANCING IN KYRGYZSTAN AND MOLDOVA

Joseph Kutzin, Melitta Jakab and Sergey Shishkin

ABSTRACT

Objective – *The aim of the paper is to bring evidence and lessons from two low- and middle-income countries (LMIs) of the former USSR into the global debate on health financing in poor countries. In particular, we analyze the introduction of social health insurance (SHI) in Kyrgyzstan and Moldova. To some extent, the intent of SHI introduction in these countries was similar to that in LMIs elsewhere: increase prepaid revenues for health and incorporate the entire population into the new system. But the approach taken to universality was different. In particular, the SHI fund in each country was used as the key instrument in a comprehensive reform of the health financing system, with the new revenues from payroll taxation used in an explicitly complementary manner to general budget revenues. From a functional perspective, the reforms in these countries*

Innovations in Health System Finance in Developing and Transitional Economies
Advances in Health Economics and Health Services Research, Volume 21, 291–312
ISSN: 0731-2199/doi:10.1108/S0731-2199(2009)0000021014

involved not only the introduction of a new source of funds, but also the centralization of pooling, a shift from input- to output-based provider payment methods, specification of a benefit package, and greater autonomy for public sector health care providers. Hence, their reforms were not simply the introduction of an SHI scheme, but rather the use of an SHI fund as an instrument to transform the entire system of health financing.

Methodology/approach – The study uses administrative and household data to demonstrate the impact of the reforms on regional inequality and household financial burden.

Findings – The approach used in these two countries led to improved equity in the geographic distribution of government health spending, improved financial protection, and reduced informal payments.

Implications for policy – The comprehensive approach taken to reform in these two countries, and particularly the redirection of general budget revenues to the new SHI funds, explain much of the success that was achieved. This experience offers potentially useful lessons for LMIs elsewhere in the world, and for shifting the global debate away from what we see as a false dichotomy between SHI and general revenue-funded systems. By demonstrating that sources are not systems, these cases illustrate how, in particular by careful design of pooling and coverage arrangements, the introduction of SHI in an LMI context can avoid the fragmentation problem often associated with this reform instrument.

INTRODUCTION

The experience of reforms in the countries that emerged following the end of the USSR (the so-called Newly Independent States, or NIS) is not yet part of the mainstream literature on health financing reforms in low- and middle-income (LMIs) countries. This chapter is an attempt to bridge this gap, focusing on reforms in two countries, Kyrgyzstan and Moldova, that are currently classified by the World Bank as low-income and lower middle-income countries, respectively (see Table 1 for some summary data on the two countries; World Bank, 2008). In many ways, these two countries have characteristics similar to LMIs in other parts of the world: relatively low levels of formal sector employment, high poverty rates, and fiscal challenges that limit the scope for public spending on health. However, there are also important differences arising from the particular historical legacies of the

Table 1. Basic Indicators on Kyrgyzstan and Moldova.

	Kyrgyzstan	Moldova
Population (2007)	5,242,827	3,792,142
Gross National Income per capita, current international $$$ (2007)	1,950	2,930
Poverty headcount ratio at national poverty line (% of population) (2005) (%)	43	29
Primary school completion rate (2006) (%)	99	98
Life expectancy at birth (2006)	68	69
U5MR (2006)	41	19

Source: World Development Indicators.

Soviet health system. In particular, both countries inherited very high ratios of health human resources and physical infrastructure per capita. Related to this, a major difference with most LMIs elsewhere in the world is that the "starting point" of their health systems in 1990 was publicly funded universal coverage that existed in reality as well as legally. The economic transition period, particularly in the first decade of independence, led to a reduction of public funding, and health systems became heavily dependent on direct payments by patients. This led to a deterioration of real coverage and an increase in regional and inter-personal inequalities (Jakab & Manjieva, 2007) Hence, a major focus of health financing reforms was to re-establish previously high levels of coverage and improve regional and inter-personal equity, concepts that were not so far from people's memories and expectations.

Compulsory social health insurance (SHI) has been widely advocated as an approach for LMI countries to improve coverage and equity (refer, e.g., Shaw & Griffin, 1995). Experience to date from countries in Africa, Asia, and Latin America with large informal economies suggests, however, that the usual manner by which this has been implemented, that is, starting with the formal sector due to ease of contribution collection and registration and then hoping for coverage expansion to the rest of the population, can actually be harmful for equity. The reason for this is that formal sector tends to be relatively well-off, and "creating health insurance" for this group typically means extending more explicit coverage to those who already have better access and financial protection than the rest of the population. Hopes that SHI would "free up" public resources for the poor have largely not been realized, nor have good intentions to gradually extend coverage by such schemes to the rest of the population. Instead, the initially covered groups advocate for greater benefits and lower contributions and through their organization and political influence are able to capture an even greater share of public subsidies (Kutzin, 1997; Gertler & Solon, 2000; González Rossetti, 2002; Lloyd-Sherlock, 2006). The result has been segmentation: the presence of an "SHI system" and a "Ministry of Health (MOH) system" in the same country, duplicating functional responsibilities and exacerbating underlying social inequalities (Londoño & Frenk, 1997). The segmented systems typically exhibit great inequalities in the level of per capita funding (and hence benefits and quality) available from these different systems.

In this chapter, we review the reforms that established compulsory SHI funds in Kyrgyzstan and Moldova. In each case, and unlike the experience of many LMIs elsewhere in the world, the reforms led to a reduction of fragmentation in the financing system and to demonstrable improvements in various measures of equity. We conclude that neither the problem nor the solution is SHI per se, but rather the manner in which reform is designed and implemented. Essential success factors for the reforms in these two countries were (a) the design of universality and equity into the system from the start, made possible by transforming the role and flow of general budget revenues in the system; (b) the elimination of fragmentation in pooling by centralizing formerly decentralized budget flows; and (c) the establishment and strengthening of a single SHI fund as the change agent for the system, enabling it to be an active purchaser of services on behalf of the entire population from its national pool. The reforms were designed to transform the entire health financing system and serve the entire population, rather than to simply create an insurance scheme. Although the specific lessons from these examples are illustrative for other NIS countries and possibly also for LMIs in other regions as well, the critical general lesson is the importance of taking a system-based rather than a scheme-based approach to health financing reform.

TRANSITION AND THE INHERITED HEALTH SYSTEM

As with most of the countries of the ex-USSR, Kyrgyzstan and Moldova suffered extreme fiscal contraction in the first half of the 1990s. By 1995, total public revenue as a share of gross domestic product (GDP) fell to 15% and 20%, respectively, from an estimated 41% in the USSR in 1989 (Cheasty, 1996). This had severe negative consequences for the ability of the government to spend on health, especially in the context of a GDP that was also contracting. It is estimated that by the mid-1990s, the real level of annual government health spending in both countries had fallen to less than half its 1990 level (Davis, forthcoming). While health care was still ostensibly free of charge for the population, early household surveys confirmed what had become apparent to both providers and patients alike: informal out-of-pocket payments had become a substantial barrier to care and a great financial burden for households that chose to seek care. Constitutional or other legal guarantees of access to care still existed, but only on paper.

Behind this was not only the fall in public spending but also the rising costs of the inherited health system. The Soviet health system was characterized by heavy reliance on physical infrastructure and specialization (Davis, forthcoming). It was possible to sustain this in the former context of high public revenues and subsidized prices for inputs such as medicines and energy. In the 1990s, however, the decline in government revenues and the increase in prices made the large infrastructure unsustainable: a large share of public spending on health was devoted to fixed costs, leaving very little to pay for treatment inputs such as medicines and supplies. In 2000, for example, over 21% of state budget health spending in Kyrgyzstan was spent on utility costs (Kutzin, 2003), while in Moldova, these expenses absorbed 27% of health spending in 2001 (World Bank, 2003). This reflected a health financing system characterized by incentives designed to meet the "needs" of the physical infrastructure (e.g., budgeting according to the number of hospital beds), rather than to the needs of the population. More specifically, the Soviet health (and health financing) system was fragmented, with each level of government funding and managing its own decentralized health system. Excess capacity was particularly marked in urban centers, where both city and provincial (*oblast*) facilities existed. As a result, health expenditures were also concentrated in urban centers.

With both the decline in public revenues and changes in relative input prices, the consequences of these structural inefficiencies became apparent, as did geographic inequities in state budget health spending and inter-personal inequities in access and financial burden arising from the growing dependence of systems on out-of-pocket payments. The changed context motivated the reform agenda in many countries, as did the political desire to move away from the "budgetary system" inherited from the past. Five of the 12 NIS countries introduced some form of "mandatory health insurance,"[1] beginning with Russia in 1993, Georgia in 1995, Kazakhstan in 1996, Kyrgyzstan in 1997, and Moldova in 2004. Only in Kyrgyzstan and Moldova did this reform lead to demonstrable positive achievements.

SHI AND HEALTH FINANCING REFORM IN KYRGYZSTAN: STEP-BY-STEP DEVELOPMENT

Beginning in 1997, Kyrgyzstan implemented profound changes to the inherited health financing system. In retrospect, three distinct phases of reform can be distinguished:

- *Phase 1 (1997–2000)*: introduction of the Mandatory Health Insurance Fund (MHIF) as a complementary funding source and development of its skills and systems as a purchaser.
- *Phase 2 (2001–2005)*: initiation and nationwide extension of the *Single Payer* reform, organized at oblast level.
- *Phase 3 (2006 to present)*: operation of the Single Payer system at national level (centralization from oblast to national level pooling).

Phase 1 (1997–2000): Establishment and Functioning of the MHIF

The MHIF was introduced in 1997. Defined covered persons were employees for whom employers a 2% payroll tax collected by a multi-purpose Social Fund (which also collected for pensions and other social benefits), pensioners funded by transfers from the pension fund, and registered unemployed persons funded by transfers from the unemployment fund. Self-employed persons were also supposed to contribute and join, but very few did. From 1997–1999, population coverage was about 30%, with almost two-third of these formal sector workers, almost one-third pensioners, and a small percentage of officially registered unemployed persons. In 2000, coverage was expanded greatly (to about 70% of the total population) by a decision to include all children under 16, funded by a transfer to the MHIF by the central state "Republican" budget (Kutzin et al., 2002).

An early and important decision made by the MHIF was not to try and provide a full package of benefits for its covered population, but rather to "top up" the revenues of the existing budget-funded health care facilities. The main reason was the low level of revenues generated: the 2% payroll tax was low to begin with and was applied to a small population base, and there was a pattern of arrears built up in transfers to the MHIF from the Social Fund of the health insurance payroll tax and the revenues on behalf of pensioners and the unemployed. By 1999, MHIF revenues constituted only about 8% of total government health spending, 14% of government spending on public hospitals, and about 25% of public spending on primary care providers. Even with the Republican budget transfers for children that began the following year, the MHIF accounted for only 10% of public spending on health in 2000 (Kutzin, 2003).

The other reason, ultimately more important for the development of the Kyrgyz health financing system, was a political decision based on the belief that Kyrgyzstan was a poor country and could not afford to have two health systems. Development of the MHIF was closely coordinated with the MOH (indeed, it was brought under the governance structure of the MOH during this period), including the introduction of a single hospital information system to support the new case-based payment mechanisms introduced by the MHIF but applied to all hospital cases. This decision was an important technical step in laying the foundation for transition to a universal health financing system.

During this first phase of health financing reform, the organization of health financing functions can be summarized as shown in Fig. 1. The underlying fragmented structure of the system remained unchanged: rayon

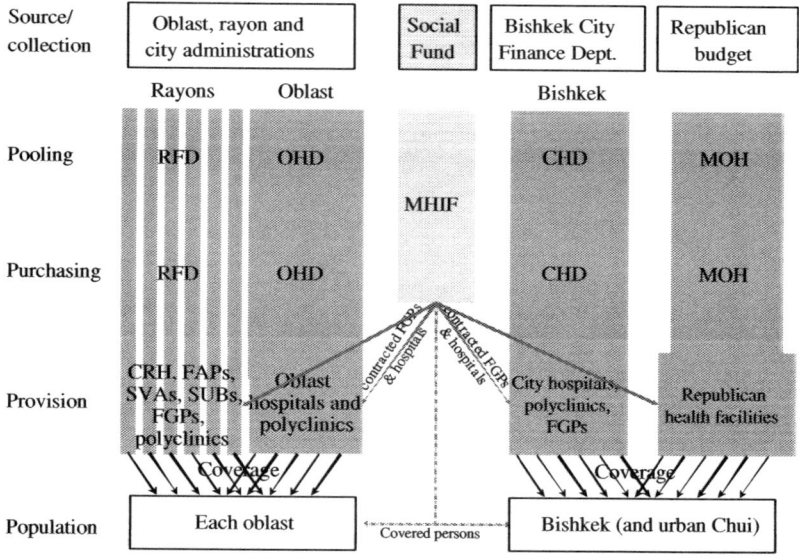

Fig. 1. Organization of Health Financing during the First Phase of Reform, 1997–2000. *Notes:* CHD, Bishkek City Health Department; CRH, Central Rayon Hospital; FAP, feldsher and midwife post; FGP, Family Group Practice (new entity for primary care introduced during this period); OHD, Oblast Health Department; RFD, Rayon Finance Department; SUB, rural hospital; SVA, rural primary care center.

(district), city, oblast, and Republican budgets funded rayon, city, oblast, and Republican health facilities in a vertically integrated manner via line item budgets. The presence of the MHIF did nothing to resolve this, but it introduced an aspect of purchaser–provider split in the system as well as population-based payment for primary care (capitation) and output-based payment for inpatient care (a case-based system that has evolved over time). Unlike the decentralized state budget structure, the MHIF operated a national pool of funds. This enabled it to promote a degree of redistribution from richer to poorer parts of the country, as shown in Fig. 2.

As shown in Fig. 2, per capita premium collections are highest in the capital, Bishkek, the richest part of the country with the largest share of the population in formal sector employment. Expenditure patterns by the MHIF mainly reflect the distribution of the insured population. Because, in 2000, well over half of the insured population were non-contributors (children under 16 and the elderly), and because the provider payment methods used by the Fund were related to population and service use, these expenditures are more evenly distributed across the country. The combination of the MHIF national pool, output-based payment, and a large share of beneficiaries who are non-contributors enabled substantial redistribution from the richer to the poorer parts of the country. The low level of MHIF expenditure in the remote Batken region in 2000 occurred because the Fund had not contracted as yet with many primary care providers in that region as yet. This problem was rectified in following years.

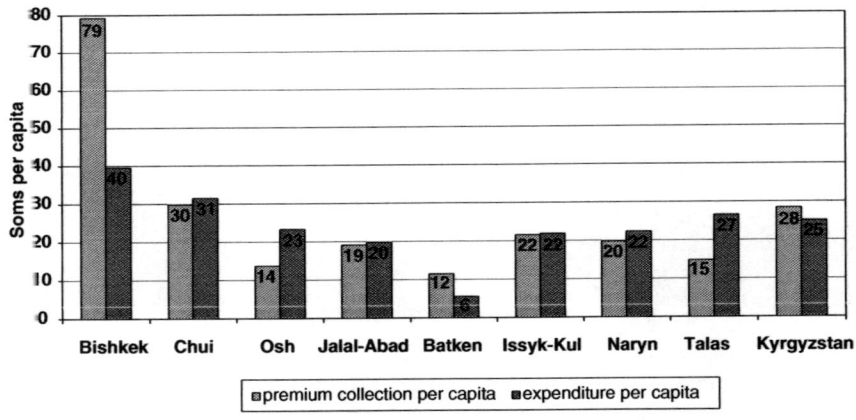

Fig. 2. MHIF Premium Collections and Expenditures by Oblast, 2000. *Source: MHIF data.*

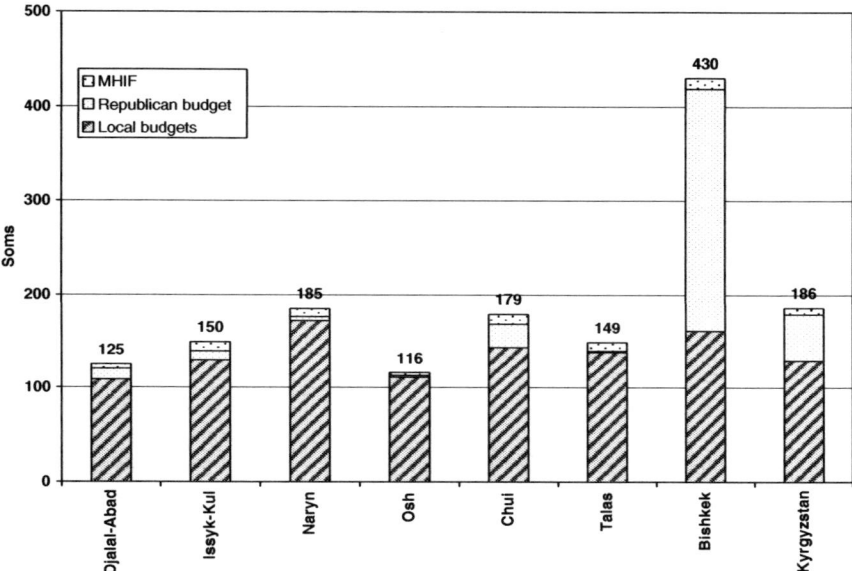

Fig. 3. Regional Distribution of Per Capita Public Spending on Health by Source, 1998. *Source*: Adapted from Kutzin (2001).

While the redistribution that occurred within the MHIF *scheme* was significant, the impact at the population level was minimal because the MHIF was only responsible for a relatively small share of public spending on health during this period. This is reflected in Fig. 3, which shows the distribution of overall government health spending by oblast.[2] Hence, while the pooling arrangements and purchasing methods used by the MHIF were effective for promoting redistribution, its equalizing effect did not have a major impact on overall resource allocation patterns in this early phase. This period was nonetheless critical for the MHIF, as it had a four years to develop its purchasing methods, information systems, and human capacity that set the stage for the next phase of reform.

Phase 2 (2001–20005): Oblast-Level Single Payer System

In 2000, the government took a decision to eliminate the oblast level of many ministries, including health. The Minister of Health responded by requesting the government to take the budget funds provided for health by local governments and put them in the oblast departments of the Health Insurance Fund. This meant that the MHIF would now manage the budget revenues for the entire population (through its oblast departments) in addition to the national pool for the insured population. Working closely together, the MoH and MHIF made plans to transform the health system by not only having the MHIF administer budget funds but also to pay providers from these funds according to the same methods it used for the insured. The existence of the unified hospital information system enabled the MHIF to simulate what each hospital would earn under the full implementation of the new system, and they then worked with the hospitals to implement downsizing plans so that they could live within these budgets. Key features of the system were the following:

- Universal coverage funded from local budget (rayon, city, and oblast) revenues with entitlement based on citizenship/residence; the contributory "SHI" benefit was complementary (rather than an alternative) to this.
- Local budget funds no longer flowed directly to the health care facilities of each local government, but instead were pooled in the oblast department of the MHIF; the MHIF pool for the insured remained national.
- From both pools, the MHIF paid providers on the basis of outputs (e.g., case-based payment) and needs (e.g., capitation), and therefore, from the provider's perspective, there was only one purchaser.
- A "state guaranteed benefit package" (SGBP) was defined, including universal free primary care and referral care with co-payment. The level of co-payment was linked to a patient's insurance and exemption status (insured pay less than uninsured). The benefit of being insured was entitlement to reduced co-payments and an additional outpatient drug benefit.
- Greater autonomy was given to providers with regard to their internal resource allocation decisions (relaxation of strict line item budget controls).
- While out-of-pocket payment became explicit with the co-payment, the reform did not involve any change in the sources of funds.

The Single Payer reform was introduced in two oblasts in 2001, two more the following year, and reached nationwide coverage during 2004. The organization of health financing functions under the oblast-level Single Payer system is shown in Fig. 4. A comparison of this to Fig. 1 reveals how this re-organization of functional arrangements addressed many of the underlying problems in the health system. The pooling of budget funds at oblast level completely eliminated the fragmentation and overlap that had

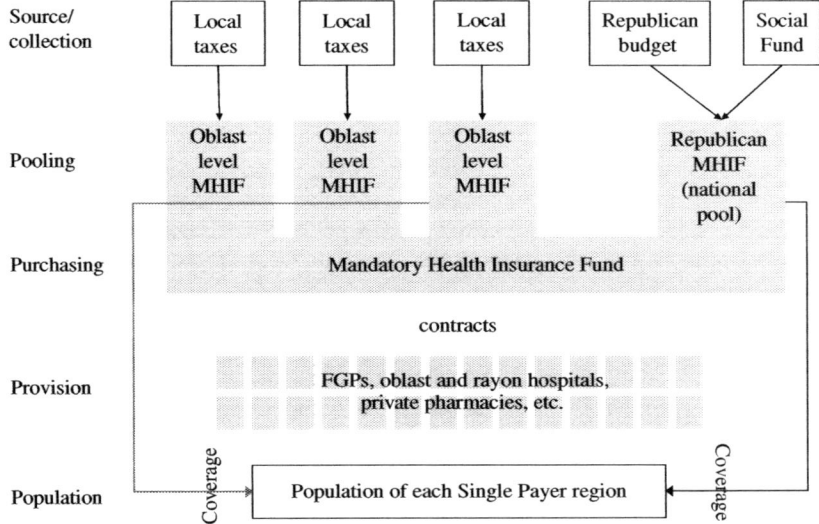

Fig. 4. Oblast-Level Single Payer System, 2001–2005.

existed *within* oblasts. The purchaser–provider split and change in payment methods shifted the incentives so that providers, particularly at hospital level, were now interested to increase productivity and reduce fixed costs. Even though the sources of funds remained the same, the role of the MHIF was transformed, and it became the key instrument for driving change in the system.

Numerous gains from the oblast Single Payer reform have been documented. In the first year of implementation, the number of hospital buildings in the two reforming regions was reduced by over 30%, and the share of public revenues devoted to patient treatment inputs (drugs, supplies, and food) in hospitals doubled. Extensive quantitative (Jakab, 2007; Jakab et al., 2005; Kutzin, 2003) and qualitative (Schüth, 2001) research shows that the reforms also were largely successful in replacing informal payments with formal co-payments and reducing patient financial burden, particularly for medicines and medical supplies, despite the fact that the total level of public spending on health did not increase very much over this period. Household survey data also show that equity in utilization improved: the richest 20% of the population used outpatient care 2.5 times more than the poorest 20% in 2000, but this fell to about 2.0 times as much in 2003. Similarly, the ratio of rich:poor utilization of inpatient care fell from 1.75 to 1.25 during the same period. The system was still inequitable, but the Single Payer reform was associated with a reduction in this inequity (Jakab et al., 2005).

Phase 3 (2006 to present): National Pooling Under the Single Payer

The third phase of financing reform began in 2006 with the pooling of all public revenues for health care at the national level. The impetus for this change originated not in the health sector but in a wider public finance reform that decentralized public financing for many public services to the level of elected self-government. For health financing, this meant either organizing the system at the level of over 400 villages plus 2 large municipalities or centralizing it to the national (Republican) level. After some political debates, health financing was further centralized rather than decentralized.

Pooling of funds at the Republican level allowed the MHIF to initiate the process of equalizing allocations for the SGBP by oblast. To ensure that the centralization and equalization process will not raise opposition from Bishkek city, the government did not reduce allocations there, but rather used incremental funds to increase funding in previously under-funded areas. This became possible as funding trends began to reverse in 2006 with a strong government commitment to increase health expenditures over the next five years and the introduction of budget support by five donors in the health sector under a Sector-Wide Approach. The resulting increase in fiscal space was used by the MHIF to increase funding in previously under-funded oblasts outside of the capital city.

The impact of centralizing pooling at the Republican level was immediate. Fig. 5 shows government health spending per capita[3] by oblast in 2005 and in 2006 relative to Bishkek. The funding gap between Bishkek and other oblasts reduced in all cases with the exception of one. In Naryn oblast, one of the poorest and geographically most challenging due to its mountainous terrain, per capita expenditures even exceeded that of Bishkek. Single financing standards formed the basis for the allocation of funds across regions, and they were adjusted through new coefficients to account for the differences in geographic and demographic characteristics of each region. This approach leads to variance in per capita expenditures by oblast, but this variance, unlike the one that existed before 2006, is expected to reflect real differences in relative need and the cost of delivering services.

The results also appear to have translated into equity gains at the individual level. As shown in Fig. 6, equity in the burden of out-of-pocket

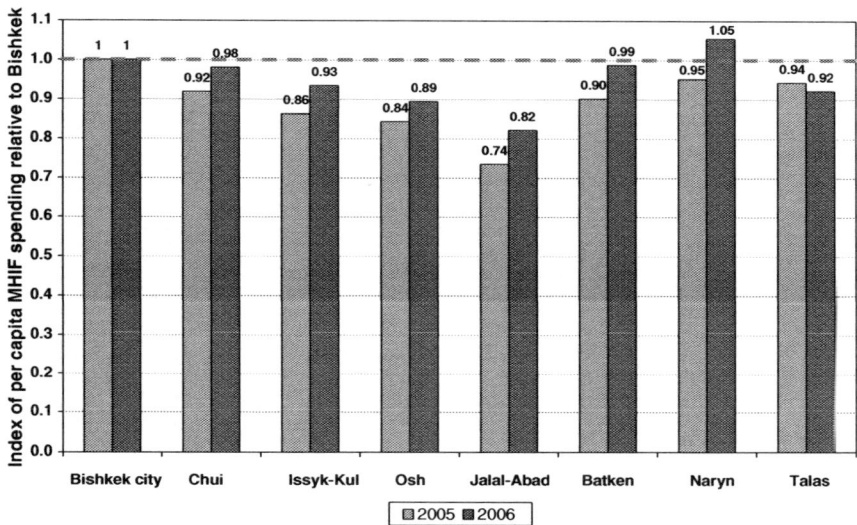

Fig. 5. Index of Per Capita Public Spending for the SGBP Relative to Bishkek.
Sources: MOH Financial Management Reports on execution of the State
Guaranteed Benefit Package and 2007 MOH Performance Indicator Report.

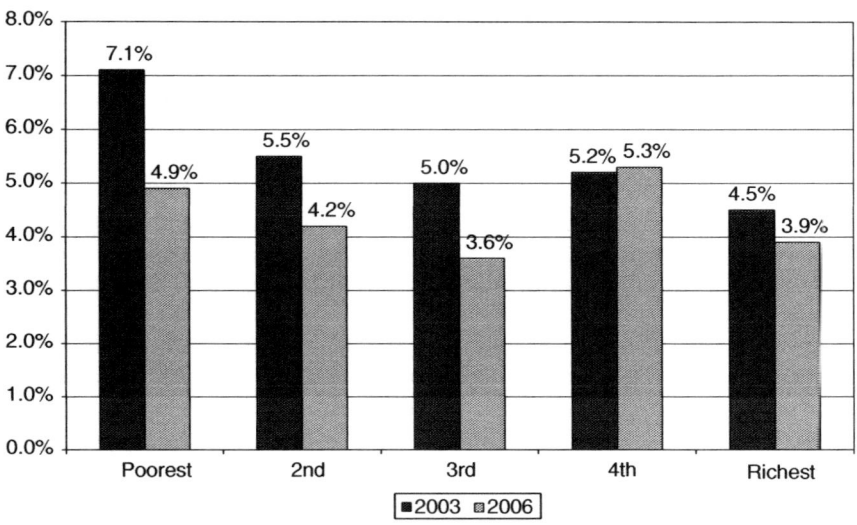

Fig. 6. Mean Out-of-Pocket Payment for Health Care as Share of Total Household
Consumption. *Sources:* National Statistical Committee, Center for Health Systems
Development, and Falkingham et al. (2007), based on the Kyrgyz Integrated
Household Survey – Health Module 2004, 2007, reported in MOH 2008.

payments improved substantially in 2006 as compared to 2003. The conclusion that the centralization reform was pro-poor is strengthened by the evidence that the utilization of services also became more equitable during this period (Falkingham, Akkazieva, & Baschieri, 2007).

SHI IN MOLDOVA: BIG BANG REFORM

Although health financing reform in Moldova was planned for several years, implementation went nationwide in 2004 following a half-year pilot in one rayon. Before this, the financing system was decentralized, with most funding and service delivery organized at rayon level, except in the large cities where there was overlapping financing and service coverage provided by different levels of government. Before reform, the system exhibited many of the inefficiencies and inequities that also existed in Kyrgyzstan. In particular, although the wider public finance system included inter-governmental transfers meant to equalize local budgets, this was not sufficient to ensure equitable funding of health care and preserved historically established disproportions. The difference between the rayons with the highest and lowest level of per capita health budget funding in 2003 was 4.6 times or 2.9 times excluding the two largest cities in the country (Shishkin, Kacevicius, & Ciocanu, 2008).

Moldova's 2004 reform addressed directly the fragmentation inherent in the previous system. A new organization, the National Health Insurance Company (NHIC), was established as the pooling and purchasing entity for health care. The financial role of rayons was eliminated as budgetary responsibility was shifted to the central government: rayons were responsible for 64% of government spending in 2003 but accounted for only 5% in 2004. The former local government health budgets were centralized and redirected to the NHIC for defined groups of the population and pooled with the revenues from the new 4% payroll tax for health insurance. Perhaps unique in a system in which entitlement is linked solely to contribution, roughly two-thirds of NHIC revenues came from budget transfers in 2004, with only about one-third coming from the payroll tax (Shishkin et al., 2008).

While the centralized system has some similarities to the post-2006 Single Payer system in Kyrgyzstan, there are also important differences. Despite the non-traditional mix of funding sources for SHI, entitlement is based on contribution, whether that contribution is made by the insured person or by the state budget on behalf of groups that are insured by statute.[4] This fundamental shift in the nature of entitlement (from the former residence/citizenship basis) created an explicitly uninsured population. This group is comprised principally of self-employed persons in agriculture, services and small commerce, and the informal sector. It is estimated that only about 7.5% of persons in these groups paid their contributions and that approximately 30% of Moldovan citizens and 13% of those living permanently in the country were uninsured in 2005 (Shishkin et al., 2008). As a result, Moldova does have the problem that confronts most LMIs that opt for SHI implementation: how to expand coverage. However, and unlike most LMIs elsewhere, the coverage of most non-contributing groups from general budget transfers has left Moldova with a relatively small percentage of the population that lacks formal[5] coverage.

The organization of the financing system following the reform is shown in Fig. 7. It is a single national pool of funds, whereas the Kyrgyz system effectively has two pools managed by the MHIF – one for the universal entitlement and the other for the additional contributory benefit on behalf of the insured population.

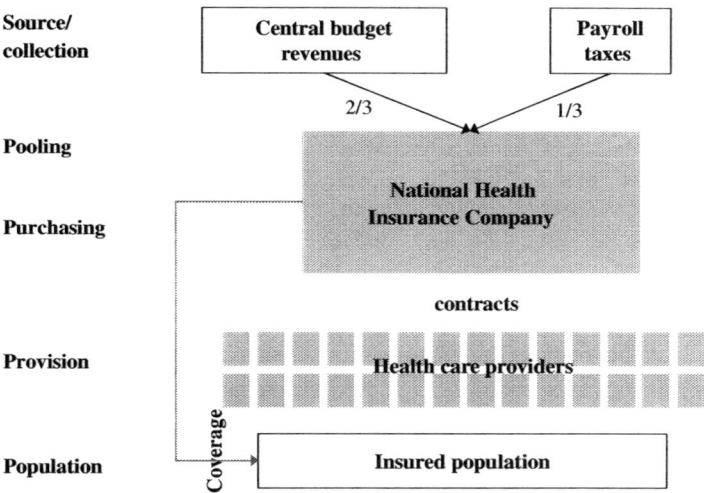

Fig. 7. Health Care Financing System in Moldova after 2004 Reform. *Note:* Self-employed persons are also meant to make contributions, but relatively few comply, and the share of NHIC funding coming from this source was less than 1% in 2004 and 2005 (Shishkin et al., 2008).

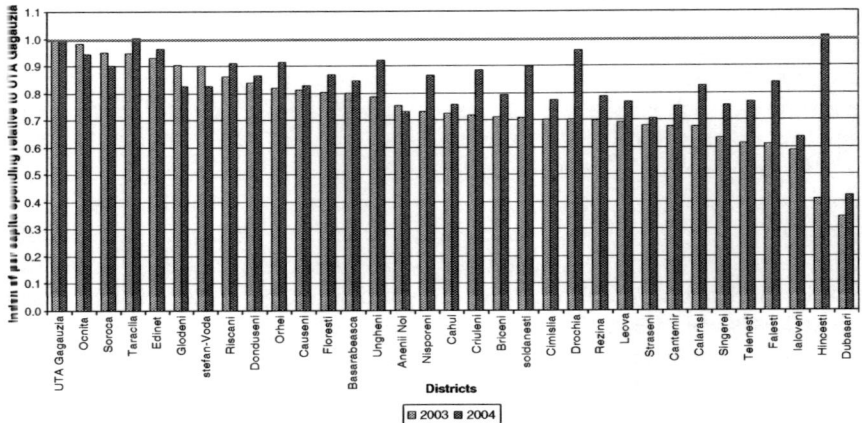

Fig. 8. Equalizing Effect of 2004 Centralization of Pooling in Moldova. *Source:* Shishkin et al. (2008). The data for 2003 reflect local budget spending per capita for each rayon, whereas for 2004, the data show per capita spending by rayon by the NHIC.

As in Kyrgyzstan, the centralization of pooling, combined with a shift from input- to output-based purchasing methods, led to improved geographic equity in government health spending per capita. This is shown in Fig. 8, which demonstrates that the variation in spending across rayons was greatly reduced in 2004 as compared to 2003.

Household survey data also suggest that equity in financing was enhanced at the individual level. The financial burden of out-of-pocket health care expenditures decreased for almost all income groups of households in 2004 (Fig. 9), and only the richest group spent sufficiently more. However, some of the reduction in financial burden for the poor may be associated with a decline in utilization experienced by the rural poor (MET, 2004).

POLICY RELEVANCE OF THESE REFORM EXPERIENCES

While reforms and their effects are always context-specific, the Kyrgyz and Moldovan cases do suggest some interesting messages for policy makers in other LMIs.

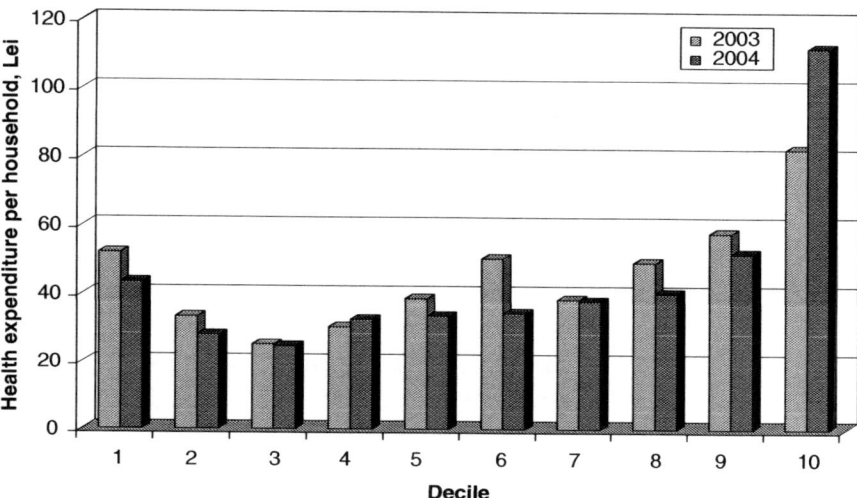

Fig. 9. Out-of-Pocket Health Expenditure by Income Deciles in 2003 and 2004.
Source: National Bureau of Statistics of Moldova (2006).

Centralizing[6] the pooling of funds was an important pre-condition for improving equity in the distribution of health spending. In both countries, a decentralized financing structure was associated with inequity, and centralization led to improvement. However, centralization alone was not sufficient to cause redistribution to occur. When this was combined with a shift from historical input-based budgeting to output-based provider payment methods, the centralized pool enabled the redistribution to occur. This, coupled with the basic logic of insurance whereby larger pools facilitate greater risk protection, calls in question the treatment of decentralization as an inherent policy objective rather than a possible means to an end that is more useful for certain objectives than for others.

In LMIs, making progress on health finance policy objectives depends critically on the role played by general budget revenues, even in the presence of a compulsory SHI fund. Because LMIs tend to be characterized by low levels of formal labor force participation, compulsory contributions (payroll taxation) can only play a limited role in promoting equity and financial protection for the population. Both Kyrgyzstan and Moldova have relatively high proportions of the population working in the informal economy; yet, they introduced a payroll tax and SHI fund and rapidly moved to universal or near-universal systems. The key to this was the role of general budget revenues, which was transformed from directly funding health facilities (subsidizing supply) to subsidizing the purchase of services on behalf of the entire population (Kyrgyzstan) or specific groups in the population (Moldova).

Universality, or the path to it, should be designed into the system from the beginning. The typical approach to SHI suggested for LMIs is to start with the formal sector and then try to incorporate more groups, gradually expanding coverage. This has proven to be very difficult, for both economic and political reasons (Savedoff, 2004; González Rossetti, 2002). The Kyrgyz and Moldovan approaches suggest that it is not necessary for developing countries to attempt to emulate the historical experience of Germany; alternatives to the gradual scaling up of coverage are possible. By using general budget revenues to fund coverage for the bulk of the (or entire) population, it is possible for rapid progress to be made.

A strong single purchaser can be a critical "change agent" for the system, and going outside the core public finance system may be necessary. While it was (and is) conceptually possible to change purchasing methods from within the core "Ministry of Health" government budgetary system, in many countries the rules governing public sector financial management may not allow the necessary flexibility or innovation. This was certainly the case in Kyrgyzstan and Moldova and perhaps provides the strongest rationale for a country to introduce a new, quasi-public pooling, and purchasing entity such as an SHI fund. It is not to "create insurance," since it is possible to ensure financial protection and access to care without such an entity, as the experience of the UK or Sweden, among others, illustrates. But as part of a comprehensive health reform agenda, a new entity may be essential for both political (to inject a new psychology into the system) and technical (to have an agency with explicit functional responsibility for pooling funds and purchasing health care services on behalf of the population) reasons.

Reducing health financing options to a choice between Beveridge and Bismarck is conceptually wrong and counter-productive. Regardless of the label attached to a country's health financing system, making effective policy requires understanding that "the devil is in the details." In any system, it is essential to address the following questions:

- What are the revenue sources and collection mechanisms?
- What are the arrangements for pooling and purchasing?
- What are the entitlements and obligations of the population, and on what basis is this entitlement determined?

- What are the connections and relationships between these aspects of the system?
- How is regulation and oversight of the entire system exercised?

Decision-makers and analysts also need to consider how to sequence the implementation of various aspects of reform. With regard to this, the evidence from Kyrgyzstan and Moldova is not definitive; these cases suggest only that such considerations are situation-specific and may depend more on leaders with the vision to seize political opportunities (e.g., Kyrgyzstan's pooling of budget funds in the oblast HIFs, Moldova's ability to make the "big bang" transformation with the centralization of budget funding) than on particular technical design issues.

Focus on the system and the entire population, not the scheme and its members. Beyond these questions, it is essential to establish goals for the health financing system at the level of the entire population, such as improving financial protection or promoting greater equity in the utilization of services. In many countries, however, design and evaluation of reforms such as the introduction of a SHI scheme have focused on the scheme itself and its members, rather than the overall system and entire population. This, we believe, is a fundamentally flawed approach. The experiences of both Kyrgyzstan and Moldova illustrate how, even in LMIs with relatively low levels of formal sector employment, a new SHI fund can transform the entire health financing system. But doing so required thinking "outside the box." Each country has a single, unified health financing system, in which mainly general budget revenues are pooled by something called an SHI fund. In other words, the focus has not been on the success of an SHI scheme, but rather on the role of that scheme (or more precisely, the SHI fund itself) in the overall health financing system. By focusing on achieving the objectives of the system, rather than that of only the scheme, both countries have demonstrated that introducing SHI in an LMI context does not inevitably worsen fragmentation and equity. Instead, because they designed and used their SHI fund to eliminate existing fragmentation in the system, great progress on policy objectives was made, particularly with regard to equity.

NOTES

1. This is the term used in the region to denote SHI.
2. In 1998, Batken was part of Osh oblast.

3. This figure is not directly comparable to Fig. 3 because it reflects only expenditure on the SGBP, whereas Fig. 3 was based on total government health spending.

4. The main groups are pensioners, children, students, and registered unemployed persons.

5. There are provisions to ensure funding of at least some services for uninsured people. Up to 50% of the SHI reserve fund resources can be used to reimburse emergency pre-hospital care in cases of major emergencies and primary health care (clinical examination by a family physician and follow-up) for uninsured people. Purchasing of these services for the uninsured is the responsibility of the NHIC. In addition, in 2005, a state budget funded and MOH managed program was created for for uninsured persons with tuberculosis, psychiatric disorders, cancers, and communicable diseases (Shishkin et al., 2008).

6. Decentralization is a very broad term that is open to interpretation. In Kyrgyzstan and Moldova, the centralization of pooling that occurred was on behalf of population sizes of about 5 and 3 million people, respectively. While the conceptual insurance logic of centralizing pooling would still apply for larger population sizes, the evidence from these two countries is not sufficient to support pool centralization for populations larger than this. But these experiences do suggest that it is certainly possible to manage a single pool for 5 million, and centralizing at least up to that level can promote redistribution while being administratively manageable.

REFERENCES

Cheasty, A. (1996). The revenue decline in the countries of the former Soviet Union. *Finance and Development, 33*(2), 32–35.

Davis, C. (forthcoming). Understanding the legacy: Health financing systems in the USSR and Eastern Europe prior to transition. In: J. Kutzin, Cashin, C., & Jakab, M. (eds.), *Implementing health financing reform: Lessons from countries in transition.* World Health Organization Regional Office for Europe and the European Observatory on Health Policies and Systems.

Falkingham, J., Akkazieva, B., & Baschieri, A. (2007). *Health, health seeking behavior and out of pocket expenditures in Kyrgyzstan, 2007.* Policy research paper 46, MANAS Health Policy Analysis Project. World Health Organization, Bishkek, Kyrgyzstan. Available at http://chsd.studionew.com/images//prp46khhs.pdf

Gertler, P., & Solon, O. (2000). *Who benefits from social health insurance in developing countries?* Berkeley, CA: University of California, Berkeley, Haas School of Business. Available at http://www.cepr.org/meets/wkcn/6/672/papers/Gertler.pdf

González Rossetti, A. (2002). *Social health insurance in Latin America.* Background paper prepared for the DFID Health Insurance Workshop. 9–10 April. London: Institute for Health Sector Development.

Jakab, M. (2007). *An empirical evaluation of the Kyrgyz health reform: Does it work for the poor.* Ph.D. dissertation, Harvard University, Cambridge, MA, USA.

Jakab, M., Kutzin, J., Chakraborty, S., O'Dougherty, S., Temirov, A., & Manjieva, E. (2005). *Evaluating the Manas Health Sector Reform (1996–2005): Focus on health financing.* Policy research paper 31, MANAS Health Policy Analysis Project. World Health Organization, Bishkek, Kyrgyzstan. Available at http://chsd.studionew.com/images/ EvaluationofHealth_financing_E_PRP31.pdf

Jakab, M., & Manjieva, E. (2007). The Kyrgyz Republic: Good practices in expanding health care coverage. In: P. Gottret, G. Schieber & H. Walters (Eds), *Good practices in health financing.* Washington, DC: The World Bank.

Kutzin, J. (1997). *Health insurance for the formal sector in Africa: yes, but ....* Current Concerns series, ARA Paper number 14. WHO/ARA/CC/97.4. Geneva, World Health Organization, Division of Analysis, Research and Assessment. Also available, under the same title. In: Beattie, A., J. Doherty, L. Gilson, E. Lambo & R. P. Shaw (Eds), *Sustainable health care financing in Southern Africa: Papers from an EDI health policy seminar held in Johannesburg, South Africa, June 1996.* Washington, DC: The World Bank, Economic Development Institute.

Kutzin, J. (2001). *A proposed plan for the redistribution of Republican health spending.* Policy research paper 4, MANAS Health Policy Analysis Project. Bishkek, Kyrgyzstan: World Health Organization.

Kutzin, J. (2003). *Health expenditures, reforms and policy priorities for the Kyrgyz Republic.* Policy research paper 24, MANAS Health Policy Analysis Project. World Health Organization, Bishkek, Kyrgyzstan. Available at http://chsd.studionew.com/images/ PER_JK_for_PRP24.pdf

Kutzin, J., Ibraimova, A., Kadyrova, N., Isabekova, G., Samyshkin, Y., & Kataganova, Z. (2002). *Innovations in resource allocation, pooling and purchasing in the Kyrgyz health care system.* Policy research paper 21, MANAS Health Policy Analysis Project. World Health Organization, Bishkek, Kyrgyzstan. Available at http://chsd.studionew.com/images/ RAP_PRP21_E.pdf

Lloyd-Sherlock, P. (2006). When social health insurance goes wrong: Lessons from Argentina and Mexico. *Social Policy and Administration, 40*(4), 353–368.

Londoño, J.-L., & Frenk, J. (1997). Structured pluralism: Towards an innovative model for health system reform in Latin America. *Health Policy, 41*(1), 1–36.

MET (Ministry of Economy and Trade of the Republic of Moldova). (2004). *Poverty and policy impact report.* Chisinau, Moldova: MET.

MOH (Ministry of Health of the Kyrgyz Republic). (2008). *Mid-term review report: Manas Taalimi health sector strategy,* 7 May. Bishkek, Kyrgyzstan: MOH.

National Bureau of Statistics of Moldova. (2006). *Results of survey of health status of population in the Republic of Moldova.* Unpublished data. Chisinau, Moldova.

Savedoff, W. D. (2004). Is there a case for social insurance? *Health Policy and Planning, 19*(3), 183–184.

Schüth, T. (2001). *Perceptions of the co-payment policy among patients and health personnel: rapid appraisal study in the pilot area of Chui and Issyk-kul oblasts.* Policy research paper 13, MANAS Health Policy Analysis Project. World Health Organization, Bishkek, Kyrgyzstan. Available at http://chsd.studionew.com/images/Second_Swiss_PRA_of_ copayment_E.pdf

Shaw, R. P., & Griffin, C. (1995). *Financing health care in sub-Saharan Africa through user fees and insurance.* Washington, DC: The World Bank.

Shishkin, S., Kacevicius, G., & Ciocanu, M. (2008). *Evaluation of Moldova's 2004 health financing reform*. Health financing policy paper. Copenhagen, Denmark: World Health Organization Regional Office for Europe, Division of Country Health Systems.

World Bank. (2003). *Moldova health policy note: the health sector in transition*. Report no. 26676-MD. Washington, DC: The World Bank, Europe and Central Asia Region, Human Development Sector Unit.

World Bank. (2008). Country groups. Available at http://web.worldbank.org/WBSITE/EXTERNAL/DATASTATISTICS/0,,contentMDK:20421402~pagePK:64133150~piPK:64133175~theSitePK:239419,00.html. Retrieved on 15 November 2008.

REFORMING "DEVELOPING" HEALTH SYSTEMS: TANZANIA, MEXICO, AND THE UNITED STATES

Dov Chernichovsky, Gabriel Martinez and
Nelly Aguilera

ABSTRACT

Objective – *Tanzania, Mexico, and the United States are at vastly different points on the economic development scale. Yet, their health systems can be classified as "developing": they do not live up to their potential, considering the resources available to them. The three, representing many others, share a common structural deficiency: a segregated health care system that cannot achieve its basic goals, the optimal health of its people, and their possible satisfaction with the system. Segregation follows and signifies first and foremost the lack of financial integration in the system that prevents it from serving its goals through the objectives of equity, cost containment and sustainability, efficient production of care and health, and choice.*

Method – *The chapter contrasts the nature of the developing health care system with the common goals, objectives, and principles of the Emerging Paradigm (EP) in developed, integrated – yet decentralized –systems.*

Innovations in Health System Finance in Developing and Transitional Economies
Advances in Health Economics and Health Services Research, Volume 21, 313–338
Copyright © 2009 by Emerald Group Publishing Limited
ISSN: 0731-2199/doi:10.1108/S0731-2199(2009)0000021015

In this context, the developing health care system is defined by its structural deficiencies, and reform proposals are outlined.

Findings – *In spite of the vast differences amongst the three countries, their health care systems share strikingly similar features. At least 50% of their total funding sources are private. The systems comprise exclusive vertically integrated, yet segregated, "silos" that handle all systemic functions. These reflect and promote wide variations in health insurance coverage and levels of benefits – substantial portions of their populations are without adequate coverage altogether; a considerable lack of income protection from medical spending; an inability to formalize and follow a coherent health policy; a lack of financial discipline that threatens sustainability and overall efficiency; inefficient production of care and health; and an dissatisfied population. These features are often promoted by the state, using tax money, and donors.*

Policy implications – *The situation can be rectified by (a) "centralizing" – at any level of development and resource availability – health system finance around a set package of core medical benefits that is made available to the entire population and (b) "decentralizing" consumption and provision of care. The first serves equity and cost containment and sustainability. The second supports efficiency and client satisfaction.*

Originality/value of chapter – *The chapter views commonly discussed problems of the health care system – a lack of insurance coverage and income protection – as symptoms of a large problem: health system segregation.*

1. INTRODUCTION

A population's health is primarily determined by socio-economic factors, notably level of education, and availability of medical resources that, in turn, also depend on these factors. Countries with "developed" health care systems optimize their population's health and satisfaction with their system by securing for their citizens universal entitlement to set medical benefits in an integrated, yet decentralized, system. These countries deal effectively with equity, cost containment, efficiency of medical and health production, and scope of consumer choice, that ultimately serve good health and client satisfaction.

Consequently, developed systems are likely to show better outcomes than countries with developing health care systems that have wide variations in coverage and levels of benefits – substantial portions of their populations without adequate coverage altogether – and are institutionally and functionally segregated and fragmented. The segmentation reflects and cultivates inequities. It also means, however, a disparate array of uncoordinated medical activity that prevents efficient production of care and health, cost containment and sustainability, and real choice. Worse, the situation is often instigated by the state as well as by donors.

Developing health care systems can exist at any level of economic development. Tanzania, Mexico, and the United States are at vastly different points on the economic development scale. Yet, their health systems can be classified as developing, segregated systems that do not live up to their potential.

In all three countries, considerable proportions of their population lack basic and orderly coverage. About 92% of Tanzania's total population of 39 million is considered to lack insurance, about 38% of Mexico's 109 million people are considered to lack insurance, and about 15% of the population of the United Sates, or 45 million Americans, are regarded as lacking insurance. The uninsured in Tanzania and Mexico have access to rudimentary state-supported care, often with some co-payment arrangements. In the United States, mainly the poor, the aged, and veterans benefit from state-supported care.

Simultaneously, there are a variety of adequate insurance arrangements for the organized portions of the population, notably civil servants and organized labor. Even when supported by state funds, these arrangements are usually exclusive, not open to the population as large, and inclusive, the membership tends to be locked in these arrangements, limiting free choice.

All three systems appear to underperform given their level of resources. Naturally rich in data and widely researched, the underperformance of the US system is well documented and established (Davis et al., 2007; Schoen, Davis, How, & Schoenbaum, 2006). As for Mexico and Tanzania, the two countries have life expectancy and infant mortality levels that are below those predicted by the level of income within their respective middle- and low-income country groups. The three systems suffer from structural problems.

This situation is reflected in these three countries by heavy dependence on private funding: out-of-pocket payments and private insurance, when available; they thus allow market imperfections and failures to dominate access to care, on the one hand, and its production, on the other.

Interestingly, in all three countries, the share of private funding is about 50% of the total, compared with the 20%–30% observed in countries with developed health care systems, the developed nations of the Organization for Economic Cooperation and Development (OECD, 2007).

Most of the discussion of health care reform in developing systems, including these of Tanzania, Mexico, and the United States, tends to be centered on the lack of access to quality care, and related income protection issues. The view taken in this chapter is that these issues, along with efficiency, cost containment, and choice questions, are symptoms as well as manifestations of a larger problem: the lack of an integrated and coherent health system. Israel, for example, introduced universal entitlement in 1995, when 96% of its population already had adequate coverage, and the country's performance indicators, including cost of care, were (and are) superior to these of the United States and most other countries. The objectives of the Israeli reform were the potential equity, cost control and sustainability, efficiency, and scope of choice dividends of an integrated health care system that eventually secures better health and greater satisfaction with the system (Chernichovsky & Chinitz, 1995).

The goal of this chapter is to define the "developing" segregated health care system, examine its structural weaknesses, and propose solutions involving the restructuring of the system, starting with its financing. The solutions are based on contrasting the developing systems with the good practices of developed ones, which represent the common objectives and principles reflected in the Emerging Paradigm (EP) in developed systems. The inevitable role of the state and leadership in implementing the EP is implied. The chapter relates to the experiences of Tanzania, Mexico, and the United States, while considering their particular levels of development and specific circumstances.

2. THE EMERGING PARADIGM IN DEVELOPED HEALTH CARE SYSTEMS

The health systems of developed countries, with the notable exception of the United States, share common objectives and principles. These guide the funding and organization of their health care systems, so as to maximize, with available resources, their populations' health as well as their satisfaction with the system. Differences between the countries reflect changing priorities combined with varying legacies and political contexts, but not in underlying values, objectives, and principles (Chernichovsky, 1995a, 2002). This remarkable consensus is termed here the Emerging Paradigm.

The EP suggests that the state strives to optimize its population's health and satisfaction with the system by efforts to balance a set of operational objectives: equity, cost containment, efficient delivery of quality care, and scope of choice.

These objectives, which have both instrumental and intrinsic values, are based on the recognition that the developed health care system contributes to people's health and satisfaction in ways that exceed the potential contribution of insurance coverage and access to care, and patients' contentment with care and service. These ways include the distribution of medical resources in the population or community, the protection of household consumption from "excessive" unforeseen medical spending, and public satisfaction with social fairness and availability of social safety nets (Richardson, Lezzi, Sinha, & Mckie, 2009).

Moreover, the funding, organization, and management of the system must contribute to the above as well as to the system's sustainability through cost containment and efficiency of health care production, as well as employment, income growth, and investment in human and non-human capital.

The basic principles underlying the EP are the following:

- Universal entitlement to a set of "core" medical benefits is based solely on medical conditions and indications and not on employment status, place of work, or the level of an individual's contributions to the system.
- Funding, to finance the core benefits and support an integrated system, is based on:
  - Public finance principles: compulsory contributions, mostly means-tested rather than risk-based, that are not necessarily generated by general taxation. Some or all contributions may be earmarked.
  - National pooling of these contributions, possibly through the regulation of the fundraising and spending of employers and local entities.
  - Allocation of pooled funds to budget or fund holders, commonly by a risk-adjusted capitation mechanism so as to give each resident or citizen an equal opportunity to realize his or her health potential.
- Private funding, out-of-pocket (OOP) payments, and voluntary medical insurance (VMI) are regulated to minimize interference with the achievement of the system's public goals.

- Institutional separation of systemic functions: (a) stewardship and oversight, (b) funding, (c) organizing and managing the care consumption (OMCC), and (d) care provision. The first two are centralized and the responsibility of the state, at least by regulation. The last two, especially provision, are decentralized and mostly non-state and private.
- OMCC responsibility is devolved to (a) budget holder(s). These can be either (a) competing non-governmental entities or plans such as Health Maintenance Organizations (HMOs) and Sickness Funds, that assume this fiduciary responsibility or (b) decentralized state authorities as in the UK National Health Service (NHS).
- Provision of care is by providers with whom budget holders contract to serve their constituents.
- Competition for enrollees among plans, when applicable, and among individual providers.
- Open enrollment opportunity for citizens to change plans, where applicable, and providers periodically.

The OMCC task of budget holders merits elaboration. OMCC involves, firstly, devising patterns for patients to realize their core benefits. These patterns mainly concern where particular care can be obtained (community, outpatient clinic, hospital, etc.), lists of providers, and referral rules. These patterns reflect the organization of care, combined with administrative directives about access and patient choice. Secondly, OMCC involves purchasing care by contracting providers to supply care in accordance with these patterns (Chernichovsky, 1995a, 1995b, 2002).

The EP suggests decentralized health care systems as opposed to fragmented ones.[1] Decentralization means (Fig. 1) (a) vertical separation of all system functions: stewardship and oversight, funding and allocation, OMCC, and provision; (b) horizontal integration of the first two pairs; and (c) horizontal separation of vertically separated provider and possibly budget holders or plans (responsible for OMMC) (Chernichovsky & Chernichovsky, 2006).

The horizontal integration or application of centralized public principles and mechanisms to stewardship plus oversight, and funding and allocation, promotes equity through universal access and income protection, and cost containment and efficiency by applying financial discipline and supporting strategic (monopsony) purchasing. Simultaneously, integration supports efficient production of care and health by minimizing cost shifting, taking advantage of economies of scale, regulating natural monopolies, efficient

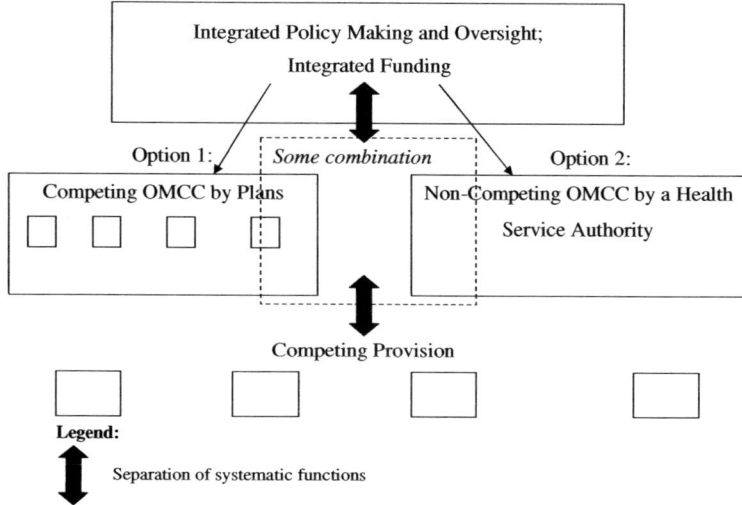

Fig. 1. EP System Design.

production of health through a coherent health policy, and coordinating personal and population care (Chernichovsky & Leibowitz, 2009).

The vertical separation and division of functions, applying decentralization and market principles and mechanisms to the OMCC and provision functions, aims to promote efficiency in the production of care, as well as accountability to clients, through competition in internal markets.

3. HEALTH SYSTEM DESIGN PRINCIPLES

We can contemplate health systems according to the funding function, on one hand, and the OMCC plus provision functions, on the other, as illustrated in Fig. 2. The sources of the funding (x-axis) reflect the extent to which funding is based on private (voluntary) or public (mandatory) principles and also serve earmarked or general purposes. The principles by which OMCC and provision are organized and managed (y-axis) reflect the extent to which the two functions are based on both decentralized and competitive market principles.

Various structural designs can be mapped by this classification.[2] On one extreme, the domain around point A, a wholly competitive OMCC and

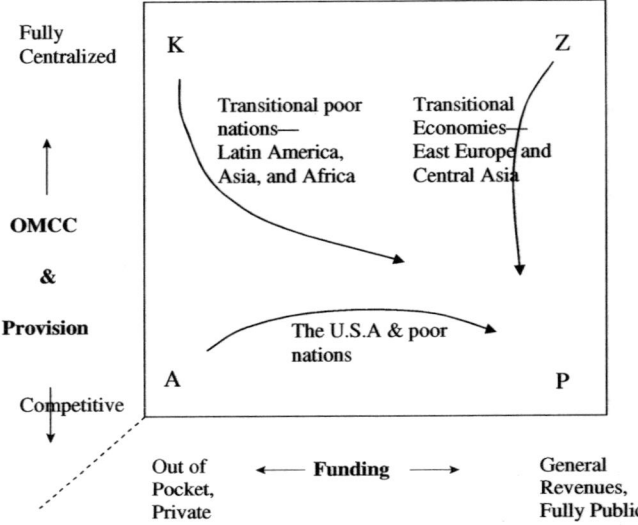

Fig. 2. Potential Structural Reform by Funding, Organizational, and Management
Principles. *Source:* Chernichovsky and Chernichovsky (2006).

provision, and funded by OOP payments and private insurance. At the other
extreme, the domain around point Z, the wholly centralized system is
funded through general revenues.

The region around point P represents the EP, whereby funding is based
on centralized public finance principles, while OMCC and provision are
based on either competitive principles that are applied in so-called internal
markets, where competing plans operate, or decentralization principles
applied to a state administration, for example, an NHS. The area around
point K is either considered a monopolistic market wherein private funding
finances monopolies or a "corrupt system" wherein private funding finances
centralized state institutions. While the domain around point K is generally
undesirable, except for cases of natural monopolies, the other domains each
have their virtues.

The funding dimension leads the discussion. At the same time, the
organizational dimension of the OMCC and provision functions cannot be
overlooked (Chernichovsky & Chernichovsky, 2006). In fact, whether the
system provides effective universal coverage and is integrated under funding
by general revenues (e.g., the UK) or under social health insurance (SHI)
(e.g., Germany), while quite important for the economy at large, may be

quite immaterial for the health care system, particularly the individual patient and his doctor. At the end of the day, it is the OMCC and provision of services that matter to contributors and beneficiaries. The institutional arrangements of those functions, as well as funding, thus matter as a single whole.

4. SEGREGATION VS. DECENTRALIZATION – THE FUNDING PERSPECTIVE

From the financing perspective, systems can be classified on a spectrum that ranges from those predominantly funded by OOP payments, through those predominantly funded by a variety of SHI arrangements, to those predominantly funded by general tax revenues. These are illustrated in Fig. 3, which represents the *x*-axis of Fig. 2. Movement rightward indicates that greater proportions of population are covered under common and shared entitlement and funding arrangements. The universal models indicate universal coverage in a decentralized system (Chernichovsky, Chernichovsky, Homann, & Schramm, 2009a).

By this classification, the health systems of concern here are those consistent with the Formal Non-Universal Non-Market (FNN) model – represented by Tanzania and Mexico – and the Formal Non-Universal Market (FNM) model – represented by the United States.

The FNN model is based on group characteristics, most notably profession, place of work, or union. Although the underlying group characteristic is attained, enrollment and exit can still be quite as prohibitive as it was in the European guilds well into the 19th century. This model is

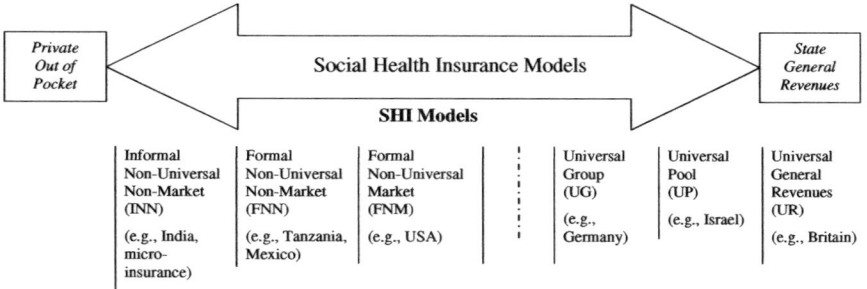

Fig. 3. Social Health Insurance Models. *Source:* Chernichovsky et al. (2009a).

probably the most prevalent today in non-national health systems, notably in Latin America and Africa, as well as in the United States. It is shown in Fig. 4 for Mexico, by the major schemes making up the Mexican system. A practically identical picture can be presented for Tanzania, starting with the National Health Insurance Fund (NHIF) for state employees in Tanzania. The United States has exclusive selective programs, notably those for the poor (Medicaid), the elderly (Medicaid), and now children (State Children's Health Insurance Program (SCHIP)). The exclusive Federal Employees' Health Benefits Program (FEHBP) includes all age groups and is supported by the federal government as an employer.

The FNM is based on market corporations rather than exclusive and inclusive groups. Enrollment is based on willingness and ability to pay the "right" premium. This model, which delineates private insurance arrangements, might be considered SHI if there is cross-subsidization among group members; some pay above their fair premium, some below it. Kaiser Permanente in the United States has age-based community rated premiums that involve cross-subsidies. Israeli sickness funds have similar arrangements for Supplemental Insurance for their membership, through community rated premiums.

The EP calls for a decentralized system – vertical separation of functions among different institutions; horizontal integration of funding and oversight,

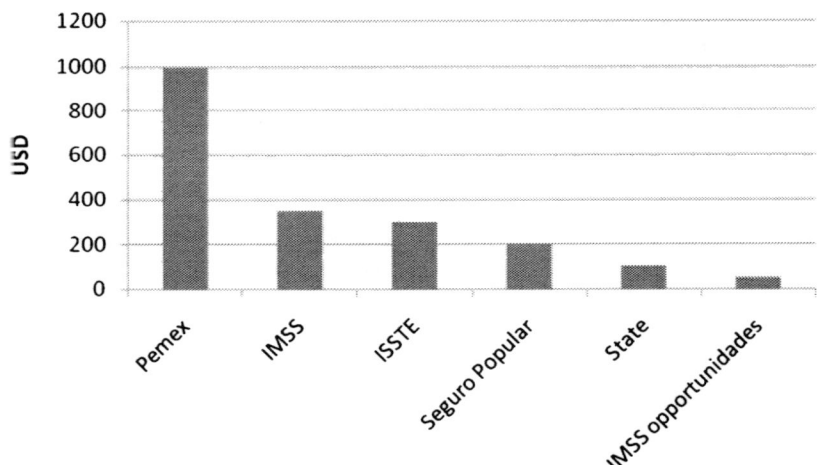

Fig. 4. Per Capita Health Care Spending by Institutions, Mexico, 2005. *Source:* SINAIS.

to form a unified system; and horizontal division of provision and possibly OMCC functions, to form one or two internal markets (Fig. 1). In contrast, developing systems are horizontally segregated and, at the same time, as in the cases of Mexico and Tanzania, highly vertically integrated. These systems comprise separate "silos" that integrate responsibilities for funding, budget-holding – OMCC, provision, and often the government functions of policy making, setting standards and regulation, monitoring, and enforcement. These silos are often closed for exit and entry.

The government and, frequently, donors in low-income countries, Tanzania being a key example, are invariably involved in the fragmented arrangements, in fact promoting them. At the outset, government employees have relatively favorable (self-serving) arrangements. The government indeed contributes in these arrangements as an employer; at the same time, it is tax money nonetheless that is used for the benefit of select exclusive groups in situations where there is no or limited coverage for considerable portions of the population.

Moreover, state programs that aim at securing coverage and related income protection to the poor and uncovered are often organized as separate, potentially stigmatized, silos segregated from other schemes that are, in themselves, often supported by government. The innovative Mexican *Seguro Popular* is independent of existing programs. The same can be argued for the Community Health Fund (CHF) program in Tanzania. To an extent, the US state-supported programs, notably the program for the poor, Medicaid, also fit this description. In the cases of Tanzania and Mexico, members cannot "graduate" into another program that is associated with the formal sector, even if they can afford the premium.[3] This does not help the credibility of these second tier programs or promote their badly needed proliferation.

In addition, governments usually exhibit vertically integrated systems, performing all system functions, especially for universal services such as maternal and child health. This is clearly the case in Mexico and Tanzania. The situation tends to be aggravated by donors who create vertical programs dealing with specific challenges, human immunodeficiency virus (HIV)/acquired immune deficiency syndrome (AIDS), and malaria being key examples.

Segmentation is reflected in structure and flows of funding. At the outset, the significant role of donors in low-income countries such as Tanzania is illustrated in Fig. 5. The financial flows among institutions organized by functions in Tanzania is illustrated in Fig. 6. All funding agencies distribute to all budget holding agencies, which, in turn, pay out to all providers. A closer look at the situation suggests a lack of transparency in the flow of

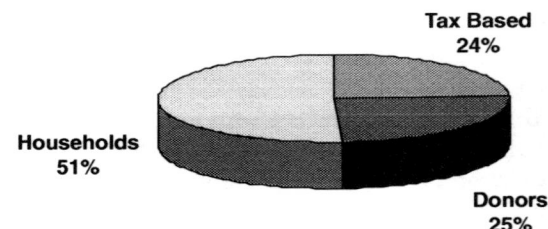

Fig. 5. Health Care Funding Sources, Tanzania, 2000. *Source:* Government of Tanzania (2001, p. 81).

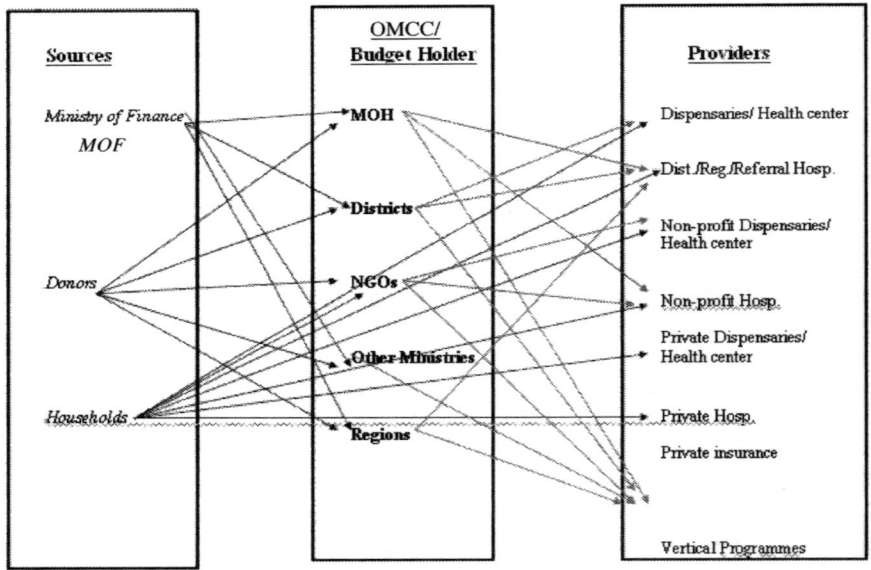

Fig. 6. Flow of Funds by Institutions and Functions, Tanzania. *Source:* Government of Tanzania (2001).

funds (Chernichovsky, Mclaughlin, Picazzo, Preker, & Tubman, 2009b). The situation is similar, albeit somewhat better, in Mexico (Martinez, Aguilera, & Chernichovsky, 2009).

Segregation adversely affects system performance, optimal health, and satisfaction with the system, by undermining cost containment, efficiency of production of care and health, and choice.

4.1. Equity

Fragmentation represents inequities and often state-led unfairness. In the case of Mexico (Fig. 4), the state oil monopoly, PEMEX, provides the most generous benefit package in Mexico to its employees and their families, while organized labor of the state and formal employers, benefit from considerably lower benefits. At the same time, the state programs, *Seguro Popular*, State, and *IMSS Opportunidades*, provide the lowest levels of benefits. Although for much lower levels of absolute benefits, a very similar picture can be presented for Tanzania, starting with the relatively generous package offered to state employees under the NHIF. And, at much higher levels of benefits, a similar picture can be depicted for the United States, starting with the FEHBP, if one is to cite a program associated with the state that applies to all age and income groups.

Worse, lacking a universal and uniform yardstick that is based on common principles for allocation of government funds in the fragmented system, it is practically impossible to allocate funds in a just and efficient way to different schemes. Even state-supported funding in the United States, such as Medicare, for the elderly, and the SCHIP that have mutually exclusive age groups, cannot be considered comparable in terms of either fairness or efficiency, one vis-à-vis the other. The problem is more serious when the allocation criteria follow different parameters, say age and income. Thus, by employing a variety of allocation criteria, similar needs and situations are liable to receive unequal amounts of public money. This is illustrated by the considerable variation in funding level, including state support, in the different states of Mexico (Table 1). It is clear from these data that the federal government in Mexico does not compensate for the relative non-availability of funding for medical care from the social security arrangements and private sources.

While segmentation reflects inequities, it also helps promote them. It is evident from the discussion earlier that the political economy "favors" those who are closer to the state budget.[4]

4.2. Cost Containment

The cost issue in the United States is well established and has been widely discussed (Davis et al., 2007; Schoen et al., 2006; Kotlikoff & Hagist, 2005). The concern is naturally the rise in cost that is associated with the relative inflation in the health care system. Since rising costs are perceived to be

Table 1.   Public and Social Security Per Capita Spending by State, 2005.

State	As a % of State GDP			Index Relative to National (= 100)		
	Public and Social Security	Social Security	Public	Public and Social Security	Social Security	Public
National	2.43	1.51	0.92	100	100	100
Aguascalientes	2.47	1.56	0.90	101	104	98
Baja California	2.11	1.58	0.53	87	104	58
Baja California Sur	3.65	2.54	1.12	150	168	121
Campeche	3.38	1.73	1.66	139	114	179
Chiapas	1.53	0.44	1.08	63	29	117
Chihuahua	2.22	1.58	0.65	91	104	70
Coahuila	2.55	2.11	0.44	105	140	48
Colima	3.19	1.88	1.30	131	125	141
Distrito Federal	6.11	4.75	1.36	251	315	147
Durango	2.32	1.42	0.90	95	94	97
Guanajuato	1.65	1.03	0.62	68	68	67
Guerrero	1.65	0.71	0.94	68	47	102
Hidalgo	1.78	0.79	0.99	73	52	107
Jalisco	2.21	1.42	0.79	91	94	86
México	1.31	0.70	0.61	54	46	66
Michoacán	2.91	1.49	1.43	120	98	154
Morelos	2.15	1.27	0.88	89	84	96
Nayarit	2.36	1.36	1.00	97	90	108
Nuevo León	2.64	2.23	0.42	109	147	45
Oaxaca	1.64	0.55	1.09	67	36	118
Puebla	1.80	1.02	0.78	74	68	85
Querétaro	1.83	1.18	0.66	75	78	71
Quintana Roo	2.10	1.36	0.73	86	90	80
San Luis Potosí	1.78	1.01	0.77	73	67	83
Sinaloa	2.27	1.50	0.76	93	100	83
Sonora	2.55	1.75	0.80	105	116	86
Tabasco	3.78	1.34	2.44	155	89	264
Tamaulipas	2.49	1.67	0.82	102	110	89
Tlaxcala	1.72	0.85	0.87	71	56	94
Veracruz	1.85	1.16	0.69	76	77	74
Yucatán	2.71	1.67	1.04	111	111	112
Zacatecas	1.94	0.90	1.04	80	60	112

Note: GDP, gross domestic product.
Source: Own elaboration with information from SINAIS.

unimportant in low-spending situations, inflationary pressures are frequently overlooked in low-income countries. However, considering their real resource constraints (human and financial resources), these pressures should be at least as great a concern in these countries as they are in developed countries. For Mexico, following a drop in the relative prices of health goods and services during 1996–1999, there has been a constant rise in health care prices. As a result, by 2006, health care prices adjusted by the Mexican Consumer Price Index were almost 15% higher than in 1995. This relative inflation in cost of care, which also probably reflects increases in its quality, signifies a minor inflation in Mexico (Martinez et al., 2009). Although in nominal US dollar terms, the increase in Tanzania from 2004 to 2005/2006 is significant – up by 43%. In real terms, adjusted using the consumer price index, the increase is only 36% (Chernichovsky et al., 2009b). However, in the absence of a price index for medical care, it is hard to assess the relative inflation in this sector. It is reasonable to hypothesize that this has been greater than the general consumer index. Like the United States, with 50% of health care financing being private, Mexico and Tanzania may also be exposed to rising inflationary pressures in their systems.

4.3. Efficiency

Inefficiencies in the fragmented system follow from the impact of segregation of all system functions. At the outset, clear government functions – policy making, setting standards and regulations, and enforcement – executed by non-government institutions led to a lack of coherent and effective policy making, quality control, and general oversight. This is particularly an issue in the vertically integrated systems of Mexico and Tanzania, where the state itself is a key budget holder as well as provider. The government – functioning both as a "plan" and a provider – is a biased policy maker, regulator, and enforcer in the system. This is bound to lead to inefficient policy making, with the government favoring its own providers.

Then, the "State within a state" status of Mexico's social security scheme (IMSS) and its Tanzanian counterpart (the NHIF) in their respective systems is rather well accepted. With time, it is likely that these vertically integrated, non-competing, and closed institutions will become bureaucratic, develop self-serving "standards", and lax enforcement. Accountability to the membership will have a tendency to drop.

Segmentation often makes it impossible to effectively coordinate individual and population health care, link personal preventive and therapeutic care, promote continuity of care, and effectively control its quality. The linking of long-term provision of personal care to population health inputs has been shown to have a substantial positive impact on health outcomes in developed countries (Kindig & Stoddart, 2003; Kindig, 2007; Marmot, 2005; McGinnis, Williams-Russo, & Knickman, 2002; Smedley & Syme, 2000).

Private insurers, where they exist as in the United States, have almost no incentive to promote the goal of long-term health development through investments in prevention and health promotion. The insurers are concerned that the benefits of prevention will accrue to clients who move on to other insurers. Fragmented systems do not encourage health investments early in the life cycle, which can prevent costly illnesses at a later age (Halfon & Hochstein, 2002; Heckman, 2007). This may be the case in Tanzania as well, where upon retirement, civil servants lose their insurance coverage through the NHIF.

The segregated systems, notably these involving multiple collection and allocation arrangements and highly specialized provider operations, as key examples, fail to take advantage of potential economies of scale from the consolidation of these operations and from the regulation of natural monopolies. Duplication exists, mostly in the cities of Mexico and Tanzania, in segmented provider services as well as in logistic infrastructure, such as the distribution of medications across a vast country.

Matters have started changing in Mexico where some states that ran (OMCC) the *Seguro Popular* program now procure care from IMSS. Similarly, the NHIF in Tanzania "procures" care from state institutions, notably hospitals. This latter arrangement gives rise to the hypothesis that this can be yet another vehicle by the NHIF to shift costs to the state while crowding out non-NHIF members from state facilities.

4.4. Choice

Open enrollment in plans, where they exist, and with providers is a fundamental principle of the EP. This principle cannot be adhered to in segregated, vertical, and exclusive arrangements. These situations give rise to issues of choice, accountability, and responsiveness to patients. Not only Tanzanian and Mexican citizens have choice and related responsiveness problems. Many insured Americans are locked into the insurance *cum* provider arrangements selected by their employers. Only half of all workers can change plans and providers at their own will today (Kaiser/HRET,

2007). The result in Mexico is that although many in the formal sector have health insurance with IMSS, they seek care elsewhere. In the United States, however, even beneficiaries of state-supported programs are allowed choice of plans and providers.

5. REFORM ARCHITECTURE

The reform outlined here follows the goals, objectives, as well as the funding, organization, and management principles of the EP. A summary of the goals, objectives, and principles of the EP is presented in Table 2, contrasting them with the situation in developing systems. The focus of the discussion is finance – specifically fundraising and allocation, in a situation based on entitlement to a core package of medical benefits.

5.1. Prelude

Rooted in labor relations and benefits, health insurance can be part of wider welfare benefits, notably pensions. This is still the situation in both Tanzania and Mexico, at least for their major health funds (IMSS and NHIF, respectively). This needs to be rectified in these two countries and others facing a similar situation. Health care and pension funding are based on distinct principles. The first is, by-and-large, funded on a "pay as you go" basis while the second is, in many cases, financed on an accrued basis. The two bases are incompatible.

Given rather endemic shortages in pension funds, health care funds can become a vehicle for subsidizing pensions. There are serious governance and accountability issues associated with such subsidies. Worse, perhaps, is the negative impact this may have on willingness to contribute to health care in systems that are trying to establish themselves by efforts to mobilize substantial informal sectors, skeptical of the state to start with.

5.2. Entitlement

The first and fundamental reform task is to:

- Define a core package of medical care benefits (CB) per standard capita, to which every citizen or resident is entitled.

Table 2. The EP and Developing Systems.

Element	EP – Developed Systems			"Developing" Systems (Tanzania, Mexico, United States)	
	Principle	Main functional goals (positive)	Public–private mix	Situation	Consequences
Entitlement	Universal, to a package of core benefits	Equity – access to care, independent of ability to pay. Protection of non-medical household consumption Satisfaction – security of access to core benefits; sense of solidarity and fairness Health – via equity	Right to voluntary procurement of core and extra benefits by out-of-pocket pay and regulated VMI	Nominal, varies by employment status, institutional affiliation, and location	Substantial proportion of the population with or without orderly access to care Variable state-supported entitlement that hinders improvement of average health of population by improving the health of low-income groups
Funding	Public finance principles: means-tested taxes and other mandated contributions, some are earmarked. 70%–80% of funding is of this nature Funds are centrally collected and pooled	Equity – removal of financial barriers to access to care; protection of income and consumption from ("catastrophic") medical expense Cost containment – budgetary discipline Efficiency – reduced costs of funding collection and administration; support of coordination of personal care, public health and health promotion; support strategic purchasing; minimize cost shifting Satisfaction – fairness of funding; transparency in case of earmarked funding; sense of contribution Health – via equity	Private pay out-of-pocket and by VMI for core and extra benefits of choice	Taxes and other means-tested mandated contributions for formal sector only Informal sector can join social health insurance arrangements voluntarily Public spending about 50% of aggregate spending Segmented management of collection and management of funds	Regressive funding because of the high share of private funding, reflecting in part out-of-pocket pay by poor segments of the population. Poor consumption protection Good budgetary cost containment mechanism but no control over about 50% of spending that is private and likely to be growing under current conditions Hinders implementation of national health policy High collection and administration cost of funding

Allocation	According to universal and uniform principles of need, independent of one's contribution to the system. Commonly a risk-adjusted prospective capitation	Equity – support of access to care as a function of need; risk adjustment to reduce risk selection; Compensation for social and infrastructural deficiencies. Cost containment – support of budgetary discipline; help with monopsony purchasing; enables prospective payment mechanisms that involve financial risk sharing among the state, plans, and providers. Efficiency – prospective pay promotes saving at the risk of cream skimming and quality of care cum service. Satisfaction – fairness in allocation. Health – by access		Two lines, via national schemes and via state administrations. Not rational or transparent variable. Largely input rather than need-based budgeting	Impossibility of conducting a unified national and regional health policy that combines personal, and public as well as health promotion initiatives. Drives variations in access to actual entitlement. Budgeting facilitates contains cost but does not promote efficiency and responsiveness. Potential for political discontent with non-transparent and not fair allocation
OMCC	Either by a non-competing but decentralized state independent authority (á la UK NHS) or by competing plans, or both. Open enrollment, in case of plans	Can be performed by for-profit as well as not-for-profit entities, when not performed by a non-competing NHS	When by competing plans, the plans may be regulated to offer VMI and OMCC privately acquired benefits, in conjunction of the OMCC of entitlement	Non-competing even when executed by plans. A mix of non-competing state administrations, not independent NHS, and plans	Impossibility of implementing a unified national and regional health policy, combining personal, and public as well as health promotion initiatives harms continuity of care. Lack of accountability

Notes: NHS, National Health Service; VMI, voluntary medical insurance.

This package is the pillar around which the system can reform and build, starting with the organization and management of finance.

Consequently, the medical services available in the system can be classified as follows:

a   The CB package
b   Supplemental benefits (SB) available through intra-group arrangements such as those available to members of existing groups or plans
c. Extra benefits (EB) acquired either entirely through individual VMI, OOP payments, or a combination of the two.

This exhaustive arrangement of benefits accommodates all possible arrangements while securing universal entitlement to CB. It also can accommodate institutionally as well as politically existing arrangements, at least for accounting purposes. Consequently, the benefit packages would look as depicted in Fig. 7 for the different programs in Tanzania. Identical arrangements can be made for Mexico and the United States (Martinez et al., 2009; Chernichovsky, 2009).

The basic idea here is to separate, initially for accounting purposes, the CB from other medical benefits, which are not to be supported by the public, yet are provided mainly by the formal sector institutions. Initially, the minimal package supported by the state – CHF in Tanzania, *Seguro Popular* in Mexico, and an arrangement based on the public programs, notably SCHIP and Medicaid, in the United States – can be declared as the CB package.

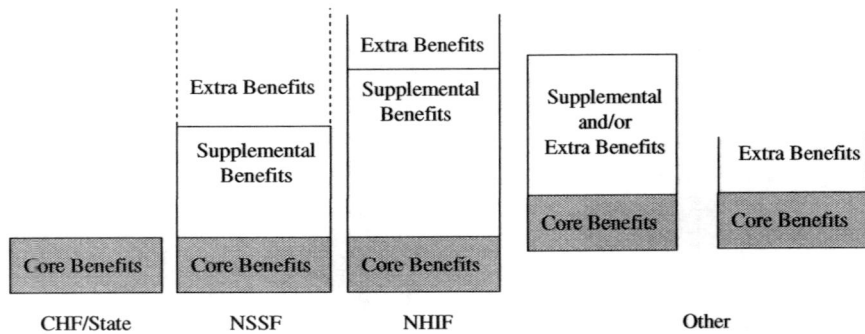

Fig. 7.   Proposed Structure of Medical Benefits by Institutions/Schemes, Tanzania.

5.3. Funding of Care

The CB would be common to all citizens and of direct financial concern to the state as well as to donors where they play a significant role, in a country like Tanzania. The CB would provide the framework for the state's financial liability in the system. Funding of care must be tailored accordingly. Consequently, the CB would be funded by:

1. Central – federal and local – state budgets.
2. A flat mandatory contribution, possibly based on age of head of household, forming an inverted U-shape by age (relatively less for children and for the aged) and size of household. Alternatively, where possible, contributions can be means tested.
3. Co-payments, where applicable.

Flat contributions are suggested for the informal sectors of Tanzania and Mexico because means testing might be impossible or costly. These contributions, while regressive vis-à-vis means tested contributions, are more equitable than OOP payments. In the United States, of course, means tested contributions can be applied as in other developed systems. Regardless, exemptions should be considered for qualifying households and individuals who can be unequivocally identified.

The mandated contributions would replace existing fee for service and possibly some co-payments. People may have to be coerced to contribute by denying them any state-supported service and eliminating the possibility of enrolling only once they become ill, as in the case of the Mexican social security system. At the same time, the system needs to be transparent and accountable. Based on earmarked contributions, a SHI system can help. Donors must play along.

While the total budget from the different sources must cover the total cost of the CB for the entire population, there should be no direct link between an individual's contribution toward funding CB, and the cost of one's entitlements or level of actual CB services he or she receives, except for an appropriate co-payment. This means fundraising by one set of criteria and distribution of funds by another.

This, in turn, requires pooling of funds, at least through accounting, at the highest state administrative, federal, level. That is, all contributions to the system become central federal through a national pool, the foundation of the integrated health system. As local authorities invariably contribute to health care from their own tax revenues, reconciliation of the funding by local and central federal authorities would be required.

Indeed, alignment and reconciliation of financial streams in the segregated system, to form an integrated pool, need distribution or allocation criteria in addition to fundraising criteria.

5.4. Allocation

The reformed system stipulates that each citizen is given an equal opportunity to access the CB by an allocation from a central pool. Considering that the allocation toward an individual must be administered through several types of collecting and budget holding institutions, a risk-adjusted capitation mechanism, based on age and gender, at least, is indispensible for a fair allocation and management of pooled funds (van de Ven & Ellis, 2000).

Once this mechanism is in place, the system has a Collection Schedule for mandated contributions for each relevant tax paying unit and a risk-adjusted Allocation Schedule for the entitled citizens. As several administrations may mediate between an individual's contribution and entitlement in financial terms, some accounting according to the two schedules is inevitable.

Here is where the fragmenting "grid" between the state vertical structures – central vs. regions and districts – and the horizontal structures of mainly national schemes such as IMSS in Mexico, the NHIF in Tanzania, and the FEHBP in the United States – comes into play. The three countries are of a federal nature. Both Tanzania and Mexico have been implementing major decentralization reforms that aim to transfer management powers over the system to local authorities. This clearly is the case in the United States, where states have considerable powers vis-à-vis the federal government. These administrations should be the overriding organizational framework of the system in relation to the national schemes or plans (to avoid a state within a state). Namely, funds should flow from the state center, the national pool, down to plans through the state administrations, branches of the national pool (Chernichovsky & Chernichovsky, 2006). This suggests reconciliation between local (state) government and central (federal) government as to the contribution of each toward the CB for the local population. This should be based on the strength of the local state economy and population. The federal or central government should have an equalizing role.

That is, states that collect from their population in mandatory contributions, by the national Contribution Schedule, more than the cost of the CB, by the national Allocation Schedule, for its population, will transfer the excess to the national pool. States that collect less from their local pool will receive a subsidy from the national pool. Hence, the local pool will have sufficient funds to secure the CB for the population.

Now schemes, usually of a national structure, come into play. They must become local cost centers for the local population – defined administratively – that they handle. If, on the one hand, they collect mandatory contributions for CB in lieu of a state edict and, on the other hand, secure benefits for their enrollees, they too have to balance positive or negative surpluses with the local pool (which in turn balances with the national pool).

The funding and allocation system described thus far, in conjunction with the CB package, creates a fair and transparent system whereby the state supports all citizens equitably. The implied zero-sum game may give more to some regions and institutions at the expense of others, but it does not fundamentally change the structure of benefit packages provided by different institutions. Funds can be provided to make the transition less painful by avoiding erosion of benefit packages supported by the state, and thus make reform more acceptable politically. In the longer term, with the growth of the formal sector, all contributions, including those for the core package by any citizens, can become means-tested, adding to the equity of the system.

Accordingly, each country needs to create a national pool for contributions for the CB – the National Health Fund – that will collect all mandated contributions in the system directly from households and employers, when applicable, and indirectly from centrally and locally collected taxes. It might be useful to establish the pool on an existing infrastructure. This notwithstanding, the state should continue to promote community and private health insurance in lieu of OOP fees paid by the population.

The pool will provide the distributional and efficiency advantages of integrated funding listed earlier, paving the way for potential gains of the integrated yet decentralized system (Table 2).

However, the proposed funding reform has several challenges. Existing schemes need to eventually give up their right to raise funds for the CB. They can at best become an arm of the state or pool for this purpose. Any excess fund collection, beyond mandated contributions transferred to the pool, becomes supplemental insurance to fund the SB. Such insurance can continue to be organized at the discretion of the group and its members. The group essentially becomes a plan responsible for OMCC and that offers supplemental insurance.

While the state may encourage the development of new plans, where competition is feasible, it should mandate open enrollment in existing plans, and see to it that cream skimming through supplemental insurance is minimized.

Donors, where they operate, must fall in line. Their contributions need to become part of the pool and their activity part of integrated national health policy and programs.

The key challenge is, however, to enlist the uninsured, converting fee-for-service payments to mandated, eventually means-tested, contributions. As discussed elsewhere, this can be aided by SHI arrangements (Chernichovsky et al., 2009a).

6. CONCLUSION

The discussion earlier relates to vastly different economies and health systems that, nonetheless, share common structural challenges. However, the difference between the systems cannot be overlooked. It might be argued at the outset that given levels of income and development, the United States can "afford" more inequity and inefficiency than Tanzania. This is a rather complex proposition that has to do with how the relatively poor, with limited access to care, feel about their relative positions in their own systems. This concerns fairness. Moreover, it appears that level of income and development might not make the challenges simpler. Vested interests in existing institutions can exert formidable political powers. That is, leadership is required, regardless.

At the same time, social, economic, and political infrastructures matter and should be considered carefully in specific reform proposals (e.g., Martinez et al., 2009; Chernichovsky, 2009). To a substantial degree, Tanzania and Mexico need to develop financial and managerial as well as civil society institutions in support of reformed health care systems. Nonetheless, even the less-developed economies have institutions they can build on to reform their systems, starting with "virtual" accounting changes that can put the house in order.

NOTES

1. The use of the term "health system" is often misguided. Most so-called systems are actually not systems or even competitive markets, which are actually systems in their own right.

2. For simplicity, without much loss of generality, we confine ourselves to two dimensions, combining the OMCC and provision functions. These two functions can be presented by separate dimensions.

3. Mexicans not in the formal sector can join IMSS, the social security scheme, when sick, and leave it thereafter. This risk selective behavior clearly discourages the scheme from enrolling them.

4. Incidence issues may aggregate the problem.

REFERENCES

Chernichovsky, D. (1995a). Health system reforms in industrialized democracies: An emerging paradigm. *The Milbank Quarterly, 73*(3), 339–372.

Chernichovsky, D. (1995b). What can developing economies learn from health system reforms of developed countries? *Health Policy, 32*(1–3), 79–91.

Chernichovsky, D. (2002). Pluralism, public choice, and the state in the emerging paradigm in health systems. *The Milbank Quarterly, 80*(1), 5–39.

Chernichovsky, D. (2009). *Adapting the Obama health care proposal to the emerging paradigm in health care systems of the U.S. Key Allies.* Israel: Ben-Gurion University of the Negev (Forthcoming).

Chernichovsky, D., & Chernichovsky, M. (2006). *Decentralization in healthcare: A framework for design and application* (Mimeo). Washington, DC: World Bank.

Chernichovsky, D., Chernichovsky, M., Homann, J., & Schramm, B. (2009a). *Social health insurance; The road to an integrated equitable and efficient healthcare system.* Israel: Ben-Gurion University of the Negev (Forthcoming).

Chernichovsky, D., & Chinitz, D. (1995). The political economy of health system reform in Israel. *Health Economics, 4*(2), 127–141.

Chernichovsky, D,. & Leibowitz, A. (2009). *Integrating public health and personal care in a reformed U.S. health care system.* UCLA Public Policy Working Paper. UCLA School of Health Policy, Los Angeles, USA.

Chernichovsky, D., Mclaughlin, J., Picazzo, O., Preker, A., & Tubman, A. (2009b). *The Tanzanian health care system and the emerging paradigm in health care systems.* Israel: Ben-Gurion University of the Negev (Forthcoming).

Davis, K., Schoen, C., Schoenbaum, S. C., Doty, M. M., Holmgren, A. L., Kriss, J. L., & Shea, K. K. (2007). *Mirror, mirror on the wall: An international update on the comparative performance of American health care.* New York: Commonwealth Fund.

Government of Tanzania. (2001). *Summary of health expenditures 1999/00.* Dar es Salaam, Tanzania: Government of Tanzania.

Halfon, N., & Hochstein, M. (2002). Life course health development: An integrated framework for developing health, policy, and research. *The Milbank Quarterly, 80*(3), 433–479.

Heckman, J. J. (2007). The economics, technology, and neuroscience of human capability formation. *Proceedings of the National Academy of Sciences USA, 104*(33), 13250–13255.

Kaiser/HRET. (2007). *Employer health benefits 2007.* Washington, DC: The Henry J. Kaiser Family Foundation and Research and Educational Trust.

Kindig, D. A. (2007). Understanding population health terminology. *The Milbank Quarterly, 85*(1), 139–161.

Kindig, D., & Stoddart, G. (2003). What is population health? *American Journal of Public Health*, *93*(3), 380–383.

Kotlikoff, L. J., & Hagist, C. (2005). *Who's going broke: Comparing growth in healthcare costs in ten OECD countries*. NBER Working Paper no. 11833. National Bureau of Economic Research, Cambridge, MA.

Marmot, M. (2005). Social determinants of health inequalities. *The Lancet*, *365*(9464), 1099–1104.

Martinez, G., Aguilera, N., & Chernichovsky, D. (2009). *The Mexican health care system and the emerging paradigm in health care systems*. Working Paper. Inter-American and Caribbean Organization of Social Security, Mexico city, Mexico.

McGinnis, J. M., Williams-Russo, P., & Knickman, J. R. (2002). The case for more active policy attention to health promotion. *Health Affairs (Project Hope)*, *21*(2), 78–93.

Organization for Economic Cooperation and Development – OECD. (2007). *Statistics and Indicators for 30 Countries*. Paris: OECD.

Richardson, J., Lezzi, A., Sinha, K., & Mckie, J. (2009). *The relative social-willingness to pay instrument: Justification and initial results*. Melbourne: Monash University (Forthcoming).

Schoen, C., Davis, K., How, S. K., & Schoenbaum, S. C. (2006). U.S. Health system performance: A national scorecard. *Health Affairs (Project Hope)*, *25*(6), 457–475.

SINAIS. Sistema Nacional de Información en Salud. Available at www.sinais.salud.gob.mx. Accessed on May 9, 2009.

Smedley, B. D., & Syme, S. L. (2000). *Promoting health: Intervention strategies from social and behavioral research*. Washington, DC: National Academy Press.

van de Ven, W. P., & Ellis, R. P. (2000). Risk adjustment in competitive health plan markets. In: J. P. Newhouse & A. J. Culyer (Eds), *Handbook of health economics* (1st ed., pp. 755–845). Amsterdam: Elsevier.